"The much-anticipated new edition of Dr. Sperry's Handbo ment of DSM-5-TR Personality Disorders is a critically r health clinician working with personality disordered clients. updated, and remarkably practical. This is one of those rare books that should be on the shelf of all mental health professionals and trainees. Dr. Sperry has offered the profession an important and much needed update to a now classic text."
    Thomas G. Plante, *PhD, ABPP, is Professor at Santa Clara University and Emeritus Adjunct Professor in Psychiatry at Stanford University School of Medicine*

"Uniquely trained as a psychologist and a psychiatrist with extensive clinical experience, Len Sperry MD, PhD is one of the top academic masters in the world in the diagnosis and treatment of personality disorders. That expertise along with his lifelong career as an educator, Len has the ability to frame cases and theory into a crystal-clear narrative for the reader in his latest edition making it a must read for all MH clinicians."
    Jon A. Lehrmann, *MD, Chair and Charles E. Kubly Professor, Department of Psychiatry and Behavioral Medicine, Medical College of Wisconsin*

"Sperry's 4th edition of *the Handbook of the Diagnosis and Treatment of DSM-5-TR Personality Disorders* effectively engages the latest theory and research in this vital and complex area of clinical practice. I consider this the essential volume on the topic because of Sperry's evidence-based insights about the full set of personality disorders integrated with a diverse range of practical treatment strategies. His case conceptualizations weave together the multi-faceted strengths of this approach and offer an excellent set of training tools. This is the key book on personality disorders to own."
    Steven J. Sandage, *PhD, LP, Boston University*

Handbook of Diagnosis and Treatment of DSM-5-TR Personality Disorders

The Handbook of Diagnosis and Treatment of DSM-5-TR Personality Disorders is a hands-on manual of the most current and effective, evidence-based assessment and treatment interventions for challenging disorders.

The beginning chapters describe several cutting-edge trends in the diagnosis, case conceptualization, and treatments. This is followed by specific chapters focusing on evidence-based diagnosis and treatment interventions for each of the ten DSM-5-TR personality disorders. Emphasized are the most recent developments from Cognitive Behavior Therapies, Dialectical Behavior Therapy, Mindfulness, Schema Therapy, Transference-Focused Psychotherapy, Mentalization-Based Treatment, and more. This fourth edition has been thoroughly updated throughout and includes new research for each chapter on DSM disorders. As in previous editions, extensive case material is used to illustrate key points of diagnosis and treatment.

This book provides essential knowledge and skills to health and mental health practitioners working with personality disordered clients, as well as to students in psychology, counseling, psychiatry, nursing, and social work programs.

Len Sperry, MD, PhD, is emeritus professor of clinical mental health counseling at Florida Atlantic University and clinical professor of psychiatry and behavioral medicine at the Medical College of Wisconsin. For more than five decades, he has treated, written about, and taught courses and workshops on the personality disorders. Among his 1,200+ professional publications are several articles, book chapters, and books on these disorders, including the recently published *Highly Effective Therapy: Effecting Deep Change in in Counseling and Psychotherapy*.

Handbook of Diagnosis and Treatment of DSM-5-TR Personality Disorders

Assessment, Case Conceptualization, and Treatment

4th Edition

Len Sperry

NEW YORK AND LONDON

Designed cover image: Makhbubakhon Ismatova © Getty Images

Fourth edition published 2025
by Routledge
605 Third Avenue, New York, NY 10158

and by Routledge
4 Park Square, Milton Park, Abingdon, Oxon, OX14 4RN

Routledge is an imprint of the Taylor & Francis Group, an informa business

© 2025 Len Sperry

The right of Len Sperry to be identified as author of this work has been asserted in accordance with sections 77 and 78 of the Copyright, Designs and Patents Act 1988.

All rights reserved. No part of this book may be reprinted or reproduced or utilised in any form or by any electronic, mechanical, or other means, now known or hereafter invented, including photocopying and recording, or in any information storage or retrieval system, without permission in writing from the publishers.

Trademark notice: Product or corporate names may be trademarks or registered trademarks and are used only for identification and explanation without intent to infringe.

First edition published by Routledge 1995
Third edition published by Routledge 2016

ISBN: 978-1-032-61790-9 (hbk)
ISBN: 978-1-032-61789-3 (pbk)
ISBN: 978-1-032-61793-0 (ebk)

DOI: 10.4324/9781032617930

Typeset in Sabon
by KnowledgeWorks Global Ltd.

Contents

Preface *viii*
Acknowledgments *x*

1 Diagnosis and Treatment of Personality Disorders Today 1
2 The Alternative Model for Personality Disorders 28
3 Case Conceptualization and Effective Treatment of Personality Disorders 38
4 Antisocial Personality Disorder 50
5 Avoidant Personality Disorder 69
6 Borderline Personality Disorder 86
7 Dependent Personality Disorder 112
8 Histrionic Personality Disorder 129
9 Narcissistic Personality Disorder 145
10 Obsessive-Compulsive Personality Disorder 164
11 Paranoid Personality Disorder 182
12 Schizoid Personality Disorder 199
13 Schizotypal Personality Disorder 214

References 229
Index 248

Preface

Today, some 64 percent of those evaluated in clinical settings meet criteria for a personality disorder, as do 11 percent of the general public (Torgersen, 2021). These disorders can greatly disrupt an individual's work, family, and social relationships. Personality disorders are associated with high rates of family conflict, separation, divorce, child custody proceedings, job termination, homelessness, substance abuse, violence, and criminal behavior. Personality disorder complicates co-occurring medical conditions, as well as the prognosis of other mental disorders. They are associated with poor treatment compliance, increased use of medical and psychiatric services, and the likelihood of relapse and premature termination (Skodol, Bender, & Oldham, 2019; Skodol, 2021a). For clinicians, treating these disorders can be extraordinarily challenging, and sometimes exasperating.

The first edition of *Handbook of Diagnosis and Treatment of the DSM-IV Personality Disorders* (1995) broke new ground as the first single authored text to address the diagnosis, case conceptualization, and treatment of the DSM personality disorders. It differed from other personality disorder books by offering a brief but thorough, user-friendly resource for clinicians and trainees in planning and implementing effective treatment of these disorders. The second edition of *Handbook of Diagnosis and Treatment of the DSM-IV-TR Personality Disorders* (2003) incorporated additional resources for diagnosing, planning and implementing effective clinical interventions. The third edition of *Handbook of Diagnosis and Treatment of the DSM-5 Personality Disorders* (2016) introduced the Alternative Model for Personality Disorders as well as some new evidence-based treatment interventions and strategies. This coincided with the rise of the accountability era wherein clinicians were increasingly expected to provide evidence-based treatment to all their patients, including the personality-disordered.

This fourth edition of the *Handbook of Diagnosis and Treatment of the DSM-5-TR Personality Disorders* comes at a time when attitudes of clinicians about the treatability of the personality disorders are changing. This in itself is a welcome and necessary development. For perspective it is important to recall that for decades many clinicians and instructors assumed that most personality disorders were untreatable, and that even milder personality disorders might require years of intensive psychotherapy. This attitude held firm despite the results of a number of clinical trials demonstrating that shorter-term treatment were effective with severe personality disorders. Among these was the publication of a prospective study in 2010, which reported that 87 percent of nearly 300 individuals diagnosed and treated for Borderline Personality Disorder (BPD) over a ten-year period achieved symptom remission and 50 percent achieved total recovery (Zanarini, Frankenburg, Reich, & Fitzmaurice,

2010). Yet even clinicians who knew of the study tended to ignore or downplay its implications. The observation that "(t)herapeutic nihilism has yielded to widespread, but very inconsistent, use of the spectrum of potentially valuable treatment modalities" (Skodol, Bender, Gunderson, & Oldham, 2014, p. 868) was a chilling commentary.

For those who were skeptical about these ten-year follow-up statistics, it was harder to dismiss the 20-year follow-up data in which some 60 percent achieved recovery and for those who did not, it was due primarily to their inability to work or go to school on a full-time basis. Furthermore, recurrence of BPD was found to be relatively rare (Zanarini et al., 2018; Pucker, Temes, & Zanarini, 2019). Other studies have reported similar findings (Kvarstein et al., 2023). In short, effective treatment of what is arguably the most severe PD can no longer be ignored. This is a major development.

Another key development is the availability of more evidence-based personality disorders treatments and their impact on treatment outcomes, as well as increased training opportunities in these approaches. Accordingly, more clinicians are utilizing highly effective evidence-based treatments which increase the likelihood of successful treatment among individuals with these disorders.

Perhaps the most important development of all has been the increasing awareness and adoption of the dimensional model which is gradually replacing the DSM categorical model of personality disorders. Since ICD-11 has now embraced the dimensional model, it is not just American clinicians that are transitioning to this model. "Clinicians throughout the world are asked to utilize a dimensionalized method of diagnosis and assessment.... The PD field is now embracing a dimensionalized approach to understanding personality pathology" (Huprich, 2022, p. 4). Given the importance of this model, a new chapter entitled "The Alternative Model for Personality Disorders" has been added to this edition.

This fourth edition describes these and other developments in the treatment of personality disorders. It focuses on how clinicians can increase their effectiveness and efficacy in working with personality-disordered individuals by adopting a focused and tailored treatment strategy. A basic premise underlying of this book is that the most effective treatment is tailored treatment that addresses the underlying maladaptive pattern as well as the degree of severity of the disorder.

It emphasizes the increasing applicability and effectiveness of a variety of evidence-based interventions with personality-disordered individuals. These include Cognitive Behavior Therapies, Dialectical Behavior Therapy, Cognitive Behavior Analysis System of Psychotherapy, Pattern-Focused Therapy, Mindfulness, Schema Therapy, Structured Treatment Interventions, Transference Focused Psychotherapy, Mentalization-Based Treatment, and Developmental Therapy.

The book is intended as a reader-friendly, "hands-on" manual for practicing clinicians as well as clinicians-in-training. It offers clinicians a hopeful perspective on the treatability of these disorders and provides highly effective diagnostic and treatment interventions for achieving positive treatment outcomes. My hope is that this revised edition will further foster an attitude of confidence and a measure of competence in clinicians when working with personality-disordered individuals, and that it will make a difference in their lives.

Len Sperry

Acknowledgments

It is most important to acknowledge individuals who have greatly influenced me and encouraged my development as a researcher and clinician. One of the great pioneers in the personality disorders field was the late Theodore Millon, Ph.D. Ted was both a mentor and colleague. Our relationship began in 1984, when he was a visiting professor at the University of Wisconsin Medical School, where I was completing a fellowship. Over the years he was gracious and generous with his time and feedback. I am forever appreciative of his back cover endorsement for the first edition of this book, which appeared in 1995, and for the Foreword he wrote for the second edition, which appeared in 2003. The expectation was that he would write a Foreword for this third edition. Unfortunately, he passed away just weeks before the revision was completed.

I am most grateful to my colleagues at the Medical College of Wisconsin for their friendship and wonderful feedback and encouragement over the years. They are Harry Prosen, M.D., Laura Roberts, M.D., past chairs, and Jon Lehrmann, M.D., current chair of the Department of Psychiatry and Behavioral Medicine. All of you have enriched my career and supported my research and writing.

Finally, I would be remiss in not acknowledging staff at Routledge/Taylor & Francis over these many years. Endless gratitude to my long-term publisher, editor, and friend, George Zimmer, Ph.D. Among the many other publications in which we were involved, George contracted and guided the first three editions of this book to completion. Heartfelt thanks to my editors Sarah Rae and Ellie Broadhurst for your wonderful help and support with this fourth edition.

Chapter 1

Diagnosis and Treatment of Personality Disorders Today

The first chapter of the first edition of *Handbook of the Diagnosis and Treatment of DSM-IV Personality Disorders* (Sperry, 1995) likened the paradigm shift occurring with the personality disorders beginning the early 1990s to the paradigm shift that already had occurred with the depressive disorders. Until the mid-1970s, many clinicians felt relatively ineffective in treating depressive disorders, and until the early 1990s, this same sentiment was shared by many clinicians about treating personality disorders. I insisted that such a paradigm shift involving the personality disorders would require a major change in the way clinicians conceptualize, assess, and treat these disorders. I predicted that while such a change in attitude and practice patterns might be resisted by some, most clinicians would respond to the challenge. Such a shift would mean relinquishing the then prevailing view that the personality disorders were essentially "untreatable" conditions. With some trepidation, I ended the chapter with a quote conveying the sentiment that clinicians might even come to consider that personality-disordered patients would "become our most welcome clients in the new century, clients who are deeply troubled, but whom we can help with confidence" (*Clinical Psychiatry News*, 1991, p. 26).

Some thirty years and three editions later, much has changed in clinician attitudes and practice patterns. Indeed, the paradigm has shifted. While not every clinician believes that they can help every personality-disordered individual "with confidence," there is, nevertheless, an increasing consensus among clinicians that many patients can be helped with current treatment interventions, even those meeting DSM-5-TR criteria for Borderline Personality Disorder (Huprich, 2022a).

This chapter provides an introduction and overview to the diagnosis and treatment of the personality disorders. It begins with a description of changes in DSM-5-TR, emphasizing those involving the personality disorders. Next, it details several recent trends in diagnosis, treatment, and research. Finally, it concludes with an overview of the structure of Chapters 4–13.

DSM-5-TR and the Personality Disorders

While there were some minor changes in diagnoses and diagnostic criteria in DSM-5-TR, each diagnosis underwent a text revision for all disorders. This involved an added subsection entitled Associated Features and updates of subsections on prevalence, culture-related diagnostic issues, differential diagnoses, sex- and gender-related diagnostic issues, and development and course of the disorder (American Psychiatric Association, 2022).

DOI: 10.4324/9781032617930-1

Retained in DSM-5-TR is the earlier DSM definition of a personality disorder as an "enduring patterns of inner experience and behavior that deviates markedly from the expectations of the individual's culture, is pervasive and inflexible, has an onset in adolescence or early adulthood, is stable over time, and leads to distress or impairment" (American Psychiatric Association, 2022, p. 733). While DSM-IV-TR diagnostic criteria have been retained, there has been some updating of descriptions of the various disorders. However, there is one notable change. The diagnosis of Personality Disorder Not Otherwise Specified (NOS) has been replaced with Other Specified Personality Disorder and Unspecified Personality Disorder (American Psychiatric Association, 2022, p. 778).

Alternative Model for Personality Disorders

So, what is this alternative model? Recognizing the many limitations of the categorical model of DSM-IV, the DSM-5 Personality Disorders Work Group proposed a dimensional model to replace the categorical model. That dimensional model has two primary criteria: personality functioning and pathological personality traits (American Psychiatric Association, 2022).

With this dimensional method, it is now possible to diagnose a personality disorder based on traits. The designation: "Personality Disorder- Trait Specified" is used. Another useful feature of the Alternative Model is that it can be used to assess personality functioning and traits, irrespective of whether or not a personality disorder is present (Cain & Mulay, 2022). This increases the clinical utility of the Alternative Model because it assists clinicians to identifying clients' strengths in addition to deficits. Chapter 2 of this book provides a more detailed discussion of this Alternative Model.

Trends in the Diagnosis of Personality Disorders

Assessment and diagnosis is critical in effective treatment of the personality disorders (Dowgwillo, Molina & Forche, 2022; Sharp, Cano, Bo & Hutsebaut, 2022). This section describes a number of recent clinical and research trends that are and will continue to impact the assessment and diagnosis of personality disorders. These include: attachment styles, temperament, culture, emotional abuse and neglect, and functional impairment.

Attachment Styles and Personality Disorders

Attachment refers to the emotional bond that develops between child and parent or caregiver and subsequently influences the child's capacity to form mature intimate relationships in adulthood. It is an inborn system of the brain that influences and organizes motivational, emotional and memory process that involve care givers. The impact of the process of attachment on development cannot be underestimated since the "patterning and organization of attachment relationships during infancy is associated with characteristics processes of emotional regulation, social relatedness, access to autobiographical memory, and the development of self-reflection and narrative" (Siegel, 1999, p. 67).

Attachment researchers insist that early life relational deficits lead to both neurophysiological brain deficits as well as psychological deficits (Siegel, 1999). A sensitive and responsive parent helps grow the connections in the orbitofrontal cortex of the infant's brain by communicating—or "collaborating" with the baby, via eye contact, facial expression, gestures, tone of voice, and so on. The gurgling, smiling infant is picked up and "answered" by the parent's with a smiling and joyful expression and words. Or, the baby cries in pain or frustration and the parent soothes and consoles it, or calms down the overexcited child at bedtime. These routine and continuous interactions serve to stimulate the growth of synapses in the orbitofrontal cortex of the brain which enable children to modulate their frustration, rage, and fear, and to respond flexibly to others. Research indicates that securely attached children develop neural pathways for resilience. Even when their parents are upset or impatient, their brain's wiring "knows" from experience that they won't be abandoned and will reconnect after the storm has passed. Unfortunately, children with insecure attachment styles do not experience such reciprocal parental attention, and consequently they tend to be more vulnerable to emotional assaults, i.e., they are less able to modulate rage and aggressive affects, calm and soothe their anxieties and sadness, as well as tolerate high levels of pleasure and excitement (Ainsworth et al., 1978). Needless to say, they are also less likely to correctly interpret others' social cues because of deficits in their orbitofrontal cortex which further complicates interpersonal relationships.

Types of Attachment Styles

Distinct patterns or styles of attachment in early life tend to persist into adulthood (Main & Solomon, 1990; Bartholomew & Horowitz, 1991; Hazen & Shaver, 1990). Reflecting Bowlby's (1973) concept of working models of self and others, Bartholomew (1990) developed a four-category system of adult attachment that organizes a person's working models along two dimensions: (1) the distinction between self and others; and (2) valence—positive vs. negative evaluation. Based on these dimensions, Bartholomew derived four prototypical styles of adult attachment: The four attachment styles are: **secure** (positive view of self and others), **preoccupied** (negative view of self and others), **dismissing** (positive view of self, negative view of others), and **fearful** (negative view of self and others).

Subsequently, based on clinical experience, an additional style, the **disorganized** (fluctuating positive and negative views of self and others) style was added (Main and Solomon, 1990; Main and Goldwyn, 1998).

Accordingly, personality disorders can be viewed as the outcome of insecure working models that have become self-confirmatory. These working models of self and other have become relatively inflexible and closed to new information, and as a result, the individual experiences significant distress in social, occupational, and relational functioning. It is possible to characterize the various personality disorders in terms of this dimensional model of self and others. It should be noted that Bartholomew (1990) does not assume that "all individuals are expected to exhibit a single attachment style" (p. 162). Instead, these attachment styles are conceptual prototypes, and thus, it is more appropriate to view adult attachment in a multidimensional way, with individuals exhibiting one or more style types as predominant. Accordingly, the DSM-IV personality disorders can be categorized in the following adult attachment style designations (Lyddon & Sherry, 1999).

Preoccupied Attachment Style. The preoccupied attachment dimension is characterized by a sense of personal unworthiness and a positive evaluation of others. These individuals tend to be very externally oriented in their self-definitions. Personality disorders that seem to exemplify this adult attachment style include the dependent, obsessive-compulsive, and histrionic personality disorder.

Fearful Attachment Style. Individuals with a fearful attachment style exhibit a sense of personal unworthiness combined with an expectation that other people will be rejecting and untrustworthy. They trust neither their own internal cognitions or feelings nor other's intentions. While they believe themselves to be special and different from others, they guard against threats and unexpected circumstances since they cannot trust that others will protect them. The personality disorder most characteristic of such a fearful adult attachment style is the paranoid personality disorder.

Dismissing Attachment Style. Individuals with a dismissing attachment style are characterized by a sense of self that is worthy and positive as well as a low and negative evaluation of others which typically manifests as mistrust of others. Because they believe they are emotionally self-sufficient while other are emotionally unresponsive, they dismiss the need for friendship and contact with others. The personality disorder most characteristic of such a preoccupied and fearful adult attachment style is the schizoid personality disorder.

Preoccupied—Fearful Attachment Style. Individuals with a self-view that is negative and other- view that vacillates between positive and negative exhibit a composite preoccupied and fearful style of attachment. Their avoidance is based on the desire to be liked and accepted by others, while at the same time fearing of rejection and abandonment. The personality disorder most characteristic of such a preoccupied and fearful adult attachment style is the avoidant personality disorder.

Fearful—Dismissing Attachment Style. Individuals with a view of others that is negative and a self-view that vacillates between positive and negative exhibit a composite fearful–dismissing style of attachment. They tend to view themselves as special and entitled but are also mindful of their need for others who can potentially hurt them. Accordingly, they use others to meet their needs while being wary and dismissive of them. Personality disorders that are characterized by such a fearful-dismissing adult attachment style are the antisocial, narcissistic and schizotypal personality disorders.

Disorganized Attachment Style. Individuals with a vacillating views of both self and others exhibit the disorganized attachment style. "Disorganize attachment develops from repeated experiences in which the caregiver appears frightened or frightening to the child" (Siegel, 1999, p. 117). This style is associated with dissociative symptomatology which increases their proneness to posttraumatic stress disorder. The borderline personality disorder is characterized by unstable personality structure that seems to shift among the various insecure attachment styles creating a disorganized profile.

Temperament and Personality Disorders

Like attachment, temperament is a construct that appears to have both research and clinical utility. Temperament refers to "the characteristic phenomena of an individual's emotional nature, including his susceptibility to emotional stimulation, his customary strengths and speed of response, the quality of his prevailing moods, and the peculiarities and fluctuation and intensity of moods; these phenomenon being regarded as dependent on constitutional makeup and therefore largely hereditary in origin" (Allport, 1937, p. 54). Although proposed over 60 years ago, Allport's definition is remarkably consistent with many contemporary formulations of the construct. Reflecting the clinician's view that temperament and attachment styles are related, temperament is viewed as "a filter of personality through which information is processed, attachments evolve, and emotions are experienced and expressed" (Graybar & Boutilier, 2002, p. 156).

While clinicians seem convinced that temperament influence attachment–and vice versa, researchers are still trying to clarify the exact nature of the relationship between the two constructs. This is largely part because both constructs represent different origins and different research agendas. While temperament represents a biological determinant of personality (nature), attachment style represents an environmental determinant of personality (nurture). As in other nature–nurture discussions, the relationship is seldom "either-or" but usually "both-and." Currently, the research consensus seems to be that attachment and temperament are *modestly* related and that "both will influence the formation and expression of personality and self-concept as these are assembled during early childhood" (Vaughn & Bost, 1999, p. 221).

Temperamental traits and patterns are evident from birth. For instance, while some infants are quite sensitive to light and loud sounds, others are not; and while some are calm and placid, others are very active or very fussy. Three main temperament patterns are styles have been observed infants: *easy* (usually predictable and in a good mood), *slow to warm* (more likely to be resistant to attention and moody), and *difficult* (typically unpredictable and with irritable moods) (Thomas & Chess, 1977). A child's temperament tends to be reflected in adult patterns. For example, optimism and consistency of effort are more common in adults who have easy temperaments, while negativity and suspiciousness associated with the "difficult" temperament, and passivity and over dependency with the "slow to warm up" temperament. Several other temperament traits or descriptors have been identified in adults including: impulsivity, irritability, hypersensitivity to stimulation, reactivity, emotional lability, inhibition, reflectivity, mood constriction, hypervigilance, and intensity are noted.

Before 1980 personality disorders were typically conceptualized in "character language," such as the oral character or obsessive character. Although there was a biological tradition in the study of personality that emphasized temperament, the psychological tradition that emphasized character was in vogue for most of the 20th century. Descriptions of personality disorders in DSM-I and DSM-II reflected this emphasis on character and psychodynamics. Within the psychoanalytic community, character reflected specific defense mechanisms. Accordingly, from a character perspective, the obsessive-compulsive personality would be characterized by the defenses of isolation of affect, intellectualization, and rationalization.

Currently, personality disorders are conceptualized in a broader perspective that include both character *and* temperament (Stone, 1993; Cloninger, 2005). Character refers to the learned, psychosocial influences on personality. Character forms largely because of the socialization process, particularly regarding cooperativeness, and the mirroring process that promotes the development of self-concept and a sense of purpose in life (i.e., self-transcendence and self-responsibility).

Temperament

Temperament refers to the innate, genetic, and constitutional influences on personality. Whereas character and schema reflect the psychological dimension of personality, temperament or trait (or style, as it is used synonymously in this book) reflects the biological dimension of personality. Cloninger (2005) contends that temperament has four biological dimensions (novelty-seeking, harm-avoidance, reward-dependence, and persistence), whereas character has three quantifiable dimensions (self directedness or self-responsibility, cooperativeness, and self-transcendence). Other researchers would describe impulsivity and aggressivity as additional dimensions of temperament (Costello, 1996). Another widely known of the temperament-based models is the Five Factor Model with its trait dimensions of netuoticsm ectrvesion, openiess, agreeableness, and conscientiousess (Cosata & McCrae, 1990). Section III of the DSM-5 provides a dimensional approach to the personality disorders that is based on these and other models. It consists of five temperament domains: negative affectivity, detachment, antagonism, disinhibition, and psychoticism (American Psychiatric Association, 2013). Accordingly, from a temperament perspective, the obsessive-compulsive personality would be characterized by inhibited emotional expression, behavioral inhibition, cognitive rigidity,and overconscientiousness.

Temperament and character can be assessed by interviews and self-report instruments. The relevance of distinguishing character and temperament for treatment planning is significant. Whereas insight-oriented psychotherapy might be focused on the character dimensions, psychotherapy can have little or no impact on temperament dimensions. However, the addition of focused skill training may sufficiently regulate or modulate temperament or style features such as emotional dysregulation, impulsivity, and distress intolerance.

Attachment, Temperament, Culture, and Personality Disorders

As already indicated, research strongly suggests that insecure attachment influences the development of personality disorders (Brennan & Shaver, 1998). But what about the influence of temperament and culture on the development of personality and personality disorders? Brennan and Shaver (1998) believe that the same environmental conditions that contribute to the development of insecure attachments and subsequently personality disorders, also interact with an individual's temperament. "In addition, cultural variations in the extent to which particular traits (e.g., independence, eccentricity) are also likely to result in cross-cultural differences in the expression of personality" (p. 868).

Unfortunately, there is currently little research on the cultural aspects of personality disorders to offer specific guidelines for clinical practice (Mulder, 2012). Nevertheless, DSM-5 does offer some general guidelines regarding diagnosis. It states that personality disorders "should not be confused with problems associated with acculturation following immigration or with the expression of habits, customs, or religious and political values based on the individual's cultural background or context.... It is useful for the clinician, especially when evaluating someone from a different background, to obtain additional information from informants who are familiar with the person's cultural background" (American Psychiatric Association, 2022, p. 736).

Neuroscience and Personality Disorders

Advances in neuroscience are increasing our understanding of the role of brain circuitry, neuroanatomy, and trauma in the regulation of normal and pathological behavior. Individual differences in the regulation and organization of cognitive processes, emotional reactivity, impulsivity, and anxiety can have a profound influence in the development of a personality disorder (Siever & Weinstein, 2009; Herpertz & Bertsch, 2022; Möhler, 2022).

Changes in brain circuitry have a particular impact. For example, low threshold for impulsive aggression is related to excessive amygdala reactivity, reduced prefrontal inhibition, and diminished serotonergic facilitation of prefrontal controls. Emotional instability may be mediated by excessive limbic reactivity in gabaminergic, glutamatergic, and cholinergic circuits, resulting in an increased sensitivity or reactivity to environmental and emotional stimuli seen in borderline, antisocial, histrionic, and narcissistic personality disorders. Disturbances in cognitive organization and information processing may contribute to being detached, out-of-sync with environment cues, and cognitive and perceptual distortions seen in paranoid, schizoid, and schizotypal personality disorders. A low threshold for anxiety may contribute to the worry and apprehensiveness seen in the avoidant, dependent, and obsessive compulsive personality disorders (MacNamara, Phan, Schmahl & Friedel, 2018).

Neuroanatomical research reports that the orbitofrontal cortex also plays a role in emotion regulation. Along with the anterior cingulate cortex, the orbitofrontal cortex inhibits aggression and has a regulatory influence on the amygdala by inhibition (Möhler, 2022; Herpertz & Bertsch, 2022). Mounting research also indicates how trauma, abuse, neglect, and adverse childhood experiences (ACE) influence the development of personality disorders. Trauma, particularly sexual abuse, physical abuse, and emotional neglect are significant factors. Up to 85 percent of patients with emotional instability reported childhood abuse, 70 percent report physical abuse, and 67 percent report sexual abuse (Möhler, 2022; Herpertz & Bertsch, 2022).

Most of the research on the neurobiological correlates on personality disorders has focused on four specific disorders. Additional information on these correlates is available for the antisocial personality disorders (Baliousis, Khalifa & Völlm, 2018), for the avoidant personality disorder (Wilberg & Silk, 2018), for the borderline personality disorder (Friedel, Schmahl & Distel, 2018), and for the schizotypal personality disorder (Rosell & Siever, 2018), but less so for the other six DSM personality disorders (McCommon, Sowislo, & Caligor, 2022). In short, individual differences in brain circuitry, neuroanatomy, and trauma significantly impact health and wellbeing. Not surprisingly, changes in individuals' neurobiology influences not just their level of impairment, but also how they will respond to therapy (Siever & Weinstein, 2009; Herpertz & Bertsch, 2022).

Trends in the Treatment of Personality Disorders

Compared to conventional psychotherapy approached in the treatment of personality disorders, treatment methods today tend to be considerably more focused and effective (Huprich, 2022a). Many of these treatment approaches and intervention strategies are theory-based and have been researched in clinical trials in comparison with other treatment approaches and modalities (Huprich, 2022b). These include the Cognitive Behavior Therapies, Dialectical Behavior Therapy, Cognitive Behavior Analysis System of Psychotherapy, Pattern-Focused Psychotherapy, Mindfulness, Schema Therapy, Structured Treatment Interventions, Transference Focused Psychotherapy, Mentalization-Based Treatment, and Developmental Therapy.

Cognitive Behavior Therapies

For the past three decades, Behavior Therapy, Cognitive Therapy, and CBT were the treatment of choice for the psychosocial treatment of the personality disorders. While research did not consistently support the efficacy of these traditional approaches, it has for newer, more focused approaches such as Dialectic Behavior Therapy (DBT, Cognitive Behavior Analysis System of Psychotherapy (CBASP), and Mindfulness-Based Cognitive Therapy

(MBCT). Interestingly, DBT, CBASP, and MBCT constitute what is being called the "third wave" of behavior therapy (Hayes, Follette, & Linehan, 2004).

The first wave refers to traditional behavior therapy, which endeavors to replace problematic behaviors with constructive ones through counterconditioning and reinforcement. Cognitive therapy is the second wave of behavior therapy. It works to modify problem behaviors by changing the thoughts that cause and perpetuate them. In the third wave, treatment tends to be more experiential and indirect and utilizes techniques such as mindfulness, dialectics, acceptance, values, and spirituality. More specifically, third wave approaches are characterized by "letting go of the attempts at problems solving, and instead standing back to see what it feels like to see the problems through the lens of non-reactivity, and to bring a kindly awareness to the difficulty" (Segal, Williams, Teasdale, & Williams, 2004, p. 55). Unlike the first and second wave, third wave approaches emphasize second-order change, i.e., basic change in structure and/or function, and are based on contextual assumptions including the primacy of the therapeutic relationship. These approaches appear to be particularly germane to treating personality disorders. Extended discussions of standard DBT and Radically Open DBT in the treatment of a wide range of personality disorders appears in Chapters 3 and selectively referenced in Chapters 4–11.

Dialectical Behavior Therapy

Originally developed for the treatment of borderline personality disorder (Linehan, 1993), Dialectical Behavior Therapy (DBT) has been modified and extended for use with other personality disorders as well as Axis I or symptom disorders such as mood disorders, anxiety disorders, eating disorders, and substance use disorders (Marra, 2005; Lynch & Cuper, 2012). DBT is an outgrowth of behavior therapy but is less cognitive than traditional CBT since DBT assumes that cognitions, per se, are less important than affect regulation (Nelson, Cawood, Suzuki, Chapman & Lusk, 2022). Accordingly, DBT places more emphasis on emotion regulation rather than maladaptive thought processes. While it recognizes that cognitions are a factor in behavior, they are not a necessary mediating factor. Rather, cognitions are more likely to serve as a way to make sense of behavior and emotional events after the fact (Marra, 2005).

Theory

There are numerous similarities between DBT and traditional CBT, particularly cognitive therapy. Both require a collaborative stance between client and therapist. Both utilize learning principles, analyze triggers and environmental prompts, explore schemas and emotions, and utilize modeling, homework, and imagery. Furthermore, both recognize the importance of empathic responding.

There are a number of differences between cognitive therapy and DBT in the treatment of personality disorders. Essentially, cognitive therapy posits that the same techniques used in eliciting and evaluating automatic thoughts during depression or anxiety disorders are used in treating personality disorders (Beck et al., 2015). While cognitive therapy contends that dysfunctional feelings and behaviors are due to schemas that produce consistently biased judgments and a tendency to make cognitive errors through attributional bias, DBT focuses instead on how schemas are initially formed. Accordingly, therapists utilizing DBT explore schemas and the underlying dialectic conflicts that produced them rather than performing "collaborative experiments" to prove their limited usefulness. Rather than utilizing cognitive restructuring, the DBT therapist attempts to connect belief systems to underlying affect and need, and then assist clients to reinterpret their belief systems based upon greater awareness of their feelings and needs.

Instead of utilizing "guided discovery" to dispute and revise maladaptive beliefs, AYDBT analyzes both the affective and cognitive inference processes to determine how the schema was formed in the first place. This involves identifying deprivational emotional states in early development that could have produced fixation or perseveration and attentional constriction that could serve protection from threatening internal or external cues, as well as broadly examining the effects of negative reinforcement through emotional escape and avoidance strategies or inadequate psychological coping skills that could have been rewarded through the partial reinforcement effect (Marra, 2005, p. 141).

Finally, DBT differs from the cognitive therapy of personality disorders by adopting a nonpejorative interpretation of pathology. Instead, the DBT therapist sees behavior and strategy as operant behavior. Like others, the personality-disordered client is attempting to avoid harm and seek pleasure but has difficulty successfully obtaining the desired outcome, owing to the emotional vulnerability. Nevertheless, the DBT therapist assumes that inadequate compromises between competing and contradictory needs and desires form the basis of their personality structure and helps them achieve their needs in a non-pejorative way.

Treatment

Linehan (1993; 2015) specified four primary modes of treatment in DBT: individual therapy; skills training in a group, telephone contact, and therapist consultation (Linehan, 1993; 2015). While keeping within the overall model, group therapy and other modes of treatment may be added at the discretion of the therapist, providing the targets for that mode are clear and prioritized. The individual therapist is the primary therapist, and the main work of therapy is carried out in the individual therapy sessions. Between sessions the client should be offered telephone contact with the therapist, including out of hours telephone contact, although the therapist has the right to set clear limits on such contact. The purpose of telephone contact is not psychotherapy but rather to give the client help and support to clients to find ways of avoiding self-injury as well as for relationship repair where the client feels that she has damaged her relationship with her therapist and wants to put this right before the next session. To avoid reinforcing self-injury calls after the client has injured herself are not acceptable and, after ensuring her immediate safety, no further calls are allowed for the next twenty-four hours. DBT therapists are encouraged to participate regularly in therapist consultation groups. These groups provide both emotional support for therapists dealing with difficult clients as well as for ongoing training in DBT methods (Nelson, Cawood, Suzuki, Chapman, & Lusk, 2022).

Skills training is usually carried out in a group context, ideally by someone other than the individual therapist. In the skills training groups clients are taught skills considered relevant to the particular problems of personality-disordered individuals. There are four groups of skills: core mindfulness skills, interpersonal effectiveness skills, emotion modulation skills, and distress tolerance skills (Linehan, 2015).

Stages of Treatment. Following an initial period of pre-treatment involving assessment, commitment and orientation to therapy, DBT consists of four stages of treatment (Linehan,

2015). Stage 1 focuses on "severe behavioral dyscontrol." The goal of this stage is to increase behavioral control and targets suicidal behaviors, self-harm, and severe therapy interfering like substance abuse. Stage 2 focuses on "quiet desperation" with the goal of increasing emotional experiencing in those dealing with issues like post-traumatic stress and other residual disorders not addressed in Stage 1. Stage 3 focuses on "problems of living." The goal of this stage is to work through concerns of ordinary happiness and unhappiness. Stage 4 focuses on "incompleteness" where the work is on increasing the capacity for joy, freedom, and spiritual fulfillment. The targeted behaviors of each stage are brought under control before moving on to the next phase. Therapy at each stage is focused on the specific targets for that stage which are arranged in a definite hierarchy of relative importance.

Core Strategies. The core strategies in DBT are 'validation' and 'problem solving'. Attempts to facilitate change are surrounded by interventions that validate clients' behavior and responses in relation to the client's current life situation, and that demonstrate an understanding of their difficulties and suffering (Nelson, Cawood, Suzuki, Chapman & Lusk, 2022). Problem solving focuses on the establishment of necessary skills. Other treatment modalities include contingency management, cognitive therapy exposure-based therapies, and medication.

Practicing DBT. The provision of DBT therapy is easier to accomplish in an inpatient, partial hospitalization or residential treatment setting rather than in outpatient practice. The reason is that as described by Linehan (1993), DBT is best implemented with a treatment team in which one therapist provides psychosocial skill training, another provides individual therapy, others can provide a consultation function, and the therapists have access to a therapist consultation group for support. Recently, Marra (2005) has offered suggestions to adapt DBT treatment in private practice settings. While he recommends that skills training be provided by another therapist, he offers guidelines when that is not possible. Nevertheless, he encourages any private practice clinician who anticipates utilizing DBT to have access to a psychotherapy consultant if involvement in a therapist consultation group is not possible.

Research Support. Finally, empirical support exists for the effectiveness of DBT. Several randomized controlled trials that evaluate the overall effectiveness of a comprehensive DBT treatment have been published (Linehan et al., 1991; Koons et al., 2001; Linehan et al., 2002; Verheul et al., 2003; Bohus et al., 2003; Linehan et al., 2006). When evaluated against treatment-as-usual control conditions, DBT was superior. While most of this research focused on borderline personality disorders in females, some studies modified DBT for use in other populations and in various settings. These include studies with adolescents and adults in inpatient and forensic settings with various disorders including binge eating disorder, bulimia, anorexia nervosa, chronic depression, and other personality disorders. However, there is very little research on the use of DBT with males or minorities (Lynch & Cuper, 2012).

Cognitive Behavior Analysis System of Psychotherapy

Cognitive Behavior Analysis System of Psychotherapy (CBASP) is a form of CBT that was developed by McCullough (2000) and further elaborated (McCullough, Schramm, & Penberthy, 2015). Basic to this approach is a situational analysis which combines behavioral, cognitive and interpersonal methods to help clients focus on the consequences of their behavior and to use problem solving for resolving both personal and interpersonal difficulties. CBASP was initially targeted for the treatment of clients with chronic depression. A national, multi-site study launched CBASP as an effective treatment. Clients who met criteria for chronic unipolar depression, usually meeting criteria for both major depressive disorder and dysthymic disorder, were randomly assigned to one of three treatment groups: medication only (nefazodone with the trade name of Serzone), psychotherapy (CBASP) only, or a combination of medication and CBASP. While clients in all three treatment conditions improved significantly, those receiving the combined treatment improved the most. Over the 12-week study period, 55 percent of the medication-only group reported a positive response, and 52 percent of the CBASP-only group experienced a treatment response, whereas 85 percent of those who took both medication and received CBASP had a positive response to treatment (Keller et al., 2000).

Theory

A basic assumption of CBASP is that clients can learn to analyze specific life situations and then manage daily stressors on their own. The basic premise of CBASP is simple and straightforward: a therapist assists clients to discover why they did not obtain a desired outcome by evaluating their problematic thoughts and behaviors. In short, therapists assist clients in determining which thoughts and behaviors have gotten in the way of achieving what they wanted. Since there is often a mismatch between what a client wants and what actually occurs in the client's life, the CBASP approach can be utilized with a variety of distressing problems and presentations ranging from child behavior problems and couple's conflict to anxiety disorders and personality disorders, including borderline personality disorder (Driscoll, Cukrowicz, Reardon, & Joiner, 2004). Interestingly, McCullough (2002) noted his reservations to utilizing CBASP with adults with severe borderline personality disorder, particularly those with comorbid chronic depression.

Treatment

The overall goal of CBASP treatment is to identify the discrepancy between what clients want to happen in a particular situation and what has happened or is actually happening. By examining their specific circumstances, clients gradually discover problematic themes and patterns in their lives as well as ways in which they can achieve what is desired.

There are two phases in CBASP treatment: elicitation and remediation. The elicitation phase consists of six steps which are framed by specific questions: How would you describe the situation? How did you interpret the situation? Specifically, what did you do and what did you say? What did you want to get out of the situation, i.e., what was your desired outcome? What was the actual outcome of this situation? And, finally: Did you get what you wanted?

During the remediation phase, behaviors and interpretations or cognitions are targeted for changed and revised so that the client's new behaviors and cognitions will contribute and result in their desired outcome. First, each of the client's interpretations of the situation is assessed to determine whether it helped or hindered the achievement of the desired outcome. Next, each of the client's behaviors is similarly analyzed to determine whether or not it helped or hindered in the attainment of the desired outcome (Driscoll, Cukrowicz, Reardon, & Joiner, 2004).

A modified version of this approach (Sperry, 2005, 2006, 2014) is particularly useful in working with personality-disordered individuals, particularly those who are assessed as low in learning from experiences. Such individuals have not had sufficient experience in learning from their mistakes because they too often engage in emotional thinking rather than in consequential thinking. This modified intervention strategy works by increasing consequential thinking. It focuses the individual's attention on the link between how their negative or self-defeating thoughts and behaviors result in the negative consequence (actual outcome) they end up with instead of the desired outcome that they really want. The strategy includes nine steps which begin with a cognitive and a behavioral analysis and proceed to processing their interpretations and behaviors in terms of their desired outcome or consequence.

Pattern-Focused Therapy

Pattern-Focused Therapy was developed by Len Sperry (Sperry, 2016; 2021). It is derived from Biopsychosocial Therapy which emphasizes pattern identification and pattern change (Sperry, 1998, 2000, 2006), Cognitive Behavioral Analysis System of Psychotherapy (CBASP) (McCullough, 2000), and Motivational Interviewing (MI) (Miller & Rollnick, 2002). Both CBASP and MI are identified as empirically supported treatments by the Society of Clinical Psychology (Division 12) of the American Psychological Association.

Theory

Pattern is the predicable, consistent, and self-perpetuating style and manner in which individuals think, feel, act, cope, and defend themselves (Sperry, Brill, Howard, & Grissom, 1996; Sperry, 2006). Patterns can be maladaptive or adaptive. Maladaptive patterns tend to be inflexible, ineffective and inappropriate, and cause symptoms, impairment in personal and relational functioning, and chronic dissatisfaction (Sperry, 2010). If such a pattern is sufficiently distressing or impairing it can be diagnosed as a personality disorder. In contrast, an adaptive pattern reflects a personality style that is flexible, appropriate, and effective, and is reflective of personal and interpersonal competence (Sperry & Sperry, 2020).

Pattern-Focused Therapy is based on four premises. The first is that individuals unwittingly develop a self-perpetuating, maladaptive pattern of functioning and relating to others. Subsequently, this pattern underlies the client's presenting issues. The second premise is that pattern change is an essential component of evidence-based practice. The third premise is that effective treatment involves a change process in which the client and practitioner collaborate to identify the maladaptive pattern, break it, and replace it with a more adaptive pattern. At least two outcomes result from this change process: resolution of the client's presenting issue and increased well-being and (Sperry & Sperry, 2020). The fourth premise is that *replacing* non-productive thinking and behaviors with more productive ones, is likely to effectively and quickly lead to therapeutic change than might otherwise occur with directly *restructuring* cognitions or *modifying* behavior.

Practice

Pattern–Focused Therapy begins with establishing a collaborative relationship and educating the client in the basic premises of this approach. Central to the assessment and case conceptualization process is the identification of the maladaptive pattern, and then planning treatment that focuses on pattern change. Other key factors considered in planning treatment are level of readiness for change, severity, skill deficits, and strengths and protective factors (Sperry, 2021).

A basic therapeutic strategy in the change process is to analyze problematic situations reported by clients in terms of their maladaptive pattern. Clients are first asked to describe the situation and their resulting interpretations (thoughts) and behaviors. Then, they are queried about their expected outcome in contrast to the actual one that resulted. As therapy begins, clients inevitably report that they did not achieve their expected outcome. Parenthetically, a marker of subsequent therapeutic change is that clients increasingly experience, as a result of shifting to a more adaptive pattern, when they are achieving their expected outcome. They are then asked about their interpretation and if each *helped or hurt* them in getting what they expected. If not, they are asked what alternative interpretations would have helped them achieve. Their reported behaviors are analyzed as to whether they helped or hurt in achieving their expected outcome. If not, the focus is on identifying alternative behavior which could achieve that end. Finally, the client's *level of importance* of changing the maladaptive pattern and *level of confidence* in doing so are assessed and therapeutically processed.

In short, this therapeutic strategy focuses on identifying and changing a maladaptive pattern to a more adaptive one primarily by *replacing* the non-productive interpretations and behaviors that underlie the maladaptive pattern (Sperry, 2021). Other modalities including cognitive restructuring, behavioral activation, exposure, skills training, reframing, interpretation, etc., might also be employed as adjunctive treatments.

Mindfulness

Mindfulness is a form of awareness in which an individual can focus on thoughts, feelings and experiences in the present moment with an attitude of acceptance and without analysis or judgement. The practice of mindfulness can diffuse negativity, aggression and compulsivity without suppressing emotions or indulging them (Marlatt & Kristeller, 1999). While mindfulness derives from the Buddhist tradition, it has recently been incorporated into medicine and psychotherapy. Since it is associated with developing an awareness of alternative perspectives and reducing habitual response patterns, mindfulness has been proposed as a common factor across various therapeutic systems (Martin, 1997). Linehan (2015) describes the application of mindfulness techniques as a way of integrating acceptance into psychotherapy, emphasizing its association with intentional rather than automatic information processing as well as the non-judging, non-evaluative nature of mindfulness attention. Not surprisingly, mindfulness is incorporated into Linehan's dialectical behavior therapy of borderline personality disorder. Recently, mindfulness approaches have been incorporated in several cognitive and cognitive behavioral treatment interventions including depression (Teasdale, Segal & Williams 2000; Segal, Williams, & Teasdale, 2002), substance abuse (Marlatt, 1994), borderline personality disorder Linehan,1994), panic disorder (Kabat-Zinn et al., 1992), binge eating (Kristeller & Hallet, in press), generalized anxiety disorder (Roemer & Orsillo, 2002), and obsessive compulsive disorder (Schwartz & Begley, 2002). There is mounting research evidence that mindfulness is effective in these disorders as well as medical conditions such as stroke and Tourette's syndrome (Schwartz & Begley, 2002). The extent to which mindfulness has become the core strategy in Teasdale's approach to depression and other disorders is reflected in the name of his approach: "mindfulness-based cognitive therapy" (Teasdale, Segal, & Williams 2000). It is also interesting to note that

Young, Klosko and Weishaar's *Schema Therapy* (2003) has incorporated mindfulness as a key strategy in the treatment of personality disorders.

Schema Therapy

Schema Therapy is an elaboration of cognitive therapy that has been developed by Young (1990; 1999; 2003) specifically for personality disorders, and other difficult individual and couples problems. It integrates elements of Adlerian psychology, behavior therapy, object relations, and gestalt therapy into a systematic approach to treatment. Recently, it has incorporated mindfulness for clients sensitive to the spiritual dimension.

The most basic concept in Schema Therapy is an Early Maladaptive Schema (Farrell & Shaw, 2022). Schemas are defined as broad, pervasive themes regarding one's view of self and of others that were developed during childhood and elaborated throughout one's lifetime. They are enduring and self-defeating patterns that typically begin early in life, although they can also form in adulthood, cause negative/dysfunctional thoughts and feelings, and interfere with accomplishing goals and meetings one's needs. These schemas are perpetuated behaviorally through the coping styles of schema maintenance, schema avoidance, and schema compensation. (Young, 1999).

Young (1999; 2003) has identified 18 schemas. Schemas develop in childhood from an interplay between the child's innate temperament, and the child's ongoing damaging experiences with parents, siblings, or peers. Because they begin early in life, schemas become familiar and thus comfortable. We distort our view of the events in our lives in order to maintain the validity of our schemas. Schemas may remain dormant until they are activated by situations relevant to that particular schema.

These schemas are arranged into five broad developmental categories of schemas called schema domains. Each of the domains represents an important component of a child's core needs. Schemas interfere with the child's attempts to get the core needs met within each domain. Table 1.1 provides a capsule description of these schemas and domains.

Schema Therapy involves identifying maladaptive schemas, deciding on the appropriate level of change, and planning interventions to effect this level or degree of change. Differing levels of schema change are noted: schema reconstruction, schema modification, interpretation and schema camouflage. Schema reconstruction, i.e., maladaptive replacing the schema with a more functional one, is the most extensive level of transformation and often involves long-term treatment, whereas schema camouflage is the least extensive and may be more appropriate goal in shorter-term treatment (Young, 1999; 2003; Farrell & Shaw, 2022).

Structured Treatment Interventions

Unlike schemas that reflect the psychological dimension of personality, temperament, i.e., the innate, genetic, and constitutional aspect of personality reflects its biological dimension. Temperament plays an important role in the regulation and dysregulation of an individual's affective, behavioral and cognitive styles (Sperry & Sperry, 2016). While research shows that medication can modulate or normalize dysregulated behaviors, a similar modulating effect has also been noted for social skills training (Lieberman, DeRisi & Mueser, 1989). Thus, it appears that social skills training is a relatively potent bottom-up treatment strategy for normalizing such limbic system mediated behaviors as impulsivity, aggressivity, and mood lability, to name a few. Sperry (2015) contends that personality-disordered individuals typically exhibit significant skill deficits, and that structured skill training interventions are useful and

Table 1.1 Maladaptive Schemas and Schema Domains

Disconnection and Rejection

- **Abandonment/instability:** The belief that significant others will not or cannot provide reliable and stable support.
- **Mistrust/Abuse:** The belief that others will abuse, humiliate, cheat, lie, manipulate, or take advantage.
- **Emotional deprivation:** The belief that one's desire for emotional support will not be met by others.
- **Defectiveness/Shame:** The belief that one is defective, bad, unwanted, or inferior in important respects
- **Social Isolation/Alienation:** The belief that one is alienated, different from others, or not part of any group.

Impaired Autonomy and Performance

- **Dependence/Incompetence:** The belief that one is unable to competently everyday responsibilities without considerable help from others.
- **Vulnerability to Harm or Illness:** The exaggerated fear that imminent catastrophe will strike at any time and that one will be unable to prevent it.
- **Enmeshment/Undeveloped Self:** The belief that one must be emotional close with others at the expense of full individuation or normal social development.
- **Failure:** The belief that one will inevitably fail or is fundamentally inadequate in achieving one's goals.

Impaired Limits

- **Entitlement/Grandiosity:** The belief that one is superior to others and not bound by the rules and norms that govern normal social interaction.
- **Insufficient Self-Control/Self-Discipline:** The belief that one is incapable of self-control and frustration tolerance.

Other-Directedness

- **Subjugation:** The belief that one's desires, needs, and feelings must be suppressed in order to meet the needs of others and avoid retaliation or criticism.
- **Self-Sacrifice:** The belief that one must meet the needs of others at the expense of one's own gratification.
- **Approval-Seeking/Recognition-Seeking:** The belief that one must constantly seek to belong and be accepted at the expense of developing a true sense of self.

Overvigilance and Inhibition

- **Negativity/Pessimism:** A pervasive, lifelong focus on the negative aspects of life while minimizing the positive and optimistic aspects.
- **Emotional inhibition:** The excessive inhibition of spontaneous action, feeling, or communication—usually to avoid disapproval by others, feelings of shame, or losing control of one's impulses.
- **Unrelenting Standards/Hypercriticalness:** The belief that striving to meet unrealistically high standards of performance is essential to be accepted and to avoid criticism.
- **Punitiveness:** The belief that others should be harshly punished for making errors.

necessary in successful treatment of moderate to severe personality disorders. Skill deficits can be reversed by the acquisition of requisite in individual and group sessions through practice via modeling, coaching, role-playing, and graded task assignment. Sixteen structured intervention strategies for modifying a personality-disordered individual's affective, behavioral and cognitive temperament styles are described and illustrated in *Cognitive Behavior Therapy of DSM-5 Personality Disorders, Third Edition* (Sperry & Sperry, 2016). Table 1.2

Table 1.2 Structured Treatment Interventions

1. Anger Management Training
2. Anxiety Management Training
3. Assertiveness Training
4. Distress Tolerance Training
5. Emotional Regulation Training
6. Empathy Training
7. Impulse Control Training
8. Interpersonal Skills Training
9. Limit Setting
10. Mindfulness Training
11. Problem Solving Training
12. Radical Openness Skills Training
13. Self-Management Training
14. Sensitivity Reduction Training
15. Symptom Management Training
16. Thought Stopping

lists these interventions. An extended description and illustration of these and other ultra brief cognitive behavioral interventions is provided in Sperry and Binensztok (2019).

Transference-Focused Psychotherapy

Transference Focused Psychotherapy (TFP) was developed by Otto Kernberg, M.D. and associates (Clarkin, Yeomans, & Kernberg, 2015) for the treatment of personality disorder, but initially for Borderline Personality Disorder. It is a highly structured, manualized, evidence-based treatment approach (Levy, Yeomans, & Spina, 2022).

Theory

TFP emerged in response to the failure of psychoanalysis to treat personality disorders. While psychoanalysis benefited some individuals, it was not helpful for those with severe personality disorders. In fact, many with personality disorders appeared to worsen with psychoanalysis. Instead of concluding that the treatment method itself might be the cause, many concluded that personality disorders were untreatable. The developers of TFP challenged this belief and went on to modify and tailor the traditional psychoanalytic methods to severe personality disorders.

TFP is based on object relations theory which contends that infants form internal representations of themselves ("self") and others ("objects"). Typically, these "objects" are early caregivers. These early self-object representations are connected to each other through a dominant affect or feeling. In early stages of infant development, it is posited that positively toned, self-object representations develop separately from negative-toned representations. According to Kernberg, healthy adult personality development requires these split-off, positively and negatively toned object representations to become integrated into a single, cohesive whole. On the other hand, when good and bad representations remain split-off and separate, a disintegrated personality organization, or personality disorder, is likely to result.

Once formed, these object relationship pairs (dyads) serve as a map or template by which later relationships can be understood and enacted. Such internalized object relations are thought to later play out in the individual's life in important relationships. To the extent that an individual has an accurate map or template, a healthy and accurate understanding of future relationships is available. In contrast, when the individual has an inaccurate, "split-off" and polarized map or template, interpersonal problems result. This also applies to the relationship with a therapist. Accordingly, the therapist is able to identify the nature of the problem and its repair (Levy, Yeomans & Spina, 2022).

Treatment

In Transference-Focused Psychotherapy (TFP) the relationship that forms between the therapist and patient is the mechanism of change. This means that the therapeutic relationship itself provides the means to identify and then correct the problematic personality structure. The goal is to provide patients with a corrected template of relationships. This correction becomes possible through the process of "transference" which occurs because the patient draws upon the faulty relationship template formed during childhood. As transference occurs during therapy sessions, the therapist uses this experience as a framework for identifying, understanding, and updating these internal representations or templates. As TFP therapists recognize this transference, they assist patients to understand and to modify these internal representations.

The primary goal of TFP is to assist patients in achieving a corrective emotional experience by means of the therapeutic relationship (Levy, Yeomans, & Spina, 2022). The therapist seeks to create an empathic and soothing relational climate that enables patients to directly experience painful, contradictory, and ambivalent feelings toward the therapist. In this safe and comforting setting, patients learns to confront and tolerate the disturbing feelings that emerge when the chaotic and split-off, self-object representations are activated. This ability to tolerate these highly uncomfortable feelings was not possible as an infant or child. The purpose of this process is to assist the patient to integrate split-off representations of self-and-other into a cohesive whole. The ultimate goal of TFP is identity integration.

TFP differs from the traditional psychoanalytic treatment, in several ways. For one, there is a very specific agenda and therapy contract. The contract addresses the boundaries of the treatment, such as frequency and duration of sessions, phone calls, and procedures when crises arise. The therapist is not simply a passive listener, but instead takes on a very active role in the therapy, asking pointed, clarifying questions, and challenging self-destructive or other negative behaviors. Of particular note is that the focus of treatment is on here-and-now, relational problems. Such a focus helps patients make connections between their present relationship with the therapist, and the current problems they experience with other relationships in their life (Levy, Yeomans, & Spina, 2022).

Furthermore, patients are expected to develop a meaningful and productive life outside of therapy by finding a job, engaging in volunteer work, or continuing in school. Typically, therapy sessions are 45 minutes long and meet twice weekly. When indicated, group treatment or involvement in a 12-step program may be recommended.

Mentalization-Based Treatment

Mentalization-Based Treatment (MBT) was developed by Anthony Bateman and Peter Fonagy for the treatment of personality disorders, particularly for Borderline Personality Disorder (Bateman & Fonagy, 2007; 2009; Bateman, 2022).

Theory

MBT is primarily based on attachment theory wherein the basic premise is that infants have an inborn need to seek closeness with their caregiver. When distressed an infant's attachment behaviors (e.g., smiling, clinging, crying) are activated in an order to elicit the response of soothing from a caregiver. How the caregivers respond greatly influences the development of the child's basic sense of security. Over time, children develop an internal working model of relationships based on their interactions with caregivers, and this model influences other important relationships later in life (Bateman, 2022).

To the extent caregivers respond appropriately in soothing and comforting the child, a secure attachment is formed. As a result of secure attachments, children learn to self-soothe and self-regulate their emotions as they model their caregiver's comforting responses. To the extent the caregivers fail to respond appropriately, an insecure attachment is formed, and the child is less likely to engage in self-soothing and self-regulating behaviors.

Mentalization is the ability to reflect upon, and to understand one's own state of mind. It is the insightful understanding of what and why one is feeling. Mentalization develop because of the caregiver's empathic and insightful response to a child's distress. It is learned through the experience of a secure attachment.

Mentalization is a critical coping skill necessary for effective emotional regulation. For all practical purposes, mentalizing is like hitting the "pause" button. For example, the experience of a powerful negative feeling is usually coupled with an intense urge to act or respond. The ability to briefly tolerate that powerful feeling and to reflect on it can effectively deter one from acting on that intense urge. Since the defining characteristic of a personality disorder is relational difficulties, personality-disordered individuals typically have deficits in these critical skills. A basic premise of MBT is that mentalization must be learned to correct relational difficulties. Accordingly, a basic goal of MBT therapy is to increase the capacity for mentalization. necessary skill (Bateman, 2022).

Treatment

Typically, this is how MBT therapy works. It begins with the development of a warm and empathic therapeutic alliance which provides the context for learning the skill of mentalization. Then, the therapist actively encourages the patient to reflect upon current relational interactions. This includes interactions within therapy sessions. The mind of the patient becomes the focus of treatment in that patients come to know and understand what their minds are thinking. They also learn to identify and label the feelings associated with what they are thinking. They learn to evaluate errors and misjudgments in themselves and others that have led to negative consequences. Usually, individuals sessions are scheduled on a weekly basis as are group sessions in which group members learn from one another (Bateman, 2022).

Developmental Therapy

As increasing numbers of individuals seek or demand that psychotherapy help them to improve personal, relational or professional performance, in other words, to become more fully functioning, therapists and focused therapies will rise to the occasion. The developmental focus in psychotherapy that begin to emerge in the 1960s and 70s (Blocher, 1974;

Shostrum, 1976) and was subsequently eclipsed is now being retrieved (Cortright, 1997; Blocher, 2000; Sperry, 2002; 2016). Such a developmentally focused approach conceptualizes an individual's needs and concerns on a continuum ranging from pathological states to growth states.

The developmental perspective is particularly compatible with the treatment of personality disorders, in that it conceptualizes problem-oriented and growth-oriented needs and views in dimensional rather than in categorical terms, i.e., on a continuum from the low to high level of functioning: disordered, adequate, and optimal functioning (Sperry, 2002). Such a developmental–dimensional perspective is superior to the current DSM-5-TR categorical distinction between pathological functioning vs. normal functioning or optimal functioning. While it is true that third party payers may not easily be convinced that it is immediately in their best interest to reimburse for therapy that focuses on optimal functioning, such a developmental–dimensional conceptualization can serve to not only guide therapists' decisions for optimizing treatment but also to guide outcomes research on the cost-effectiveness of such treatment. A brief overview of these three levels of functioning for each of the ten personality styles–disorders are presented in Table 1.3.

A protocol for conducting developmental therapy focused on increasing optimal functioning is described by Sperry (2002; 2016). Other developmental approaches for fostering optimal functioning have been described by Cortright (1997) and Blocher (2000).

Medication Strategies

Traditionally, the use of medication in the treatment of personality disorders was viewed as limited. Medication tended to be utilized only for a concurrent clinical disorder such as Bipolar Disorder or a target symptom like insomnia. This view is rapidly changing. Today, a growing number of psychopharmacologists believe that psychopharmacological treatment can and should be directed to basic dimensions that underlie the personality. Psychopharmacological research on treatment of selected personality disorders has grown rapidly in the past few years (Reich, 2002; Sperry, 2003; Marin, Foster, & Goodman, 2022). Until recently, medication treatment of personality-disordered individuals has been largely empirical, that is largely trial and error. The reason is that there are still no specific drug treatments for DSM-5-TR personality disorders except for avoidantm borderline, and schizotypal personality disorder (Silk & Fuerino, 2012; Black, Zanarini, Romine, Shaw, Allen, & Schulz, 2014).

Combined and Collaborative Treatment

There is growing consensus, among all segments of the mental health community, that effective treatment of the personality disorders involves combining treatment modalities and integrating treatment approaches (Sperry, 2006; Winkeller & Schlesinger, 2021). In many treatment centers, this means individual therapy is combined with group therapy or psychoeducation groups, and it may include medication or other modalities. Combining medication with individual and group modalities tends to increase effectiveness. Such efforts to integrate various approaches, as well as to combine treatment modalities, would have been considered heretical just a few years ago. Now, integrating and combining treatments is an emerging consensus that reflects the immensity of the "paradigm shift" that is occurring (Beitman, 2003; Sperry, 2003).

Table 1.3 Developmental Levels of Personality: Optimal, Adequate, and Disordered

OBSESSIVE	
Optimal	Conscientious but spontaneous individuals who balance personal integrity with generosity, hopefulness, and kindness
Adequate	Less perfectionism and rigidity in tasks and relationships with some degree of emotional involvement
Disordered	Perfectionism and feeling avoidance that interferes with task completion and relationships; overly rigid thinking and attitudes; pessimistic and stingy
HISTRIONIC	
Optimal	Having found the love they seek within themselves, they are altruistic and giving without expecting reciprocity
Adequate	While fun loving and often impulsive, they can delay gratification and be emotionally appropriate much of the time
Disordered	Uncomfortable in situations in which he or she is not the center of attention
NARCISSISTIC	
Optimal	Energetic and self-assured without expecting special treatment or privilege
Adequate	Confident, yet emotionally vulnerable, and favor special treatment or privilege
Disordered	Manifests a grandiose sense of self-importance and demand special privilege
AVOIDANT	
Optimal	While sensitive to interpersonal cues and possessing a keen intuition about others, they are nonetheless respectful and compassionate toward others
Adequate	Maintain a reserved demeanor around others, because they are sensitive and concerned about others' opinion of them
Disordered	Avoid social and work-related activities that involve significant interpersonal contact because of fear of criticism, disapproval, or rejection
SCHIZOID	
Optimal	Deeply grounded in themselves, they are emotionally connected to the world
Adequate	Reasonably comfortable being around others, provided there are limited demands for intimacy or emotional connectedness
Disordered	Neither desires nor enjoys close relationships
DEPENDENT	
Optimal	May seek out the opinions and advice of others when making major decisions, but the decisions they make are ultimately their own
Adequate	Have the capacity to be responsible and make decisions, but still seek out and rely on others for help and advice
Disordered	Need others to assume responsibility for most major areas of their life
ANTISOCIAL	
Optimal	Have the gift of gab and easily befriend others, although they may not offer much depth to these relationships
Adequate	Earn respect by acting honorably and with compassion, by using power constructively, and by promoting worthwhile causes
Disordered	Exhibit aggressive, impulsive, self-serving and irresponsible behavior

(Continued)

Table 1.3 (Continued)

BORDERLINE	
Optimal	Sensitive, introspective, and impressionable individuals who are very comfortable with their feelings and inner impulses
Adequate	They quickly and easily engage in relationships and are sometimes hurt and rejected in the process
Disordered	Display frantic efforts to avoid real or imagined rejection and abandonment
SCHIZOTYPAL	
Optimal	Possess the unique capacity to view situations and life differently so as to benefits others
Adequate	Immersed in the unique and unusual, irrespective of whether it has any socially redeeming value.
Disordered	Exhibit odd, eccentric or peculiar behavior, thinking and speech
PARANOID	
Optimal	Highly observant and discerning, they can defend themselves without losing control or becoming aggressive
Adequate	Thin-skinned, they are rather sensitive to and hurt by criticism
Disordered	Suspicious, without sufficient basis, that others are exploiting, harming, or deceiving them

Trends in Personality Disorders Research and Training

This section evaluates the trend and developments in both research and clinical training. Overall, following the publication of the DSM-5 Alternative Model of Personality Disorders in 2013 research on personality disorders began to increase. However, training of students and clinicians in the assessment, diagnosis, and treatment of the personality disorders in both graduate programs and clinic sites did not appear to increase appreciably.

Research

Then, "personality disorder (PD) research was poised to become the vanguard of psychopathology science in an era marked by the profound influence of personality on psychiatric taxonomy, driven by transformative changes in PD diagnosis…However, today, the field presents a stagnant panorama, marked by a conspicuous lack of advancement in methodologies, conceptual frameworks, and consequential implications for therapeutic interventions" (Hopwood, Kaurin, & Pincus, 2024). Fueling the apprehension and pessimism of Hopwood and associates are two factors. First, is the lack of appeal that PD research has for young clinical scientists largely because of narrow research focus and outdated methodology. Second is the perceived limited clinical relevance of current research. (Hopwood, Kaurin, & Pincus, 2024). There are some recommended courses of action for reversing this downward trend.

The first is that future research focus and methodology would do well to "incorporate the most recent insights in the field of personality pathology development. These consist of a more comprehensive, integrative, and lifespan-informed view of personality pathology that explains the development of personality pathology and how it interdigitates with other common forms of mental illness. We suggest tailored methodological techniques that match the complexity of non- linear and reciprocal personality development, as well as interventions that focus on specific features and patterns of personality pathology that arise at different developmental epochs" (Johnson & Vanwoerden, 2021, p. 7). These authors believe that the field is "at the cusp of a new era in understanding PD development that will open the door to effective prevention efforts that stave off the burden of PDs earlier in life" (Johnson & Vanwoerden, 2021, p. 7).

Training

As to the matter of training graduate students and practicing clinicians in the effective assessment, diagnosis, case conceptualization, and treatment implementation of the personality disorders, it appears that little progress has been forthcoming. While clinicians in the past decades have become less pessimistic about the treatability of patients with personality disorders, training has neither increased nor appreciably improved. Although it is no longer common for instructors to tell students "Borderline Personality Disorder is untreatable" instructors seem more focused on teaching interventions and strategies for common symptom disorders like depression, anxiety, and PTSD than interventions and strategies for personality disorders. Such teaching too often reflects the structure of the textbooks used by these instructors, in which the Personality Disorder is placed near the end the textbook *after* the symptom disorders. This is how the DSM-5-TR is structured. Because I believe that patients' personality and personality pathology inform their clinical presentation, the chapter in my psychopathology textbooks on personality disorders comes *before* the symptom disorder.

Commenting on the importance of training students and clinicians in the effective treatment of personality disorders, Johnson and Vanwoerden (2021) concluded:

> Unfortunately, personality disorder treatment and research are not commonly taught among training programs. Given the prevalence of PDs and their costliness to society, further training and education of clinicians regarding PDs might reduce stigma, alleviate burnout, improve early detection and intervention, and lessen the overall burden of PDs on individuals, carers, healthcare providers, and society at large.
> (Johnson & Vanwoerden, 2021, p. 6)

Training research suggests that education and training must be multifaceted meaning that it occurs in graduate training and supervision as well as targeting trainees and practitioners at clinic sites. This means instituting policies and practice that modify a training program's and clinic's culture to foster positive attitudes and provide clinicians with the clinical skills and administrative support to utilize effective treatment interventions with personality-disordered patients (Klein, Fairweather & Lawn, 2022). More specifically, "this review suggest that education and training as a stand-alone strategy is unlikely to be sufficient to instill adequate and sustained changes in health practitioners' attitudes and practice in BPD. Rather, a system-wide approach to tackling structural stigma at both the macro- and micro-levels of institutions is required, including implementing coordinated and targeted changes to organizational leadership approaches, policies, culture, and practices" (Klein, Fairweather, & Lawn, 2022, p. 16). Although this research focused on BPD, the findings are applicable to other personality disorders.

So, it is not just about whether an instructor is committed and prepared to teach students how to accurately diagnose, conceptualize cases, and implement tailored treatment with personality-disordered individuals, it is as much about the training program's culture, commitment, and support of faculty who provide this instruction. Such system dynamics are powerful. Similarly, these system dynamics are operative at clinic sites, which will either encourage and support clinicians and trainees to competently and effectively collaborate with personality-disordered patients to effect needed change in their lives.

Structure of Subsequent Chapters

Each chapter is divided into five major sections: overview, description, case conceptualization, assessment, and treatment. The overview section provides a brief historical sketch of the disorder including its evolution in DSM. It also reports an incidence/prevalence data on the disorder.

The section on Description provides an extensive discussion of the particular personality disorder in biopsychosocial terms. Emphasized are aspects of temperament such as cognitive style, emotional style, behavioral style, and interpersonal style. To assist the clinician in both establishing whether the presentation is one of disorder or style, and what the profile of successful treatment of the disorder would look like, descriptions, characteristic features and case examples of both the personality style and disorder are provided. Included are DSM-5-TR descriptions, prototypic descriptions, and prevalence data. Case conceptualizations can be thought of in terms of diagnostic, clinical, cultural, and treatment formulations (Sperry, Gudeman, Blackwell, & Faulkner, 1992; Sperry & Sperry, 2020). This section represents a diagnostic formulation of the disorder.

The next section contains five different case conceptualizations of the disorder. The four dominant clinical formulations are psychodynamic, the biosocial—represented largely by Millon (1981, 1985, 1990); the cognitive—represented largely by Beck and Freeman (1990); and the behavioral–represented by Turkat (1990); the interpersonal—described by Benjamin (1993); and the integrative or biopsychosocial developed by Sperry (1990) and Sperry and Mosak (1993).

The section on assessment describes typical interview behavior manifest by the personality-disordered patient and the ease or difficult of establishing rapport. It also describes characteristic response patterns common for this personality disorder on such psychological tests as the MMPI-I, the MCMI-II, which is based on Millon's (1981, 1990) biosocial formulation and research data; and two common projective tests, the Rorschach, R-PAS, and Therapeutic Apperception Test (TAT). Since psychological testing can be particularly useful in clarifying a dimensional characterization of the patient's personality, i.e., where more than one personality disorder or clusters of traits are present, this section may be clinically relevant to psychologists and others who utilizes psychological assessment. The following section on case conceptualization can be quite useful in understanding the origins of these disorders.

Three general approaches most commonly utilized in the individual treatment of the disorder are detailed. They are the psychodynamic, the cognitive-behavioral and the interpersonal approaches. The psychodynamic approaches usually include a description of the ways the traditional analytic method has been modified for this disorder in terms of expressive-supportive terms. The cognitive therapy of personality disorder approach of Beck, Davis, and Freeman (2015) is highlighted, and complemented with the research-based behavioral approach of Turkat (1990) and others. Furthermore, Benjamin's (1993; 2006) protocol for interpersonal treatment is presented.

Other modalities of treatment relevant to the disorder are explored along with relevant research on theory indications and efficacy. A unique feature of this book is the discussion of group, marital and family, and psychopharmacology modalities for each disorder. The group treatment modality can be either homogeneous or heterogeneous, structured and time limited, or less structured and ongoing. Heterogeneous refers to the composition group being diverse in terms of functioning. Homogeneous refers to the group composition being similar in terms of personality types and level of functioning (Francis, Clarkin, & Perry, 1984). Homogeneous groups lend themselves to being structured, and time limited. Finally, specific suggestions for combining modalities and integrating or blending treatment approaches, rounds out this section and the book. Chapters 4 to 13 follow the same general format or chapter outline as noted in Table 1.4.

A key to providing effective treatment of the personality disorders is an in-depth understanding of how and why personality disorder pathology develops as well how it is experienced by the both personality-disordered individual and related others. Although the narrative of each chapter—i.e. Section II Description—provides a detailed description of a given personality disorder, a table providing a *capsule summary* of these defining characteristics is included in each chapter. Its purpose is to facilitate both initial learning about the disorder and to serve as a subsequent reference source. Table 1.5 lists these characteristics. This is followed by a brief description of each these 12 characteristics.

Triggering Event(s)

The characteristic and predictable situations, circumstances or other stimuli that initiates a characteristic maladaptive response—in family or intimate relations, in social situations, or in work settings (Othmer & Othmer, 2002) —which are reflected in the individual's behavioral, interpersonal, cognitive and emotional styles. Triggering events can be intrapersonal, such as failing an exam, or interpersonal, i.e., a narcissistic injury.

Behavioral Style

The characteristic way in which an individual reacts personally to a triggering event. Examples include: self-centeredness, impatience, defensiveness, arrogance, etc.

Interpersonal Style

The characteristic way in which an individual relates to others. Examples include: exploitive, disdainful, socially facile without empathy, pleasing, clinging, blaming, condescending, etc.

Cognitive Style

The characteristic way in which an individual perceives and thinks about a problem and then conceives and implements a solution. Examples of such styles include analytic, methodical, global or thematic, cautious, careless, etc.

Table 1.4 Chapter Format

I Overview and Background
II Description

   1 Defining Characteristics

      a Style vs. Disorder
      b Triggering Event
      c Behavioral Style
      d Interpersonal Style
      e Cognitive Style
      f Emotional Style
      g Attachment Style
      h Optimal Diagnostic Criteria

   2 DSM-5-TR Characterization
   3 Prototypic Description
   4 Associated Features

      a Prevalence
      b Differential Diagnosis
      c Development & Course
      d Culture, Sex, and Gender

   5 Alternative Model

III Case Conceptualization

   1 Psychodynamic
   2 Biosocial
   3 Cognitive-Behavioral
   4 Interpersonal
   5 Integrative

VI Assessment

   1 Interview Behavior and Rapport
   2 Psychological Testing Data

      a MMPI-2
      b MCMI-IV
      c Rorschach/R-PAS & TAT

V Treatment Approaches and Interventions

   1 Treatment Considerations
   2 Individual Psychotherapy

      a Psychodynamic Approaches
      b Cognitive-Behavioral Approaches
      c Interpersonal Approaches

   3 Group Therapy
   4 Marital and Family Therapy
   5 Medication
   6 Combined and Collaborative Treatment

Table 1.5 Defining Characteristics of a Personality Disorder

- Triggering Event(s)
- Behavioral Style
- Interpersonal Style
- Cognitive Style
- Emotional Style
- Temperament
- Attachment Style
- Parental Injunction
- Self–Other Schema
- Maladaptive Core Schema
- Optimal Diagnostic Criteria

Emotional/Feeling Style

The characteristic way in which an individual responds with various types and intensities of affects. Examples of such styles include anger, rage, elation, and mood lability.

Temperament

An inborn, characteristic response pattern reflecting an individual's energy level, emotional make-up, intensity, and tempo of response which serve as "a filter of personality through which information is processed, attachments evolve, and emotions are experienced and expressed" (Graybar & Boutilier, 2002, p. 156). Examples of such styles include inhibited, impulsive, reflective, and aggressive.

Attachment Style

The pattern of adult relating reflecting the emotional bond between parent and infant which influences affect regulation, psychological resilience, access to autobiographical memory, and the development of self-reflection and narrative. Styles are either secure or insecure (Ainsworth et al., 1987; Erdman & Caffery, 2003). Examples of Insecure styles noted in personality disordered individuals include preoccupied, fearful, dismissing, and disorganized styles.

Parental Injunction

An expressed or implied parental expectation for what a child should be or should act. Examples of such injunctions are: "you can't do it by yourself," "you must be better to be worthwhile," "never make mistakes," etc.

Self-Other Schema

This schema involves self-view and view of others. An individual's self-view or personal conception of self, including a self-evaluation of abilities, personal worth, potential, and goals. Examples of such self-convictions include: "I am defective," "I need the attention of others to feel important and worthwhile," "I am special and entitled," etc. (Sperry, 2015).

An individual's evaluative conception of others includes beliefs about human nature, the world, and other people. Examples of such convictions include: "life is a struggle," "people can't be trusted," "other are here to take care of me," etc. (Sperry, 2015).

Maladaptive Schemas

Schemas are enduring and self-defeating patterns regarding one's view of self and of the world and others developed during childhood and elaborated throughout one's lifetime. They cause negative thoughts and feelings and interfere with accomplishing goals and meetings one's needs (Young, 2003). Examples of such schemas include: defectiveness, social isolation, approval-seeking, self-sacrifice, etc.

Optimal Diagnostic Criterion

It's believed that if clinicians can remember one key criterion for each personality disorder they "could then test for the presence or absence of that criterion and quickly diagnose the personality disorder" (Allnutt and Links, 1996, p. 22). An optimal criterion is derived from three characteristics: its protypicality, i.e., having a high correlation with the sum of all criteria for that disorder, an apt behavioral description, and a high positive predictive value, i.e., the probability the individual has the criteria has the target disorder. Data on protypicality and predictive value were derived from research with the *Structured Interview for Diagnosing Personality–Revised* (Allnutt & Links, 1996).

Concluding Note

Today clinicians are considerably more confident and effective in working with personality-disordered individuals than any time in the history of psychiatry and the mental health sciences. Whereas twenty years ago, many if not most clinicians believed these disorders to be untreatable, now clinicians can point to both clinical experience and research evidence that indicates that personality-disordered individuals, including those with borderline personality disorder, can be helped to increase their functioning and well-being. As chronicled in first edition of this book, the emerging shift in the treatment paradigm of the personality disorders is now fully underway and promises to be as exciting and far-ranging as was the earlier paradigm shift in diagnosing and treating the depressive disorders.

This chapter has previewed a number of cutting-edge developments involving the conceptualization, assessment and diagnosis, and treatment of the DSM-5-TR personality disorders. Many of these developments in diagnosis and treatment are incorporated in subsequent chapters.

Chapter 2

The Alternative Model for Personality Disorders

The Alternative Model for Personality Disorders (AMPD) first appeared in DSM-5 (American Psychiatric Association, 2013) and has been retained in DSM-5-TR (American Psychiatric Association, 2022). It provides a clinically useful dimensional trait model for understanding and treating personality disorders (PD). This model allows a more accurate and clinically useful description of an individual's personality pathology than the previous DSM categorical model that first appeared in DSM-III and continued through DSM-IV-TR. In addition, this dimensional trait model has the potential to greatly facilitate the therapeutic alliance, case conceptualization and treatment planning, and treatment implementation and monitoring (Siefert, Porcerelli, Meehan & Dauphin, 2022).

This chapter begins with a short history of the development and rationale for the AMPD, followed by a description of the components of this alternative model. Next, it describes the extraordinary clinical utility of the AMPD and illustrates it with three case examples. Then, it briefly notes how the AMPD can be used in clinical practice today.

Rationale for an Alternative Model for Personality Disorders

How and why the Alternative Model for Personality Disorders (AMPD) came about is interesting and instructive. For some four decades the existing DSM categorical model garnered much criticism, particularly its limited clinical utility (Cain & Mulay, 2022). These shortcomings led to the unfortunate overuse by clinicians of the PD Not Otherwise Specified (PD-NOS) diagnostic label. While this diagnosis conveys little information about a specific patient's personality pathology, it at least identifies "that the patient 'has a personality problem,' a situation that is not particularly helpful in case conceptualization" (Krueger, 2019, p. 63). In short, these and other "problems were numerous, and they make it essentially impossible to work with the categorical PD concepts in research and in the clinic… The conceptual and practical incoherence of the DSM PD categories is the essence of what led to the creation of the AMPD" (Krueger, 2019, p. 62). So, what is the categorical model and why replace it?

Categorical Model

The categorical model assumes that each personality disorder is a distinct entity or category, and that each personality disorder is separate from the other personality disorders, as well as from "normal" personalities. Since every categorical diagnosis is characterized by specific diagnostic criteria, these criteria are used to determine if a disorder is present or absent. Three major concerns with the categorical model involve comorbidity, heterogeneity, and the construct of personality.

The concern about comorbidity is that individuals can simultaneously meet criteria for more than one disorder. For instance, it was estimated that the modal number of personality disorder diagnoses possible for an individual who meets criteria for at least one DSM personality disorder is three or four diagnoses (Gunderson, 1996). Arguably, this is problematic for case conceptualization and planning tailored interventions: if there are three diagnoses, which one should be the initial focus of treatment and why? The Alternative Personality Disorder model solves this problem through the diagnosis of Personality Disorder-Trait Specified (PD-TS). If the client is not a good match to a specific DSM-5-TR Personality Disorder, such as the Narcissistic Personality Disorder, the clinician records PD-TS and details the client's clinically important personality features. For example, a client may have features of narcissistic, histrionic, antisocial, and borderline personality disorder. Instead of recording all four diagnoses, the clinician can record PD-TS and note the mix of grandiose, attention-seeking, antagonistic, and emotional lability.

A second concern involves heterogeneity. The premise of the DSM-IV-TR Personality Disorder model was that articulating specific personality disorder categories would facilitate accurate diagnoses. Unfortunately, individuals' personality and psychopathological features seldom fit such a categorical model. For instance, individuals meeting DSM-5-TR criteria for Borderline Personality Disorder are a highly heterogeneous group. This will be quite evident in the three case examples of Borderline Personality Disorder (BPD) described later in this chapter. In fact, there are six distinctive subgroups of clients who met these criteria and these subgroups differed markedly with regard to therapeutic concerns such as past suicide attempts, antisocial behavior, and self-injury (Wright, Hallquist, Morse, Scott, Stepp, Nolf, & Pilkonis, 2013). In contrast, the Alternative Model greatly reduces this heterogeneity problem because relevant heterogeneity is specified as part of the diagnostic process. For example, a client may meet the general Borderline Personality Disorder profile but also have other clinically significant personality features, such as unusual beliefs and experiences. In this case, the diagnosis of Borderline Personality Disorder can be given while also recording the unusual beliefs and experiences.

The third concern is with the very nature of categorical diagnosis. As a categorical model it is expected to accurately determine whether an individual has or does not have a personality disorder. In many respects, such a model is not well suited for diagnosing personality disorders since personality is a continuous, multi-faceted dimension. To illustrate, consider the trait of grandiosity, a characteristic trait of the Narcissistic Personality Disorder. On a continuum from healthy self-esteem to self-centered entitlement, where does a clinician distinguish between health and disorder with regard to this trait? Utilizing a categorical model with a continuous dimension like grandiosity is akin to trying to force a round peg into a square hole.

Given these concerns, it is not surprising that many clinicians did not find this categorical model of personality disorders to be very clinically useful. As a result, many clinicians deferred making meaningful personality description in patient's charts. Many also view the model's description of these disorders as highly stigmatized, leading to further reluctance to use it.

Dimensional Model

Aware of these concerns, the DSM-5 Personality Disorders Work Group endeavored to find an alternative to the ten "official" personality disorder diagnoses that remain unchanged since categorical model was introduced in DSM-III. The Work Group's solution was to propose a dimensional model that they hoped would eventually replace the existing categorical model. In the interim they came up with a hybrid model, i.e., one that was dimensional but retained some elements of the categorical model.

However, the board of the American Psychiatric Association would not approve the replacement of the categorial model in Section II which contained the Personality Disorders diagnoses. Instead, they relegated the hybrid model to Section III. Not surprisingly, relatively few clinicians utilized the new model (Hopwood, Mulay, & Waugh, 2019). However, some clinicians did try out the new model. Soon after DSM-5 appeared, a survey of 337 psychiatrists and psychologists found the Alternative Model to be considerably more useful than the categorical model (Morey, Skodol, & Oldham, 2014). Presumably, as clinicians become more familiar with the Alternative Model, patients are more likely to receive an accurate assessments and diagnoses leading to improved clinical care.

The DSM-5-TR Personality Disorders Work Group continued to support and advocate for the dimensions model but were unable to move it to Section II. Nevertheless, they did provide the clinically useful "Associated Features" inserts in Section II (American Psychiatric Association, 2022). It is noteworthy that despite the reluctance of the American Psychiatric Association to adopt a dimensional model of diagnosis, the *International Classification of Diseases*, 11th Revision (ICD-11) did embrace the dimensional model (Herpertz, Schneider, Renneberg, & Schneider, 2022; Mulder & Bach, 2022).

ICD-11

ICD-11 refers to the 11th revision of the *International Classification of Diseases*. It is a diagnostic tool developed by the World Health Organization and has been in use globally since January 1, 2022. While DSM-5-TR was approved and became available in May 2022, it chose the older ICD-10-CM codes to identify all DSM diagnoses including the personality disorders.

Presumably DSM-5-TR chose not to adopt the new ICD-11 codes in order to maintain the older categorical system rather than embrace the dimensional model on which ICD-11 is based. However, DSM-5-TR did agree to a hybrid model for the personality disorders, called the Alternative Model for Personality Disorders (AMPD) in Section III: Emerging Methods and Models. Basically, the AMPD is a hybrid of the earlier DSM categorical model of personality disorders and the dimensional model championed in ICD-11. In short, the AMPD offers as middle-of-the-road approach that is supported by both a growing body of research and considerable promise in clinical practice (Huprich, 2022a; Mulder & Bach, 2022). Early indications are that it is well received by clinicians (Cain & Mulay, 2022).

Coding Personality Disorders in ICD-11

Once the diagnosis of a personality disorder has been established, ICD-11 requires that it be specified by level of severity. These include: 6D10.0 Mild Personality Disorder, 6D10.1 Moderate Personality Disorder, or 6D10.2 Severe Personality Disorder. An additional code: QE50.7 Personality Difficulty is not classified as a mental disorder but refers to pronounced personality characteristics that may affect treatment but do not rise to the level of severity to merit a diagnosis of Personality Disorder.

Personality Disorder and Personality Difficulty are further described using five trait domain specifiers that characterize the individual's personality which are prominent and contribute to personality disturbance. As many as necessary to describe personality functioning should be applied. These include: 6D11.0 Negative Affectivity, 6D11.1 Detachment, 6D11.2 Dissociality, 6D11.3 Disinhibition, and 6D11.4 Anankastia. An additional specifier for those presenting with the borderline pattern' is 6D11.5 Borderline pattern (Mulder & Bach, 2022).

Components of the Alternative Model for Personality Disorders

The hybrid model has two primary criteria. The first criterion, called Criterion A. focuses on Self and Interpersonal functioning. The second criterion, referred to as Criterion B, focuses on the role of 25 pathological personality facets in the expression of personality pathology that are categorized into five broad domains: Negative Affectivity, Detachment, Antagonism, Disinhibition, and Psychoticism.

Criterion A: Personality Functioning

Four elements of personality functioning are identified. There are two indicators of self-functioning: which are Identity and Self-direction. There are also two indicators of interpersonal functioning: Empathy and Intimacy. Impairment in these four elements of personality functioning is rated along a continuum from 0 to 4. Assessment of such impairment can be accomplished with the Levels of Personality Functioning Scale (LPFS) which is provided in Section III (American Psychiatric Association, 2022, pp. 895–898). The LPFS is an objective measure for quickly and accurately determining the presence of a personality disorder. It assesses four components of personality functioning in the AMPD: identity, self-direction, empathy, and intimacy (Skodol, 2021). Impairment in these four elements of personality functioning is rated along a continuum of five levels of functioning and impairment where 0 = little to no impairment; 1 = some impairment; 2 = moderate impairment; 3 = severe impairment; and 4 = extreme impairment. Moderate or greater impairment is required for diagnosis of a personality disorder. Table 2.1 is a brief summary of it.

Criterion B: Pathological Personality Traits

Personality traits are defined in DSM-5-TR as "enduring patterns of perceiving, relating to, and thinking about the environment and oneself that are exhibited in a wide range of social and personal contexts" (American Psychiatric Association, 2022, p. 735). The AMPD identifies five broad trait domains that are derived from the Five-Factor Model of Personality and contain 25 specific personality trait facets. These domains and facets can be assessed with psychometric tests such as Personality Inventory for *Diagnostic and Statistical Manual of Mental Disorders, Fifth edition*, Brief Form (PID-5-BF), It is a 25-item self-report questionnaire that measures the severity of the trait domains and facets (Gomez, Watson & Stavropoulos, 2020).

Table 2.1 Levels of Personality Functioning

0 No Impairment. These individuals functionally optimally in all spheres of life. They have a well-integrated sense of self and of the world. They experience a mostly positive and appropriately regulated emotional life. They are goal-directed and possess the capacity to function productively in society. They easily empathize with other and can form mutually reciprocating and satisfying relationships.

1 Mild Impairment. These individuals have a relatively intact sense of self and of the world and can lessen clarity about boundaries in the face of strong emotions or mental distress. They may be overly goal-directed or goal-inhibited or have somewhat unrealistic personal standards. They tend to have some difficulty appreciating and understanding others' perspectives, and my not consistently be aware of the effect of their behavior on others. Although they can form intimate and reciprocal relationships, they may be somewhat limited in their ability to respect and to cooperate with others.

2 Moderate Impairment. These individuals have a compromised sense of self and of the world, along with some difficulty maintaining boundaries. Their self-appraisal tends to be inflated or deflated and can experience difficulty in emotional regulation. Threats to self-esteem may engender strong emotions such as rage and shame. Goals are more often a means of gaining external approval than self-generated, and thus may lack coherence and stability. Their capacity for empathy is somewhat limited. While they can form relationships, they are superficial and not always reciprocal. They cooperate with others primarily for personal gain.

3 Severe Impairment. These individuals have an impoverished sense of self. Their self-appraisal ranges from self-loathing to self-aggrandizing. They have considerable difficulty in emotional regulation. They have a weak sense of autonomy, and may experience a lack of identity, or emptiness. Boundaries are poorly defined or rigid. They have difficulty establishing and achieving personal goals. Their ability to reflect upon and understand their inner experiences is quite limited, and their capacity for empathy is limited. Their relationships are unstable and are viewed as means of meeting their needs. Cooperative efforts are often disrupted, owing to the perception of slights from others.

4 Extreme Impairment. These individuals have a greatly impoverished, disorganized, weak, ineffective, and/or conflicted sense of self. They have a propensity to negative and significantly dysregulated emotions. Their capacity for empathy is significantly limited, and they cannot consider alternative perspectives, or are threatened by different perspectives. They lack the capacity for adaptive and cooperative interpersonal functioning and social behavior.

The five trait domains and their polar opposites are: Negative Affectivity vs. Emotional Stability; Detachment vs. Extroversion; Antagonism vs. Agreeableness; Disinhibition vs. Conscientiousness; and Psychoticism vs. Lucidity. They are listed in Table 2.2.

It is noteworthy that the polar opposite side of each trait domain does not imply a healthy adaptive response. For example, the opposite of disinhibition is conscientiousness but extreme conscientious represents rigid perfectionism which is pathological indicator of the obsessive-compulsive personality disorder. Similarly, extreme agreeableness equates to gullibility which predisposes an individual to easy manipulation and abuse. Accordingly, the key to healthy personality and adaptive functioning is flexibility meaning that appropriate responding varies according to the demands of each situation.

Six specific personality disorders are listed in the AMPD in Section III: Antisocial Personality Disorder, Avoidant Personality Disorder, Borderline Personality Disorder, Narcissistic Personality Disorder, Obsessive-compulsive Personality Disorder, and Schizotypal Personality Disorder. That means that four of the ten in Section II are not included, presumably because of limited research to support their inclusion. They are: Dependent Personality

Table 2.2 Trait Domains and Trait Facets

Negative Affect
- Emotional Lability
- Anxiousness
- Separation Anxiety
- Submissiveness
- Hostility
- Perseveration

Detachment
- Withdrawal
- Intimacy Avoidance
- Anhedonia
- Depressivity
- Restricted Affect
- Suspiciousness

Antagonism
- Manipulativeness
- Deceitfulness
- Grandiosity
- Attention Seeking
- Callousness
- Hostility

Disinhibition
- Irresponsibility
- Impulsivity
- Distractibility
- Risk Taking
- Rigid Perfectionism

Psychoticism
- Unusual Beliefs And Experiences
- Eccentricity
- Cognitive And Perceptual Dysregulation

Disorder, Histrionic Personality Disorder, Paranoid Personality Disorder, and Schizoid Personality Disorder.

This or another dimensional model is expected to become the "official" diagnostic approach for personality disorders at some point in the future. In the meantime, clinicians may wish to familiarize themselves with the hybrid model. They can also choose to use this dimensional model now.

Clinical Utility of the Alternative Model for Personality Disorders

Clinical utility of a conceptual model or framework refers to the ease and value with which that framework might be used for diagnosis, case conceptualization, treatment selection, outcomes monitoring, clinical decision making, as well as communicating with others. That research shows that clinicians seldom consult categorical personality disorder criteria when making diagnoses which suggests that the categorial framework has limited clinical utility (Rodriguez-Seijas, Ruggero, Eaton, & Krueger, 2019).

In contrast the emerging literature on the clinical utility of the Alternative Model is quite promising. Several articles outline the ways in which the Alternative Model can be used to inform case conceptualization and subsequent treatment planning. Increasingly, research also "suggests that the information in the AMPD is considered more useful by clinicians and corresponds with actual treatment decision-making; and data suggest that maladaptive personality constructs might provide information about differential treatment response" (Rodriguez-Seijas et al., 2019 p. 288).

Treatment Planning and Implementation

Besides facilitating a more precise diagnosis, the AMPD can facilitate an accurate case conceptualization and a tailored treatment plan. Decisions about the choice of treatment interventions are best informed by the diagnosis and case conceptualization (Sperry, 2022).

For instance, various interventions like behavioral activation, exposure and response prevention can be particularly useful when the primary trait profile involves High Negative Affectivity. Relational Interventions are indicated when the focus of treatment is on increasing interpersonal effectiveness. Treatment for elevations in traits related to the Disinhibition domain that include contingency management and motivational interviewing and to increase commitment cab be quite useful. For presentations characterized by High Psychoticism, a clinical focus on confrontation of Active Perceptual Dysregulation and the development of skills aimed at increasing rational understanding of the self and impact on one's environment may be indicated. Similarly, for elevations in Antagonism and Detachment behavioral activation and skills training intervention as in Dialectical Behavior Therapy (DBT) have been found to be effective (Hopwood, 2018).

DBT is described in detail in Chapter 1. It was developed by Linehan (2015) for the treatment of Borderline Personality Disorder. Its four set of skills: emotional regulation skills, interpersonal skills, distress tolerance skills, and core mindfulness skills, are also valuable in targeting treatment to other personality disorders characterized by any of the five trait domains and many of the trait facets. Table 2.3 visualizes the treatment targets of Criterion A and Criterion B and DBT interventions. It is should not be too surprising that DBT is utilized in the three cases of BPD described in the next section.

Using AMPD to Plan and Gude Treatment

The clinical utility and value of the Alternative Model is evident in the following three cases that have the same DSM-5-TR categorical diagnosis of BPD. All three utilized the Level of Personality Functioning Scale (LPFS), and the Personality Inventory for the DSM-5 (PID-5) or its Brief Form (PID-5-BF) to diagnose, plan treatment, and monitor treatment progress. Yet the cases could not be more different. Case #1 involves a young person with acute presentation no comorbidities, a short history of BPD, and successful treatment outcomes in 18 months. The other two cases involve individuals with longer histories of BPD, chronic comorbidities that complicates treatment, two separate therapeutic approaches, and prescribed medication. Treatment continues into the third year for Case #2 and Case #3. Both are actual cases described by Bliton and colleagues (2022) in which some therapeutic

Table 2.3 AMPD Focused Treatment for Borderline Personality Disorder with DBT

BPD: Criterion A and Criterion B	DBT: Individual and Group Interventions
IMPAIRED SELF-FUNCTIONING a identity disturbance OR b self-direction	Validation & identity development [DBT individual therapy]
IMPAIRED INTERPERSONAL FUNCTIONING a empathic deficits OR b intimacy deficits	Interpersonal Skills [DBT group]
PATHOLOGICAL PERSONALITY TRAITS DOMAINS 1 Negative Affect 2 Disinhibition 3 Antagonism	Emotion Regulation Skills [DBT group] Distress Tolerance Skills [DBT group] Core Mindfulness Skills [DBT group]

progress continues to be reported. In short, all three cases demonstrate the clinical utility of AMPD in planning and guiding treatment.

Case #1: Ms. A

Ms. A is a 19-year-old single white female who presented with emotional dysregulation, fear of abandonment, threats of hurting herself, and a recent history of wrist-cutting. She describes herself as angry, impulsive, and overly sensitive. She reports "never really be sure who I am" and has been living with her parents until she figures out what to do with her life. Recently she became convinced that her boyfriend was cheating on her. She reported "I became unhinged and threatened to hurt myself if he left me." This is her first treatment.

Ms. A met the DSM-5-TR categorical criteria for Borderline Personality Disorder (BPD). Criteria A: LPFS at the intake was 3. Criteria B: Ms. A struggles with identity disturbance and exhibited the following traits: Emotional lability (Negative Affect), Separation insecurity (Negative Affect), Impulsivity (Disinhibition), and Hostility (Antagonism). DBT was offered as the treatment of choice with impaired self and interpersonal functioning as well as pathological personality traits as the treatment targets (See Table 2.3). Ms. B agreed to participate in twice weekly structured individual Dialectical Behavior Therapy (DBT) sessions, one-on-one telephone consultation, and a DBT-based skills group.

Treatment progress was monitored. In terms of Criterion B: No trait facets identified. With regard to Criterion A, her level of functioning level improved over the 18 months of treatment. Her LPFS was 3 before starting treatment. After 6 months of treatment, the LPFS was 2, while at termination her LPFS was 1. The final DSM-5-TR diagnosis was that Ms. A no longer met categorical criteria for the diagnosis of BPD.

The course of treatment and its outcome were also monitored. After 12 months Ms. A completed the skills group. She continued with individual therapy sessions and telephone consultation on a biweekly basis another three months before successfully terminating treatment. As a result of this treatment experience, she was able to develop a more stable self-image and identity. She exhibited significant improvement in distress tolerance, and emotional regulation, while being better able to maintain stable relationships. Her pattern became more adaptive in relating to others with more realistic demands of them without engaging in self-harmful behaviors. In short, significant BPD symptom relief and much needed self-validation occurred.

Case #2: Ms. B

Ms. B is a 55-year-old White female with a long history of treatment-resistant depression and anxiety related to difficulties maintaining relationships and employment. She met categorical criteria for Borderline Personality Disorder with dependent and narcissistic traits, as well as Generalized Anxiety Disorder and recurrent, moderate Major Depressive Disorder.

With regard to Criterion A, Ms. B struggled with empathy, specifically with an inability to see beyond the immediacy of her own affective needs which left her therapist feeling dismissed and ineffective. For Criterion B, she presented as anxious and emotional dysregulated. Treatment consisted of individual Transference Focused Psychotherapy and Dialectical Behavior Therapy skills group. It targeted emotional dysregulation, anxiety, hostility, and an overall internalizing style with high levels of dependency and fears of being deprived and abandoned. Treatment consisted of individual Transference Focused Psychotherapy, medication management, and Dialectical Behavior Therapy skills group. She has continued in therapy for almost three years and believes her life has improved.

Case #3: Mr. D

Mr. D is a 25-year-old White male with a history of impulsive gambling, substance abuse, and difficulty maintaining employment. After several hospitalizations Mr. D was referred for individual psychotherapy. He presented with concerns related to affective lability, substantial impulsivity, dysfunctional relationships, suicidal ideation, and difficulty following through on goal-oriented behaviors. He met categorical criteria for Borderline Personality Disorder with antisocial traits, Substance Use Disorder, and recurrent, moderate Major Depressive Disorder.

With regard to AMPD Criterion A, Mr. D's difficulty in observing and tolerating the impact of his behavior on others tended to leave his therapist feeling parentified. His LPFS was 3. For Criterion B, his presentation would be characterized as impulsive and irresponsible. Accordingly, his treatment targeted irresponsibility, risk-taking, externalizing, and greatly feared exposing incompetence and flaws. Treatment consisted of individual Transference Focused Psychotherapy, medication management, and Dialectical Behavior Therapy skills group. He has continued in therapy for more than three years and, like Ms. B, he believes his life has improved.

Case Commentaries

Despite sharing the same diagnosis and the same basic DBT treatment, AMPD guided each treatment based on the unique trait facet and intensities that were the target of treatment. Overall, the Alternative Model better accounted for each patient's distinct borderline presentations, with much greater specificity than the categorical diagnostic criteria. Although all three patients were diagnosed with BPD at intake, the Alternative Model shed light on their distinctive core deficits in functioning and style of presentation. Accordingly, the treatment process was targeted to their distinct deficits, challenges to the treatment process were anticipated, and the likelihood of achieving positive treatment outcomes increased. This contrasts with the categorical model. Again, It bears repeating that DBT that is guided by AMPD was not applied in a generic fashion. Rather, specific DBT interventions were tailored to the unique trait facet profile of each of the three patients. It is this tailoring that increases the likelihood of positive treatment outcomes.

Using the AMPD in Everyday Clinical Practice

The diagnostic category Personality Disorder-Trait Specified (PD-TS) in Section III replaces the traditional Personality Disorder Not Otherwise Specified (PD-NOS) category in Section II. While the PD-NOS diagnosis provides relatively little specific information about an individual's personality pathology, the inclusion of maladaptive traits in AMPD describes the specific features of the individual's personality pathology. Accordingly, it provides immediate information pertinent to case conceptualization and treatment planning which is largely absent in the PD-NOS diagnosis.

With the hybrid model, it is now possible to diagnose a personality disorder based on traits. The designation PD-TS allows clinicians to specify the presence of a personality disorder without requiring a specific diagnostic name for it. In addition, AMPD can be used to assess personality functioning and traits, irrespective of whether or not a personality disorder is present. This increases the clinical utility of the hybrid model because it assists clinicians in identifying an individual's strengths in addition to deficits. This offers a great deal more flexibility and descriptive information than the current categorical approach. Another advantage is eliminating the need for vague and overused diagnoses such as Other Specified and Unspecified Personality Disorder.

Concluding Note

The AMPD was developed to provide a diagnostic system for personality disorders that corresponds with empirical evidence regarding the nature of normal and maladaptive personality. Diagnosis using the AMPD provides comprehensive information about the individual's presenting pathology that can easily be incorporated in clinical practice and aligns with actual clinical decision-making. Further, several publications have demonstrated how information from the AMPD can be incorporated in clinical assessment, diagnosis, case conceptualization, and treatment planning. In short, the AMPD provide a clinically useful means of assessing personality pathology and choosing appropriate treatment interventions. Presumably the three case examples in this chapter illustrated its clinical utility. Finally, the literature further suggests that information from the AMPD is also useful in planning and treating non-personality psychopathology.

Chapter 3
Case Conceptualization and Effective Treatment of Personality Disorders

In this age of accountability, effective clinical practice presumes that clinicians will conduct a focused clinical assessment and develop a compelling case conceptualizations based on it. The case conceptualization then becomes the basis for making informed clinical decisions about treatment tailored to the individual's circumstances and level of functioning. In other words, the case conceptualization is central to achieving effective treatment outcomes with difficult-to-treat individuals, particularly those with personality disorders.

This chapter describes the clinical value of an integrative case conceptualization. It defines and describes case conceptualization and its components and elements. It makes the case for the centrality of the case conceptualization as the bridge that links assessment with treatment, and particularly in informing treatment goals and interventions. It is argued that effective case conceptualizations are those with high levels of explanatory power and predictive power, and which focus on replacing maladaptive patterns with more adaptive ones. Examples of case conceptualizations for three of the most common personality disorders in clinical practice today are presented. Case material illustrates the discussion.

Case Conceptualization

While the term "case conceptualization" is relatively new, clinicians and researchers have used the term "case formulation" for more than 50 years (Tarrier, 2006; Sperry, 1989). Common to most case conceptualization models, including the analytic, constructivists, interpersonal, psychodynamics, cognitive behavioral, and systemic approaches is the element of "pattern." This is not to suggest that all approaches to case conceptualization are the same. However, while there are elements that are unique in every approach, there are also some elements, such as pattern, that are common among nearly all approaches (Eells, 2007; 2010). The remainder of this chapter describes an integrative approach to case conceptualization that emphasizes common elements and can incorporate unique elements as well (Sperry & Sperry, 2020; Sperry & Sperry, 2022).

Definition

A case conceptualization is a way of summarizing diverse information in a brief, coherent manner for the purpose of better understanding and treating of the individual. Furthermore, a case conceptualization consists of four components: diagnostic formulations, clinical formulations, cultural formulation, and treatment formulations (Sperry, 2010; Sperry & Sperry, 2020; 2022).

Components

An integrative case conceptualization consists of four components: diagnostic, clinical, cultural, and treatment formulations (Sperry, 1992; Sperry & Sperry, 2020).

Diagnostic Formulation. A diagnostic formulation is a descriptive statement about the nature and severity of the individual's psychiatric presentation. The diagnostic formulation aids the clinician in reaching three sets of diagnostic conclusions: whether the patient's presentation is primarily psychotic, characterological, or neurotic; whether the individual's presentation is primarily organic or psychogenic in etiology; and, whether the individual's presentation is so acute and severe that it requires immediate intervention. In short, diagnostic formulations are descriptive, phenomenological, and cross-sectional in nature. They answer the "What happened?" question (Sperry & Sperry, 2012; 2020). For all practical purposes the diagnostic formulation lends itself to being specified with DSM-5-TR criteria.

Clinical Formulation. A clinical formulation, on the other hand, is more explanatory and longitudinal in nature, and attempts to offer a rationale for the development and maintenance of symptoms and dysfunctional life patterns. Clinical formulations answer the "Why did it happen?" question. Just as various theories of human behavior exist, so do various types of clinical formulations exist: psychoanalytic, Adlerian, cognitive, behavioral, biological, family systems, biopsychosocial, or some combination (Sperry & Sperry, 2012; 2020). In this book, Cognitive Behavioral case conceptualizations are emphasized.

Cultural Formulation. A cultural formulation is a systematic review and explanation of cultural factors and dynamics that are operative in the presenting problems. It answers the "what role does culture play" question. More specifically, it describes the client's cultural identity and level of acculturation. It provides a cultural explanation of the client's condition, as well as the impact of cultural factors on the client's personality and level of functioning. Furthermore, it addresses cultural elements that may impact the relationship between the individual and the therapist, and whether cultural or culturally sensitive interventions are indicated (Sperry & Sperry, 2012; 2020).

Treatment Formulation. A treatment formulation follows from the diagnostic, clinical, and cultural formulations and serves as an explicit blueprint governing treatment interventions. Rather than answering the "What happened?" or "Why did it happen?" questions, the treatment formulation addresses the "What can be done about it, and how?" question (Sperry & Sperry, 2012; 2020).

The most useful and comprehensive case conceptualizations are integrative ones which encompass all four components: diagnostic, clinical, cultural, and treatment formulations (Sperry & Sperry, 2020; Sperry & Carlson, 2014). The format of the following chapters of this book will highlight integrative conceptualizations. The diagnostic formulation will emphasize DSM-5 criteria. The clinical formulation will emphasis Cognitive Behavioral explanations, while the treatment formulations will suggest Cognitive Behavioral treatment goals and methods.

Basic Premises

In the opinion of many clinicians and researchers, case conceptualization is one of the most challenging clinical competencies to master (Eells, 2010; Sperry & Sperry, 2022). The perceived difficulty in developing an effective case conceptualization may be one reason why many therapists neither develop nor use case conceptualizations, or they lack confidence in their ability to conceptualize cases. My experience is that both experienced therapists and trainees can easily and confidently begin to master this competency in as little as 2–3 hours of formal training (Sperry & Sperry, 2022). The training approach involves learning an integrated model of case conceptualization based on common and distinctive elements, and that emphasizes the element of pattern, i.e., maladaptive pattern. Two basic premises underlie this integrative model.

Maladaptive Pattern. The first premise is that individuals unwittingly develop a self-perpetuating, maladaptive pattern of functioning and relating to others. Inevitably, this pattern underlies the individual's presenting issues. Effective treatment always involves a change process in which the client and therapist collaborate to identify this pattern, break it, and replace it with a more adaptive pattern. At least two outcomes result from this change process: increased well-being and resolution of the client's presenting issue.

Pattern Recognition and Change. The second premise is that pattern recognition and pattern change is at the heart of the case conceptualization process. Pattern is the predictable, consistent, and self-perpetuating style and manner in which individuals think, feel, act, cope, and defend themselves (Sperry, Brill, Howard & Grissom, 1996; Sperry, 2006; (Sperry & Sperry, 2022). Pattern change involves three processes: (1) identify the maladaptive pattern; (2) relinquish the maladaptive pattern and replace it with a more adaptive pattern; and (3) maintain the adaptive pattern (Beitman & Yue, 1999).

Elements

The integrative case conceptualization described in this chapter is comprised of 8 elements. They are: Precipitant, Presentation, Predisposition, Pattern, Protective Factors, Perpetuants, Plan, And Predictive Factors (Sperry, 2024a). Table 3.1 provides brief descriptions of each. Accurately identifying these elements is essential in conceptualizing cases that are relatively complex.

Centrality of Pattern

Figure 3.1 visualizes the interrelationship of these eight elements. Note that Pattern is central to all other elements. Pattern is the main target for therapeutic change (Sperry, 2024b).

Case Conceptualization: Strengths and Protective Factors

This integrative case conceptualization model accounts for strengths and protective factors as well as deficits, and risk factors (Sperry, 2014b; Sperry & Sperry, 2020). The influence

Table 3.1 Case Conceptualization Elements

P-1: PRECIPITANT	Triggering event that activates Pattern and is expressed as Presentation
P-2: PRESENTATION	Symptomatic expression of the Pattern
P-3: PREDISPOSITION	Biological, psychological, social and family factors that underlie and drive the Pattern. Included are: particularly culture/acculturation; gender; self-regulation; relational skills; health status; family history; temperament; previous treatment
P-4: PROTECTIVE FACTORS	Personal strengths and positive external factors that foster well-being, resilience and decrease the likelihood of negative outcomes
P-5: PATTERN	Consistent, self-perpetuating way of thinking, feeling, behaving and coping. Pattern change involves shifting from a maladaptive to a more adaptive pattern
P-6: PERPETUANT	Factors that maintain or reinforce the Pattern
P-7: PLAN	Goals and treatment interventions
P-8: PREDICTIVE FACTORS	Anticipated treatment challenges and obstacles based on the Pattern

of client strengths and protective factors—specified as one aspect of Predisposition—is of considerable clinical value in a case conceptualization because it both "balances" strengths and protective factors with deficits and risk factors and provides a tangible basis for estimating prognosis.

Case Conceptualizations: Explanatory, Tailoring, and Predictive Power

A clinically useful case conceptualization has three characteristics. First, it provides a high level of *explanatory power*. Explanatory power means that the case conceptualization provides a compelling explanation for the presenting problem that answers the question of why the individual acted the way he or she did. Second, it provides a high level of *tailoring power*. Tailoring power refers to the selection of treatment interventions that are the "best fit" to the individual's style and functional profile, and extent of symptom severity, level of functioning, and whether it is an internalizing or externalizing disorder. The selected interventions must also match the presenting problem and the clinical, diagnostic, and cultural formulations and have a high likelihood of being successful for effecting change. Third, a clinically useful case conceptualization also provides a high level of *predictive power*.

Figure 3.1 Relationship of Eight Case Conceptualization Elements

Predictive power is the anticipation of both the most likely obstacles and facilitators to treatment success (Sperry & Sperry, 2012). All three are essential for effectively and competently planning and guiding the treatment process.

Case Conceptualization: Full-Scale vs. Concise Case Conceptualizations

Full-scale case conceptualizations include all eight elements, hereafter referred to as the 8Ps. In contrast, a concise case conceptualization includes as few as five elements (5Ps): Presentation, Precipitant, Predisposition, Pattern, and Plan (Sperry, 2023). The clinical utility of incorporating Protective Factors, Predictive Factors, and a high level of severity, i.e., LPFS, are key factors in determining whether a full-scale or concise case conceptualization is indicated. The concise case conceptualization does not include Protective Factors and Predictive Factors.

Clinicians would do well to utilize a full-scale case conceptualization for patients who meet the criteria for one or more personality disorders and have a high level of severity, i.e., a LPFS of 2, 3, or 4 (Sperry & Sperry, 2022). The presence of a comorbid psychiatric and/or medical conditions is another reason for utilizing the full-scale case conceptualization.

In contrast clinicians might choose a concise conceptualization for patients who do not meet personality disorder criteria but have identifiable personality traits and a low level of severity, i.e., a LPFS of less than 2 (Sperry & Sperry, 2022). While a concise case conceptualization provides explanatory power, it does not provide tailoring power or predictive power because of the absence of two key Ps: Protective Factors and Predictive Factors.

By definition, personality disorders are inflexible, maladaptive, and impairing patterns (American Psychiatric Association, 2022). Accordingly, knowledge of a patient's LPFS and Protective Factors and Predictive Factors can be of considerable clinical value in planning and implementing treatment. In my experience, a full-scale case conceptualization is both necessary and clinically useful in working with any personality-disordered individual because of its explanatory power, tailoring power, and predictive power.

Case Conceptualization: Case Examples

The process of constructing an integrative case conceptualization is illustrated in three case examples. Each consists of background information, a table that summarizes the 8Ps, and a full-scale case conceptualization statement which integrates this information in a coherent narrative.

Case of Geri

Geri is a 41-year-old African American female who works as an administrative assistant. She is single, lives alone, and was referred by her company's human resources director for evaluation and treatment following three weeks of depression and social isolation. Her absence from work prompted the referral. Z's symptoms began soon after her supervisor told her that she was being considered for a promotion. As a child, she reports isolating and avoiding others when she was criticized and teased by family members and peers. She is highly acculturated and reports having no best friend as a child and only one coworker with whom she feels comfortable being around. Besides a paternal aunt, she has limited contact with her family. It is noteworthy that despite the experience of being a college graduate and

Table 3.2 Case of Geri

PRESENTATION	Discouraged reaction of Increased social isolation and depressive symptoms
PRECIPITANT	News of an impending job transfer and promotion and perceived loss of her coworker and only friend
PREDISPOSITION	Her style of relating with others mirrors the avoidant manner in which she related to family members to avoid criticism and unreasonable demands. She views herself as inadequate and defective as a person and views life and others as demanding, harsh, arbitrary, and critical. Therefore, she found her place by avoiding most relationships, socially isolating, and overly investing in those that she deems as trustworthy. As a result, she has limited relational skills. Also, she is highly acculturated
PROTECTIVE FACTORS	Trustworthy and supportive work friend; qualifies for an Americans (ADA) job accommodation
PATTERN	Avoid relationships and withdraw whenever she feels unsafe
PERPETUANT	Her pattern is self-reinforcing as the price she pays for feeling "safe" is loneliness, limited relational skills, and unlikely to have the close intimate relationship she desires
PLAN	*Goals:* return to work. decrease depressive symptoms and enhance relational skills *Interventions*: medication evaluation; behavioral activation, interpretation; skills training group; job accommodation
PREDICTIVE FACTORS	Likely to "test" the therapist initially; resist engaging in relational skills group; premature termination

working for several years in an office setting, she continues to have significant skill deficit in assertive communications, friendship skills, and problem solving skills. Furthermore, she lacks confidence in being around others whom she cannot fully trust.

Diagnosis. She meets criteria for Avoidant Personality Disorder with Obsessive-Compulsive traits, and Major Depressive Disorder, Single Episode, Mild. Level of severity on the *LPFS* was assessed as 2: moderate Impairment. Table 3.2 summarizes the elements of an integrative case conceptualization in the case of Geri.

Case Conceptualization Statement. Geri's increased social isolation and depressive symptoms [**Presentation**] seem to be her discouraged reaction to news of an impending job transfer and promotion and the perceived loss of her only friend and co-worker [**Precipitant**]. Given her history of critical and demanding people in her life, she avoids most relationships and has a history of isolating throughout her childhood. Geri's presenting problems are understandable when viewed from the perspective of her life style. As a psychologically only child, her style of relating with others mirrors the tentative and avoidant manner in which she related to family members. All she wanted was to safely connect without being criticized or having unreasonable demands from them. She views herself as inadequate and defective as a person, and views life and others as demanding, harsh, arbitrary, and critical. Therefore, Geri found her place by avoiding most relationships, socially isolating, and overly investing in those that she deems as trustworthy [**Predisposition**]. Fortunately, she has one close, trusting friend at work and qualifies for an ADA job accommodation which could facilitate her return to work. She is highly acculturated and neither gender nor culturally sensitive interventions appear to be indicated now. [**Protective Factors**]. In short, her avoidant pattern is to distrust and avoid new relationships and withdraw whenever she feels unsafe [**Pattern**]. This pattern is self-reinforcing and the price she pays to feel "safe" is high: she is lonely, has limited relational skills and experiences, and so she is unlikely to develop the close intimate relationship she so desires [**Perpetuants**]. A medication evaluation was completed, and antidepressants were not indicated. Mutually agreed upon treatment goals included (1) decreased discouragement and depressive symptoms; (2) enhanced relational skills, and (3) return to work. Returning to work is likely to be problematic unless her protective factors are activated: she can remain with her trusted work colleague; and the therapist facilitates an ADA job accommodation. Behavioral activation will target depressive symptoms, and assertiveness/shyness skill training group will increase relational skills, and interpretation to modify her faulty convictions of avoidance to feel safe [**Plan**]. It is anticipated that Geri may engage in "testing" behaviors in therapy and initially resist involvement in a relational skills group unless adequately prepared [**Predictive Factors**].

Clinical Outcome. In this composite case (Sperry & Sperry, 2020) twenty individual and ten group treatment sessions were pre-approved. The physician performing the medication evaluation concluded that medication was not indicated at the time. Therapy initially focused on the first treatment goal as well as preparing Geri for entry in the skills group. Addressing the third goal of returning to work greatly facilitated treatment success. The therapists consulted with Geri's supervisor and with the "leverage" afforded by ADA job accommodation provision, the company agreed that Geri could return to work in her same supportive office setting with a raise and minor promotion. This arrangement allowed her to maintain a relationship with her trusted coworker, which facilitated her progress in individual and group sessions.

Case of Kiera

Kiera is a 33-year-old never married female who was first diagnosed with Borderline Personality Disorder after some 20 years of psychotherapy and drug treatment. During this time, she experienced mood instability, unstable relationships, and life-threatening behaviors, including wrist cutting and overdosing, which lead to several hospitalizations and ongoing outpatient therapy.

Growing up she describes herself as overly sensitive and emotionally dysregulated. Reportedly, her childhood was marked by demanding, critical, and emotionally distant parents. Her parents divorced when she was about 4 years old, presumably become of her father's alcoholism. Her mother is described as "invalidating" meaning that she denied, disregarded, and erratically responded to Kiera's concerns and experiences. Kiera was also blamed for not meeting her mother's high expectations and standards for achievement and propriety. Over the years, she has been involved in several intense, short-term relationships as well as many jobs, all of short duration.

She also reports a history of sexual abuse initially by a babysitter at age six, which may be related to her hypersexuality throughout her adolescence and early adulthood. Her first suicide attempt was at age 12, leading to one of her many hospitalizations. Since then, she has engaged in various self-harming behaviors including wrist cutting. She began substance use at age 14 which escalated until her early 20s. Reportedly, she has been sober for ten years with ongoing AA and NA involvement. Kiera describes being involved in "every form

Table 3.3 Case of Kiera

PRESENTATION	Mood instability, unstable relationships, and life-threatening behaviors
PRECIPITANT	Situations which elicit feelings of victimization, jealousy, and anticipated abandonment
PREDISPOSITION	Oversensitivity, distress intolerance, and emotional dysregulation; demanding, critical, invalidating, and emotionally distant mother. She views herself as helpless and vulnerable and views others as dangerous and uncaring. Biologically vulnerable to substance abuse, distress intolerance, and impulsivity
PROTECTIVE FACTORS	Validation and support of Raymond and consistent work environment during DBT treatment
PATTERN	Drives others away with unrealistic demands for closeness
PERPETUANT	driving others away and self-harming behaviors when faced with increasing distress and fear of abandonment further reinforce her maladaptive pattern
PLAN	*Goals:* reduce distress, abandonment fears, and self-harming behaviors shift to a more adaptive pattern of effectively relating to others without self-harm. *Interventions*: DBT group skills training, individual DBT sessions, and telephone consultation
PREDICTIVE FACTORS	Expect emotional reactivity, impulsivity, and self-injury; termination preparation should be strategic and supportive because of abandonment sensitivities

of therapy" with several therapists for nearly 20 years for moodiness, substance abuse, and self-harmful behavior before beginning individual and group DBT.

Despite several risk factors that seemed to fuel her distress and self-harming behavior, there have also been some protective factors. These include the validation and financial and emotional support of Raymond, her mother's ex-boyfriend, and a consistent and supportive work environment for the time Kiera during the course of DBT therapy appear to have been significant factors in her recovery. Kiera's description of her relational pattern as a cycle of accusing, arguing, crying, and self-harming behavior was quite useful in framing the case conceptualization.

Diagnosis. Her DSM-5 diagnoses were Borderline Personality Disorder. Level of severity on the *LPFS* was assessed as 3-severe Impairment. Table 3.3 summarizes this case information.

Case Conceptualization Statement. Kiera presented with mood instability, unstable relationships, and life-threatening behaviors (**Presentation**), which were her reactions to feelings of victimization, jealousy, and anticipation of abandonment (**Precipitant**). Her oversensitivity to distress and emotional dysregulation, her demanding, critical, and emotionally distant parents. Particularly her mother's "invalidating" response to her. She views herself as helpless and vulnerable and views others as dangerous and uncaring. Kiera is particularly sensitive and finds it very difficult to tolerate such negative emotional states. She is also biologically vulnerable to substance abuse, distress intolerance, and impulsivity (**Predisposition**). The validation and support of Raymond, her mother's ex-boyfriend and her consistent work environment during the course of Dialectical Behavior Therapy

(DBT) appear to have greatly facilitated her recovery (**Protective Factors**). Her relationship difficulties involve the cycle of accusing, arguing, crying, and then more accusing. This results in Kiera driving others away, owing to unrealistic demands for closeness. It is a strong externalizing pattern designated as "severe impairment" on the *Level of Personality Functioning Scale* (**Pattern**). Her response to increasing distress and fear of abandonment is to drive others away and self-harming behaviors further reinforce her maladaptive pattern (**Perpetuants**). DBT with group skills training in mindfulness, emotion regulation, distress tolerance, and interpersonal effectiveness are interventions that, together with individual DBT and telephone consultation is the treatment mutually agreed upon. Goals are to decrease Kiera's distress intolerance and increase her sense of self-control, emotional balance, and resilience. Treatment will further (1) decrease her suicidal and self-harming behaviors, while achieving safety; (2) work through her emotional and traumatic experiences and learn to survive them; (3) work through problems of daily living and maintain gainful employment; (4) increase her capacity for experiencing a fulfilling life and sustaining relationships; and focus on shifting to a more adaptive pattern of effectively relating to others without self-harm (**Plan**). Emotional reactivity, impulsivity, and self-injury are likely treatment challenges. Given here abandonment sensitivities preparing for termination should be strategic and supportive (**Predictive Factors**).

Clinical Outcome. Kiera respond positively to a full course of DBT and continuing care. An intensive course of twice weekly individual and group DBT were effective in ending her distress, mood instability, unstable relationships, and life-threatening behaviors. After a year she was in remission of her personality disorder, and over the next two years increasingly began to experience a more fulfilling life.

Case of Aimee

Aimee is a 30-year-old single mother of two boys, aged 12 and 11. She's currently employed as a limousine driver and attends graduate school part time. Her stated reason for seeking therapy was to learn to deal with anger and resentment toward her mother. She describes herself as passive and hides her anger and resentment, but manifest these feelings "by beating myself up, running myself ragged" which means she continually focuses on meeting the needs of others and not relaxing nor enjoying life. Aimee is very careful and circumspect in talking with her mother, fearful she will hurt her mother's feelings. Essentially, Aimee was abandoned by her mother as a child and raised by her maternal grandmother. She indicated that she was and is very close to her grandmother and remains much closer to her father than to her mother.

She also reported that her ex-husband had been verbally and physically abusive to her and that he is being released from prison soon. In anticipation of his release, she worries for her safety and that of her children. Aimee reports that she remains very close to her father but quite emotionally distant from her mother. On the intake form she stated, "I have very angry feelings about her." No current medical problems are reported, although she does report having somewhat severe headaches, anxiety, depression, trouble with sleeping, and bad dreams. Psychological testing reveals a high need to please and being a victim. She reports that her greatest worry is being alone. While Aimee had been involved in therapy previously, she indicated that while she understood her situation better, no positive changes occurred.

Table 3.4 Case of Aimee

PRESENTATION	Depression, fatigue, insomnia, anger at her mother; worries
PRECIPITANT	Increased demands to care for others; anticipation of her ex-husband's release from prison
PATTERN	Meet others' needs but not her own and be overly conscientious
PREDISPOSITION	Biological. family history of alcohol and substance abuse
	Psychological. *personality style:* dependent and obsessive-compulsive; *Skill deficits:* assertiveness; self-care; negotiation, *Self-view:* nice but deficient; *world view:* demanding and critical
	Social. neglectful, overly demanding, self-absorbed parents; teased, belittled by peers; abusive ex-husband
	Cultural. highly acculturated; no obvious acculturative stress
PROTECTIVE FACTORS	Bonded with grandmother; successfully left abusive husband; success in work and raising children on her own
PERPETUANT	Maintained by the approval of others, her schemas and skills deficits
PLAN	Reduce depressive symptoms, fatigue, insomnia; increase self-care; Shift to a more adaptive pattern of meeting the needs of both herself as well as others, in a more natural way
PREDICTIVE FACTOR	Overly agreeable; perfectionistic—procrastination with homework; resist efforts to increase independence; difficulty with termination; very good prognosis as she succeeded in leaving an abusive marriage

There were some key strengths and protective factors. Among these were the fact that she bonded to a caring maternal grandmother who effectively raised her when her own abusive mother was absent for long periods of time. Although it was quite difficult, Aimee was able to leave abusive husband knowing that her father would protect her from him. She is also articulate, hardworking and perfectionistic. She also has notable skill deficits in assertiveness and self-empowerment.

Diagnosis. Her DSM-5 diagnoses was Dependent Personality Disorder, Obsessive-Compulsive Personality traits, and Other Specified Depressive Disorder. On the *Levels of Personality Functioning Scale* (American Psychiatric Association, 2022), her impairment was assessed as 2-Moderate Impairment. Table 3.4 summarizes this case information.

Case Conceptualization Statement. Aimee presented with depression, fatigue, insomnia, anger at her mother, and worries about her children and ex-husband (**Presentation**), which were her reactions to the increased demands to care for others and the anticipation of her ex-husband's release from prison (**Precipitant**). Her maladaptive pattern involves focusing on meeting others' needs in a perfectionistic and overly conscientious manner while ignoring her own needs. Doing so allowed her to feel needed and worthwhile (**Pattern**). The origins of this pattern include an upbringing in which her parents were self-centered, highly critical, and overly demanding while emotionally absent; as well as skill deficits in assertive communication and self-care. It also included maladaptive beliefs about herself as being nice but deficient, and a view of the world as demanding, critical, and conditional (**Predisposition**). Despite it all, Aimee bonded with her grandmother and was successful at leaving an abusive domestic relationship as well as raising two children on her own (**Protective Factors**). Her maladaptive pattern was reinforced and maintained by the need from approval from others, her negative self-world schemas, and her skills deficits (**Perpetuants**). Treatment would initially be focused on decreasing symptoms of depression, fatigue and insomnia. The longer-term goal was to balance meeting the needs of others and her own needs in a reasonably conscientious manner, which was a more adaptive and life-giving pattern. Six planned treatment sessions were mutually agreed upon (**Plan**). Overly agreeable, perfectionistic, and procrastination are likely treatment challenges. She may resist efforts to increase independence, and because of dependency on therapist and therapeutic process she might experience difficulty with termination. Nevertheless, her prognosis is very good prognosis given her success in leaving an abusive marriage (**Predictive Factors**).

Clinical Outcome. In the last of her six planned session treatment, Aimee indicated that she achieved all her treatment goals. In a subsequent interview seven years after therapy was completed, Aimee indicated that she not only maintained the treatment gains but also extended these gains to other areas of her life (Sperry & Carlson, 2014).

Commentary on the Cases

Treatment driven by integrative case conceptualizations were illustrated for three of the most common personality disorders in clinical practice today: Avoidant, Borderline, and Dependent Personality Disorder It may be useful to step back and reflect on the successful outcomes of these three cases.

Like many individuals presenting for psychological treatment with personality disorder diagnoses, Geri, Kiera and Aimee all experienced considerable early childhood abuse and neglect. Troubling symptoms and skill deficits were common to allow. However, all three had notable protective factors and strengths that were not only recognized but also "incorporated" as therapeutic adjuncts to the treatment process by their therapists. For Kiera this included the support and validation of Raymond as well as supportive coworkers were important in her recovery. Similarly, having the experience of being raised by a caring grandmother and then later leaving her abusive marriage were obvious strengths and protective factors for Aimee. For Geri, it was a trusting and supportive coworker. Another commonality of three cases is that treatment decisions were driven by a full integrated case conceptualization, and three highly effective therapists.

While the case of Geri is a composite case, the cases of Kiera and Aimee are actual cases. Kiera's case is reported in her autobiography, entitled *The Buddha and the Borderline: A Memoir* (Van Gelder, 2010). It provides a first-hand account of the development of the Borderline Personality Disorder and response to a full course of DBT. Aimee's case was reported in detail in *How Master Therapists Work: Effecting Change from the First to the Last Session and Beyond* (Sperry & Carlson, 2014). It includes session transcriptions and commentaries on each therapy session. The focused nature of the therapeutic interventions was obvious in all cases. These case conceptualization-informed interventions were effective for all three cases, whereas previous therapeutic efforts for both Kiera and Aimee had not been effective.

Concluding Note

When clinicians inform their therapy with case conceptualizations that have high levels of explanatory power, tailoring power, and predictive power, and they recognize and "incorporate" predictive factors, positive therapeutic outcomes are likely even with patients diagnosed with personality disorders. Clinician expertise is also a factor. For example, not every clinician would be able to complete therapy with Aimee is only six sessions, but it would not be unreasonable for most therapists—including interns—to have similar results in 20 sessions following the same case conceptualization informed treatment plan. In short, treatment of even severe personalities is not as hopeless or tentative as some still believe today. What is clear that an accurate and integrative case conceptualization driven treatment is likely to achieve positive clinical outcomes with patients presenting with these disorders.

Chapter 4

Antisocial Personality Disorder

Individuals with antisocial personalities commonly present with assaultiveness, impulsivity, hedonism, promiscuity, unreliability, and drug and alcohol abuse. Criminality may be involved. These individuals fail at work, change jobs frequently, tend to receive dishonorable discharges from the military, are abusing parents and neglectful spouses, have difficulty maintaining intimate relationships, and may be convicted and spend time in prison. This disorder is similar but different from the psychopathic personality disorder, which is also known as psychopathy, and sociopathy (Skodol, Bender, & Oldham, 2019; American Psychiatric Association, 2022).

This chapter describes a framework for the assessment and effective treatment of this disorder. It includes sections on diagnosis, psychological assessment, case conceptualization, and treatment interventions. It begins with background information on the disorder as well as a DSM-5-TR description, prototypic description, associated features, and the Alternative Model of Personality Disorders description of this disorder. The section on case conceptualization provides five common clinical formulations of this disorder: psychodynamic, biosocial, cognitive-behavioral, interpersonal, and an integrative conceptualization of this disorder. Several treatment approaches, modalities, and intervention strategies are also described. These includes individual psychotherapy, group therapy, marital and family therapy, medication, and integrative and combined treatment.

Description of the Antisocial Personality Disorder

The Antisocial Personality Disorder can be recognized by the following descriptors and characteristics: styles vs. disorders, triggering event, behavioral styles, interpersonal styles, cognitive styles, affective styles, attachment style, and optimal criterion.

Style vs. Disorder. The antisocial personalities can be thought of as spanning a continuum from healthy to pathological, wherein the antisocial personality style is on the healthy end, and the Antisocial Personality Disorder is on the pathological end. Table 4.1 compares and contrasts the antisocial personality style and disorder.

The following two cases further illustrate differences between the Antisocial Personality Disorder (Juan G.) and the antisocial personality style (Gordon J.).

DOI: 10.4324/9781032617930-4

Case Study: Antisocial Personality Disorder

Juan G. is a 28-year-old Cuban male who presented late in the evening to the emergency room at a community hospital complaining of a headache. His description of the pain was vague and contradictory. At one point he said the pain had been present for three days, while at another point it was "many years." He indicated that the pain led to violent behavior and described how, during a headache episode, he had brutally assaulted a medic while he was in the Air Force. He gave a long history of arrests for assault, burglary, and drug dealing. Neurological and mental status examinations were with normal limits except for some mild agitation. He insisted that only Darvon—a narcotic—would relieve his headache pain. The patient resisted a plan for further diagnostic tests or a follow-up clinic appointment, saying unless he was treated immediately "something really bad could happen."

Case Study: Antisocial Personality Style

Gordon J. is the 38 year old president of a rapidly expanding manufacturing company. He has taken over the small business that his uncle had founded after World War II and Gordon had greatly increased production, added new product lines and formed a marketing and sales group which he personally supervised in the nine years he had run the company. Prior to taking over the company, Gordon had become the youngest member of the million dollar club for selling real estate for the firm that he had worked for just three years. His father had died in a freak skiing accident when Gordon was eleven, but that didn't seem to stop Gordon from pursuing his fascination with scuba diving and hang glider flying. Gordon was invited to join the Young President's Organization (Y.P.O.) in his region soon after turning his uncles' corporation into a highly profitable enterprise. He was quite popular in the group given his magnetic personality, visionary outlook, and captivating stories of his various exploits. He had been married for nearly five years before divorcing. Since then he has not remarried, but has maintained ongoing relationships with two women.

Because individuals with Antisocial Personality Disorder, Psychopathic Personality Disorder, and Sociopathic Personality Disorder can engage in criminal behavior, some clinicians use the three terms interchangeably. Because research indicates some notable differences in behavior and in etiology, others prefer to differentiate psychopathy and sociopathy (Hare, Neumann, & Widiger, 2012; Walsh & Wu, 2008).

Table 4.1 Comparison of Antisocial Personality Style and Disorder

Personality Style	Personality Disorder
Prefer free-lancer living and live well by their talents, skills, ingenuity, and wits	Unable to sustain consistent work behavior.
Tend to live by their own internal code of values and are not much influenced by others	Fail to conform to social norms with regard to lawful behavior, performing antisocial acts or society's norms that are grounds for arrest (rule-breaking)
As adolescents were usually high-spirited hellraisers and mischief makers	Irritable and aggressive as indicated by physical fights or assaults
Tend to be generous with money believing	Repeated fails to honor financial obligation that as it is spent, more will turn up somewhere and somehow
Tend to be wanderlusts, but are able to make plans and commitment, albeit for limited time spans	Fail to plan ahead, or is impulsive as indicated by moving about without a prearranged job or clear goals
Tend to be silver-tongued, gifted in the art of winning friends	Have no regard for the truth as indicated by repeated lying, use of aliases, or "conning" others for personal profit or pleasure
Tend to e courageous, physically bold and tough; will stand up to those who advantage of them	Reckless regarding their own and other's personal safety as indicated by driving dare take while intoxicated or recurrent speeding
Tend not to worry too much about others, expecting others to be responsible for themselves	If a parent or guardian lacks ability to function as a responsible parent
Have strong libido and while may desire several partners can remain monogamous	Have never sustained a totally monogamous relationship for long periods of time
Tend to live in the present and don't experience much guilt	Lacks remorse and feels justified in having hurt, mistreated or stolen from another

Psychopathic Personality Disorder

Psychopathic personality disorder—also referred to as psychopathy—is a mental disorder characterized by amoral behavior, extreme self-centeredness, and interpersonal deficits. such as grandiosity, arrogance and deceitfulness, and global lack of empathy. Affective deficits such as lack of guilt and remorse are also noted. According to the *Psychodynamic Diagnostic Manual* (PDM) (2006), this disorder is diagnosable by the following criteria. Individuals exhibits high threshold for emotional stimulation and aggressiveness. They are preoccupied with manipulating others. Their basic emotions tend to be rage and envy. Their view of themselves is that they are omnipotent, in that they believe that they can make anything happen and control everything. Their view of others is that everyone is selfish, manipulative, or dishonorable.

Furthermore, their basic way of defending themselves is by attempting to control everything around them. Psychopaths are not common in corporate settings and may engage in elude criminal prosecution by cleverly exploiting loopholes in regulations (Babiak & Hare, 2007).

The diagnosis of Psychopathic Personality Disorder has not appeared in the DSM since the first edition; however, it reappears as a specifier: "with psychopathic features" in the Alternative Model for Personality Disorders (AMPD) (America Psychiatric Association, 2022). More on this in the AMPD section.

Sociopathic Personality Disorder

Sociopathic personality–also known as sociopathy—is a mental disorder characterized by amoral and criminal behavior and a diminished sense of moral responsibility. Individuals with this disorder tend to spontaneously act out in inappropriate ways without thinking through the consequences. They may be nervous, easily agitated, and quick to display anger. They will lie, manipulate and hurt others, but will often avoid doing so to the select few individuals they care about. Most often they can form attachments and loyalties to others. This means that they are likely to experience guilt and remorse when they should end hurt someone they care about. While they are capable of committing heinous crimes, they are unlikely to commit crimes against family or friends. Unlike the psychopathic personality, which research suggests has more genetic loading, the sociopathic personality appears to be more influenced by environmental factors such as poverty, exposure to violence, and overly permissive or neglectful parenting (Stout, 2005). The Sociopathic Personality Disorder only appeared in DSM-II.

Triggering Event. The typical situation, circumstance or event that most likely triggers or activates the characteristic maladaptive response of the Antisocial Personality Disorder (Othmer & Othmer, 2002), as noted in behavioral, interpersonal. cognitive, and feeling styles, is: "social standards and rules."

Behavioral Style. The behavioral style of antisocial personalities is characterized by impulsivity, irritability, and aggressiveness. They are likely to be irresponsible in honoring work commitments and financial obligations. Rule-breaking is typical. Antisocial Personality Disordered individuals are also noted for their impulsive anger, deceitfulness, and cunning. They tend to be forceful individuals who regularly engage in risk-seeking and thrill-seeking behavior.

Interpersonal Style. Their interpersonal style is characterized by antagonism and reckless disregard of other's needs and safety. They tend to be highly competitive and distrustful of others and often poor losers. Their relationships may at times appear to be "slick" as well as calculating. These behaviors can characterize the successful businessman, politician, lawyer, medical professional, as well as the criminal. They tend to develop superficial relationships that involve few, if any, lasting emotional ties or commitments. Furthermore, they tend to be callous toward the pain and suffering of others.

Cognitive Style. The cognitive style of the antisocial personality is described as impulsive and cognitively inflexible as well as externally oriented. They tend to be keenly aware of social cues and may be quite adept at "reading" people and situations. Because they are contemptuous of authority, rules, and social norms, they easily rationalize their own behavior. Impulsivity, irritability and aggressivity predisposes them to argumentation and even assaultive action. Recent research indicates that there tends to be significant neuropsychological Impairment in individuals diagnosed with this disorder. In particular, there is likely to be impairment in executive functioning tasks of planning ability and set shifting (Dolan & Park, 2002).

Affective Style. Their emotional or affective style is characterized as shallow and superficial. They avoid "softer" emotions such as warmth and intimacy because they regard these as signs of weakness. Guilt is seldom if ever experienced. They are unable to tolerate boredom, depression, or frustration and subsequently are sensation-seekers. Finally, they may show little guilt, shame, or remorse over their own deviant actions.

Attachment Style. Individuals with a view of others that is negative and a self-view that vacillates between positive and negative exhibit a composite fearful–dismissing style of attachment. They tend to view themselves as special and entitled but are also mindful of their need for others who can potentially hurt them. Accordingly, they use others to meet their needs while being wary and dismissive of them. The Fearful–Dismissing Attachment Style is associated with the Antisocial Personality Disorder.

Optimal Diagnostic Criterion. Of all the diagnostic criteria for the Antisocial Disorder has been found to be the most useful in diagnosing this disorder. The belief is that by beginning with this criterion, the clinician can test for the presence or absence of the criterion and more quickly diagnose the personality disorder (Allnutt & Links, 1996). The optimal criterion for this disorder is: criminal, aggressive, impulsive, irresponsible behavior.

DSM-5-TR-TR-TR Characterization

Individuals with this personality disorder are characterized by an unremitting pattern of disregarding and violating the rights of others. They disrespect and disregard laws and social norms, and regularly engage in acts that are grounds for arrest. These individuals lie, are deceitful, and will take advantage of others for pleasure or for personal profit. They are impulsive and fail to plan ahead. They are also irritable and aggressive which results in physical fights or assaults. It is not surprising that these individuals disregard the safety of others as well as themselves. Their irresponsibility is demonstrated by their failure to engage in consistent work behavior and failure to meet financial obligations. Furthermore, their lack of remorse is shown by their indifference in having hurt, mistreated, or stolen from others (American Psychiatric Association, 2022).

Alternative Model of Antisocial Personality Disorder

The Alternative Model of Personality Disorders (AMPD) offers a clinically useful description of the Antisocial Personality Disorder in terms of typical features and trait facets. Typical features are failure to comply with laws, regulations, and ethical standards, and an egocentric and callous lack of concern for others accompanied by deceit, risk taking, and/or irresponsibility. Trait facet criteria include Manipulativeness, Callousness, Deceitfulness, Hostility, Risk taking, Impulsivity, and Irresponsibility. Six or more are required. The alternative model also includes a "specifier" for *Psychopathy* which is "marked by a lack of anxiety or fear and by a bold interpersonal style that may mask maladaptive behaviors (e.g., fraudulence)" (American Psychiatric Association, 2022, p. 885). Psychopathy is characterized by lows levels of Anxiousness and Withdrawal and high levels of Attention Seeking (American Psychiatric Association, 2022).

Prototypic Presentation

A prototype is a brief description that captures the essence of how a particular disorder commonly presents. Prototypic descriptions are useful and convenient, and clinicians commonly rely on them rather than lists of behavioral criteria or core beliefs (Westen, 2012). Here is a common prototypic description of the Antisocial Personality Disorder: These individuals displayed symptoms of Conduct Disorder from early childhood, engaged in delinquent behavior as adolescents, and turned into selfish, manipulative, and ruthless adults. Their primary interest in others is what they can get from them. They manipulate, lie, cheat, and steal and have no remorse or empathy for the harm they inflict on others. They are reckless, impulsive, and engage in criminal behavior. This disorder is common among criminals and is a predictor of violence. Fortunately, by middle age these individuals can outgrow this pattern.

Associated Features

Prevalence. ASPD has been identified in 1.8 percent of the general population and 5.9 percent in clinical practice (Torgersen, 2021). However, it is greater than 70 percent in males with alcohol and substance use disorders in clinics, prison, and other forensic settings. (American Psychiatric Association, 2022).

Differential Diagnosis. ASPD must be differentiated from Substance Abuse Disorder, Schizophrenia, Bipolar disorder, and other personality disorders. ASPD should also be differentiated from antisocial behavior not due to a mental disorder, in which case the condition of Adult Antisocial Behavior is coded (American Psychiatric Association, 2022).

Development and Course. ASPD appears to develop as a result of both genetics and childhood experiences. Although this pattern must occur by age 15, this disorder cannot be diagnosed before age 18. ASPD tends to have a chronic course, it may lessen or remit by the age of 40. This is often evident with respect to criminal behavior but may include the full spectrum of antisocial behaviors and substance abuse (American Psychiatric Association, 2022).

Culture, Sex, and Gender. The diagnosis may be misapplied to individuals in which seemingly antisocial behavior is part of a protective survival strategy as in youth gangs with high rates of violence. Others who experience high rates of child maltreatment, exposure to violence, or adverse environments that evoke occasional reactive and contextual antisocial behavior would not meet criteria for ASPD. Those from socially oppressed groups may be at higher risk of over diagnosis or misdiagnosis because they are more likely to have been misdiagnosed with Conduct Disorder in adolescence. ASPD is three times more common in males than females (American Psychiatric Association, 2022).

Conceptualizations of the Antisocial Personality Disorder

Psychodynamic Case Conceptualizations

Psychoanalytic writers describe the antisocial personality as similar to the narcissistic personality. While both form a pathological grandiose self, the antisocial individual's self is based on an aggressive introject, called the "stranger self-object" (Meloy, 1988). This self-object reflects an experience of the parent as a stranger who cannot be trusted and who harbors bad will toward the infant. Not surprisingly, this threatening internalized object derives from experiences of parental neglect or cruelty. Combined with an absence of a loving maternal object is a lack of basic trust and a fixation in the separation-individuation process so that object constancy does not occur. Since the mother is experience as a stranger or predator, the infant's emotional attachment to her is derailed leading to a detachment from all relationships and affective experiences as well as sadistic attempts to bond with others through destructive and controlling behaviors.

As a result, the antisocial individuals do not perceive others as separate individuals. Hence, they cannot develop the capacity for guilt and depressive anxieties based on how their action hurt others. A corollary is that they are incapable of true depression. Kernberg (1984) notes that these antisocial individuals are similarly stunned in superego development, except for sadistic superego precursors manifest by cruel and sadistic behaviors. Higher functioning antisocial individuals are noted to have some development of consciousness with circumscribed areas—called superego lacunae—where they superego does not seem to function. Furthermore, antisocial individuals show little interest in rationalizing or morally justifying behavior, or adherence to a value system other than the exploitive, aggressive exercise of power (Kernberg, 1984; Meloy, 1988).

Biosocial Case Conceptualization

There is mounting evidence that biological factors influences the development of the antisocial personality. Low levels of the neurotransmitter serotonin have been noted in individuals prone to aggressive and impulsive behavior. Meloy (1988) suggests that antisocial individuals often have histories of childhood abuse or neglect. They are likely to have had a difficult infant temperament (Thomas & Chess, 1977) meaning they were difficult to soothe and comfort, which may have interfered with the normal attachment process further increasing the probability of childhood abuse or neglect. Millon and Everly (1985) suggests that low thresholds for limbic system stimulation is likely in antisocial individuals. Meloy (1988) adds that antisocial individuals have been found to be autonomically hyperactive, possibly because of their inability to learn from experience, and thus manifest less anticipatory anxiety to deter them from ill-advised behavior.

Environmental factors such as parental hostility, deficient parental role modeling, and reinforcement of vindictive behavior appears to interact with these biological predisposing factors. Parental hostility may result from the child's disruptiveness with the parents, from the perception that these children are ill-tempered, or because these children are used as a scapegoat for the parents' or family's frustration. Deficient parental modelling such as when there is little or no parental guidance or an absence of any authority or a father figure in the home. Without such an authority figure to model and feeling abandoned or rejected, these children often become streetwise and hardened to the world around them. From these experiences they learn that "the end justifies the means", "it's a dog-eat-dog world", and "you've got strong and crafty to survive". Not surprisingly, this defiant behavior is met with social disapproval which farther reinforces their self-reliance and hardened outlook. As a result, they learn not to trust others and anticipating that others intend to exploit or humiliate them they strike out at others with vindictive behaviors.

This personality pattern is self-perpetuated through consistent perceptual distortion, a demeaning attitude toward affection and cooperation and antagonistic and vindictive behavior that breeds antagonism in return. Further, this pattern is perpetuated by their fear of being used and forced into an inferior, dominated position (Millon & Everly, 1985).

Cognitive-Behavioral Case Conceptualizations

According to Beck (2015) the behavior of individuals with this disorder is persistently irresponsible. They hold various core, conditional, and instrumental beliefs. Their *core beliefs* are that they must look out for themselves and be aggressive so as not to be victimized by others. They also believe they are entitled to break rules. They believe that their thoughts and feelings are always accurate, and that their choices are always right and good. In addition, they believe that feelings make facts which means they are in the right because they feel right about their actions. Their *conditional belief* is that if they don't manipulate, exploit, or attach others, they will never get what they deserve. Their *instrumental belief* is to get others before they get you and take what you need since you deserve it. Underlying these various beliefs are their beliefs about self and the world (Mitchell, Tafrate, & Freeman, 2015).

These individuals tend to view themselves as strong, clever, self-sufficient, and invulnerable. They tend to view others as either weak and vulnerable, or stupid and exploitable. Accordingly, they have two strategies: the will openly attack, defraud, and victimize others, or the will more subtly "con," deceive, and manipulating them (Beck, 2015). Furthermore, they are likely to dismiss unsolicited counsel from others as irrelevant to their purposes. Finally, they tend to be present-oriented, with absolutely no concern for future outcomes.

From a more behavioral perspective, Turkat (1990) describes three subtypes of this disorder: the clear sociopath—meaning the individuals clearly and obviously meets DSM-5-TR-TR criteria; the clever sociopath—wherein these individuals feign psychological symptoms usually to avoid legal responsibility for their actions; and the hurting sociopath, who meets the DSM criteria but is sincerely and genuinely distressed. For all three types, the core behavioral deficits are in managing impulses and anger. Of the three, only the hurting sociopath is considered amenable to behavior therapy.

Interpersonal Case Conceptualization

For Benjamin (1996), persons with Antisocial Personality Disorders typically have developmental histories of harsh, neglectful parenting. The adult consequence of this is that the antisocial individual neglects and is insensitive to others needs or exploits others. This unpredictable pattern of parenting tends to result in under modulated parental control and blaming. The result is that as an adult, the antisocial individuals fiercely protects their autonomy. Furthermore, this pattern of inept parental caring can be internalized by the antisocial individual as substance abuse, criminal behavior or parental dereliction of duty. The antisocial-to-be is likely to "take over" parental responsibilities since no one else did. As a consequence of this inappropriate parental role taking, the antisocial individual is likely to continue controlling others as an end in itself, without emotionally bonding with those being controlled. In short, a sustained pattern of inappropriate and unmodulated desire for control of others is prominent. There is also a strong need for independence, and for resisting being controlled by others who are typically held in contempt. Unbridled aggressivity is frequently utilized to sustain control and independence. Finally, antisocial disordered individuals may present friendly and sociable, albeit in a somewhat detachment, since they have little regard for others.

Integrative Case Conceptualization

The following integrative formulation provides a biopsychosocial explanation for how this personality is likely to have developed and how it is maintained. Biologically, antisocial personalities manifested "difficult child" temperaments (Thomas & Chess, 1977). As such their patterns were unpredictable, tended to withdraw from situations, showed high intensity and had a fairly low, discontented mood. This ill-tempered infantile pattern has been described by Millon (1981) as resulting in part, from a low threshold for limbic stimulation and a decrease in inhibitory centers of the central nervous system. Their body types tend to be endomorphic (lean) and mesomorphic (muscular) (Millon, 1981).

Psychologically, these individuals have a unique view of themselves, others, and the world. They tend to view themselves with some variant of the theme: "I am cunning and entitled to get whatever I want." In other words, they see themselves as strong, competitive, energetic, and tough. Their view of life and the world is variant of the theme: "Life is devious and hostile, and rules keep me from fulfilling my needs." Not surprisingly their life's goal has a variant of the theme: "Therefore, I'll bend or break these rules because my needs come first, and I'll defend against efforts to be controlled or degraded by others." Acting out and rationalization are common defense mechanisms used by the antisocial personality.

Socially, predictable parenting styles and environmental factors can be noted for this disorder. Typically, the parenting style is characterized by hostility and deficient parental modeling. Or the parents might have provided such good modeling that the child could not or refused to live up to high parental standards. The parental injunction is that "The end justifies the means." Thus, vindictive behavior is modeled and reinforced. The family structure tends to be disorganized and disengaged. The antisocial pattern is confirmed, reinforced, and perpetuated by the following individual and systems factors: The need to be powerful and the fear of being abused and humiliated leads to a denial of "softer" emotions plus uncooperativeness. This, along with the tendency to provoke others, leads to further reinforcement of antisocial beliefs and behaviors (Sperry & Mosak, 1996; Sperry, 2015).

Table 4.2 summarizes the characteristics of this disorder.

Assessment of Antisocial Personality Disorder

Several sources of information are useful in establishing a diagnosis and treatment plan for personality disorders. Observation, collateral information, and psychological testing are important adjuncts to the patient's self-report in the clinical interview. This section briefly describes some characteristic observations that the clinician makes and the nature of the rapport likely to develop in initial encounters with specific personality disordered individuals. Characteristic response patterns on various objective (i.e., MMPI-2 and MCMI-IV) and projective tests (i.e., Rorschach and TAT) are also described.

Interview Behavior and Rapport

Interviewing the Antisocial Personality Disordered individual can be particularly challenging. While it is easy to communicate with them as long as the clinician plays along, they become angry and critical when the clinician resists their manipulations. It is very difficult to have them focus on their impulsivity, irresponsibility or the negative consequences of their actions. Such lack of genuineness and sincerity limits rapport.

Table 4.2 Characteristics of Antisocial Personality Disorder

Triggering Event(s)	Social standards and rules
Behavioral Style:	Self-reliant, cunning, and forceful
	Risk-taking and thrill-seeking
	Glib and shallow
Interpersonal Style:	Deceitful
	Irritable and aggressive
	Reckless disregard for others
	Lacks empathy
	Distrustful of others
Cognitive Style:	Impulsive
	Externally oriented and realistic
Feeling Style:	Avoid "softer" emotions which connote weakness
	Show little guilt, remorse, or shame
Temperament:	Il-tempered infantile pattern and an aggressive, impulsive adult pattern
Attachment Style	Fearful and dismissing
Parental Injunction	"The end justifies the means"
Self-View:	"I'm cunning and I'm entitled to get what I want"
World View:	"Life is devious and hostile and rules keep me from fulfilling my needs. Therefore, I'll bend or break them because my needs come first, and I'll defend any efforts to be controlled or degraded."
Maladaptive Schemas	Mistrust/Abuse; Entitlement; Insufficient Self-Control; Defectiveness; Emotional Deprivation; Abandonment; Social Isolation
Optimal Diagnostic Criteria	Criminal, aggressive, impulsive, irresponsible behavior

Nevertheless, these individuals crave attention, and the clinician can stimulate discussion by encouraging them to display their accomplishment (Ackley, Mack, Beyer, & Erdberg, 2011). By avoiding a judgmental or accusatory tone, the clinician may be able to encourage cooperation and explore they negative consequences of their actions. When they are unwilling to cooperate, answer questions, or adopt a complaining or hostile posture, the clinician does well to display indifference or initiate termination of the interview. Both of these strategies may quickly reverse their behavior. However, while they are seldom remorseful about their deceit and mistreatment of others, they can be made to realize that things are going poorly for them, and they are ruining their lives. The clinician can establish rapport and review their difficulties free of distortions and lies by showing empathy for the consequences of their behavior and failures. Only when they perceive the clinician as a non-punitive ally who will support their constructive goals and shows understanding of their inability to follow social forms, can they begin to form a therapeutic alliance (Othmer & Othmer, 2002).

Psychological Testing Data

The Minnesota Multiphase Personality Inventory (MMPI-2), the Millon Clinical Multiaxial Inventory (MCMI-IV), the Rorschach Psychodiagnostics Test, and the Thematic Apperception Test (TAT) can be useful in diagnosing the Antisocial Personality Disorder, as well as the antisocial personality style or trait (Groth-Marnat, 2009).

On the MMPI-2 the 4-9/9-4 (Psychopathic Deviant-Hypomania) profile is considered the classic profile of the Antisocial Personality Disorder. While the "9" represents the activator energizer of acting-out behavior, the 4 represents the cognitive component of the psychopathy (Graham, 2011). Two patterns of antisocial personality or psychopathology have been noted (Megargee and Bohn, 1979). The primary psychopath is easily provoked to violence, and thus a spike on scale 4 (Psychopathic Deviant) with elevators on 6 (Paranoid) and 8 (Schizophrenia) are likely. The 4-9/9-4 profile is more suggestive of secondary psychopathy as is the 2-4/4-2 (Depression-Psychopathic Deviant) profile (Meyer, 1995).

On the MCMI-IV elevation on scale 5 (Narcissistic) and 6 A (Antisocial) are most likely (Millon et al., 2016). Because alcohol and drug abuse are common in antisocial individuals, elevations in B (Alcohol use disorder) and/or T (Drug use disorder) are expected. Since Antisocial individuals are usually not highly distressed, elevations on A (Generalized anxiety disorder), D (Dysthymia disorder) and H (Somatic symptom disorder) are not common (Choca & Denburg, 1997).

Projective techniques can be very helpful in assessing the antisocial patient's object relations and superego development. Although these individuals are more likely to deceive a clinician during a clinical interview by simulating guilt or remorse, they are less likely to do so with ambiguous stimuli such as Rorschach blots where there are no "correct" answer (Gabbard, 2000).

On the Rorschach, Antisocial individuals tend to produce only a low to average number of responses, and they even reject cards that they could clearly handle cognitively. There is often a delayed reaction to the color cards, but then they may respond with C (Pure Color) responses in a fairly primitive and impulsive manner. They tend to give a high number of A (Animal) and P (Popular) responses, and a low number of M (Human Movement) and W (Whole) response. An absence of shading (Y, YF, and FY) and a (OW Form plus (F+%) responses (Wagner and Wagner, 1981). The newer Rorschach Performance Assessment System (R-PAS) is an improved method for scoring and interpreting the Rorschach Inkblot Test. Besides being evidence-based and internationally normed, it increases clinical utility and is easier to use than Exner's Comprehensive System (Mihura & Meyer, 2018).

On the TAT, their stories tend to be juvenile and sophomoric. And, while the protagonist may be caught in a negative act, there is usually no mention of the consequences of the negative act (Bellak, 1997).

Treatment Approaches and Interventions

Treatment Considerations

This diagnosis is reserved for individuals with a history of disregarding and violating the rights of others from the age of 15. The differential diagnosis for Antisocial Personality Disorder includes other personality disorders such as the Narcissistic Personality Disorder, the Paranoid Personality Disorder, and the Borderline Personality Disorder where it tends to be misdiagnosed in females. The most common symptom disorders associated with it are Substance Use Disorders, Bipolar Disorder, Delusional Disorders, and Factitious Disorders.

In terms of treatment goals, these individuals are usually not interested in presenting for treatment or are resistant to treatment if they are forced by the courts, employers, or other agencies. This is probably because they appear to suffer little or no personal distress, see little wrong with their behavior or attitudes, and consent to treatment only if it is in their best interest, such as when it might improve their chances when seeking parole or probation (Hare, Neumann, & Widiger, 2012).

Individual therapy, in and of itself, has proved to be remarkably ineffective with these individuals. This is particularly the case when therapy is insight-oriented or focuses on developing empathy, conscience, or interpersonal skills. However, special residential treatment programs have shown some promise (Harris & Rice, 2006). If the antisocial personality is able to engage in psychotherapy, a clear sign of progress is noted with the appearance of depressive features (Sperry, 2015).

Individual Psychotherapy

Hatchett (2015) recently conducted an in-depth literature review regarding treatment options for antisocial personality disorder. While he concluded that there does seem to be some benefit to psychosocial interventions to remediate antisociality and reduce criminal recidivism, the picture is muddy and complex. Research has not yet identified any interventions that clearly meet the standard for treatment efficacy, in his analysis. Because of this, he concludes that there is no basis to support the clinical utility for any psychosocial intervention for the treatment of this disorder. However, this doubt is not universally held. This section reviews the psychodynamic, cognitive-behavioral and interpersonal approaches of individual psychotherapy with Antisocial Personality Disordered individuals.

Psychodynamic Psychotherapy Approach

There is relatively little literature on successful treatment outcomes of individual dynamic psychotherapy with Antisocial Personality Disordered individuals. In fact, there is widespread pessimism that dynamic psychotherapy can change the antisocial pattern (Valliant & Perry, 1985). A number of explanations have been offered for this seeming failure. These explanations involve both patient selection and therapeutic stance and interventions. However, some of the newer psychodynamic approaches may change that view (Yeomans, Clarkin & Levy, 2021).

Gabbard (1990) indicates that the clinician's task at the outset of treatment is to determine which patients are "worth" the time, energy, and money required by a long-term therapy process with an uncertain outcome. Meloy (1988) has identified five contraindications for psychotherapy with antisocial patients. They are: a history of sadistic, violent behavior toward others; total absence of remorse for such behavior; a long standing incapacity to develop emotional attachments; high or low intelligence that can thwart the therapeutic process; and the clinician's intense countertransference fear for their personal safety. In short, the more the patient resembles the dynamic profile of the pure psychopath, the less likely they are to respond to dynamic psychotherapy.

On the other hand, antisocial patients with narcissistic features may be somewhat more amenable to psychotherapy. They may reveal some dependency in the transferences, and their internal "ideal object" may be somewhat less aggressive than in the pure psychopath (Meloy, 1988). The presence of major depression may reflect amenability to psychotherapy (Woody et al., 1985). Turkat (1990) notes that the "hurting sociopath" who is sincerely and genuinely distressed, has potential for profiting from psychotherapy. However, the most important predictor of treatment success is the ability to form a therapeutic alliance. Gertsley et al. (1989) showed a significant association between the ability to form a therapeutic alliance and treatment outcome in their study of 48 methadone—maintained male opiate addicts who meet criteria for Antisocial Personality Disorder.

Parenthetically, a study of sex difference in treatment recommendations for antisocial personality is thought provoking. A survey was undertaken involving 119 clinical psychologists who responded to case histories depicting either a male or female with Antisocial Personality Disorder and somatization. Results showed that clinicians were less likely to diagnose Antisocial Personality Disorder correctly for female than for male patients. Females were consistently given better prognosis and more likely to be recommended for insight-oriented psychotherapy than males who were given poorer prognoses and more likely to be recommended for group therapy and legal constraints (Fernbach et al., 1989).

Therapeutic stance and intervention strategy and techniques are other important factors in the treatment outcome equation. The traditional dynamic stance of neutrality is contraindicated. Gabbard (2000) contends that neutrality is tantamount to silent endorsement or collusion with the antisocial patient's actions. Instead, the recommended therapeutic stance is active and confrontative. The clinician will need to repeatedly confront the patient's minimization and denial of antisocial behavior. Furthermore, confrontation must focus on here-and-now behavior rather than analyzing unconscious material from the past.

From a dynamic perspective, it is crucial for the clinician to assist the patient in linking actions with internal states. Finally, the clinician's expectation for therapeutic change must be starkly realistic. Gabbard (1994) cautions that antisocial patients take delight in thwarting the clinician's wishes for them to change.

Needless to say, countertransference issues are important in working with antisocial patients. Two common forms are disbelief and collusion (Symington, 1980). Disbelief involves the clinician's rationalization that the patient is not really "that bad". Collusion is perhaps the most problematic type of countertransference. Gabbard insists that the clinician be stable, persistent and thoroughly incorruptible, as these patients will do whether necessary to corrupt the clinical into dishonest or unethical behavior. Through simulated tearfulness, sadness, or remorse, they can manipulate the clinician into empathizing with them.

As noted previously, there are studies of dynamic treatment with antisocial patients. One study of severe personality disordered individuals, including those with Antisocial Personality Disorder, found that significant split self-representation were present in the 27 patients studied. Relaxation exercises and a merging intervention were utilized to reduce the amnestic barriers that maintained this compartmentalization. Results showed the 24 patients responded with reduced resistance, increased treatment compliance, and improved daily functioning (Glantz & Goisman, 1990).

Meloy & Yakeley (2010) point out that many of the more recent therapeutic approaches to antisocial individuals have been largely behavioral in nature. These include relapse prevention classes, social skills groups, and other such efforts at changing surface behaviors and symptoms while overlooking the changes to antisocial individuals' internal mental states. One exception to this trend is Bateman & Fonagy's mentalization-based treatment (McGauley, Yakeley, Williams, & Bateman, 2011). Sometimes referred to as "mentalizing," this is the process by which individuals interpret their own subjective cognitions, behaviors, and emotions, as well as those of others. Many antisocial individuals exhibit deficits in this ability, particularly with respect to reflect the feelings of others. This rudimentary capacity for mentalization is combined with difficulty tolerating internal states of anxiety, resulting in the type of aggressive behavior that is a hallmark of this disorder. Malancharuvil (2012) also provides a psychodynamic formulation for empathy deficit in antisocial personality disorder. It is important to note that developing the capacity to mentalize without also increasing empathy may serve to make the antisocial individual a more effective predator rather than achieving the treatment's intended goal.

Cognitive Behavioral Therapy Approaches

Beck, Freeman and Associates (2004) provide an extended discussion of the Cognitive Therapy approach to Antisocial Personality Disordered individuals. They note that it is particularly difficult to develop a collaborative working relationship with these patients. These patients are difficult to work with because they are likely to distrust the therapist, are uncomfortable accepting help, and have little motivation because of therapist's countertransference. Establishing rapport requires the therapist to avoid, or disengage from, positions of control or power struggles with them, as well as to admit vulnerability to their manipulativeness. Since these individuals are likely to lie, the therapist can avoid entrapment in the role of being arbiter of truth by admitting that it could happen. To avoid premature termination, it is suggested that the therapist work gradually to establish trust, explicitly acknowledge the antisocial individual's strengths and capabilities, and refrain from pressing the individual to acknowledge weaknesses. Premature termination also may occur if the individual's distress, i.e., depression or anxiety symptoms, are quickly alleviated. In such instances Beck suggests pointing out that continuing in therapy is in the individual's best interest and identifying any remaining distress that the individual may be denying or minimizing.

Mitchell, Tafrate, & Freeman (2015) note that, contrary to the dramatic and confrontational depictions of therapy with antisocial individuals found in popular media, a more collaborative approach is needed. Confrontation leads to loss of momentum and premature termination. Therapist qualities like warmth, empathy, and the willingness to reward are especially important to this population. Techniques such as Motivational Interviewing (Miller & Rollnick, 2013), reviewing signs and symptoms of the disorder to raise awareness of potential consequences and offer the choice to change, and focusing on the patient's strengths and values are specific ways to engage antisocial individuals in treatment. Selecting appropriate treatment goals can be challenging with this disorder and considerable time must be spent exploring these with this population. For those who experience negative symptoms of anxiety or depression, symptom relief is a primary motivator. They see themselves as suffering, and the consequence of not acting is harmful to them alone. On the other hand, those who do not experience negative symptoms may see their antisocial behavior as rewarding and ego syntonic. In this case, motivation for change is minimal or outright resistant, as it is others who suffer and not the individual. Regardless of the individual's preferences, reducing criminal behavior should remain an overarching goal of treatment because of the harm caused to others and society as a whole.

After treatment goals have been agreed upon, focusing on specific problem situations with problem solving and behavioral strategies is suggested (Fowler, Orme, & Hart, 2021).

If impulse control, acting out or inappropriate expression of anger, impulse control and anger management strategies are advised. As these individuals become better able to control impulses and anticipate consequences of their actions, shifting the therapeutic focus to automatic thoughts and underlying schemas is possible. This transition from a largely behavioral focus to a more cognitive one gradually allows these individuals to become less vulnerable and more comfortable in disclosing thoughts and feelings. As planned termination of treatment approaches, the focus shifts to the social pressures the individual faces to continued antisocial behavior. Relapse prevention strategies are useful in sensitizing these patients to people, places, and circumstances that are potential triggers for antisocial thinking and behaviors. Presuming that the individual has learned sufficient social skills to fit in with prosocial group, the likelihood of effective coping in the face of social pressures is increased. Beck notes that group and family therapy can be useful adjunct to individual treatment.

Furthermore, Freeman et al. (1990) believe that cognitive therapy can be effective in not only reducing antisocial behavior, but also in assisting the individual to adopt a more prosocial lifestyle. They caution that these individuals often terminate treatment prematurely unless they experience sufficient distress from their symptom disorder, that provides an incentive for continuing to work in treatment.

An exploratory randomized controlled trial of cognitive behavioral therapy for violent men with antisocial personality disorder was conducted by Davidson and colleagues (2009). A total of 52 adult men with acts of aggression within the past six months were randomized to "treatment as usual" (TAU) plus CBT or TAU alone. A 12-month follow-up indicated that there were no significant outcome differences in the two groups. Both groups reported decreased frequency of aggressive acts; however, trends in the data favored the CBT in the areas of problematic drinking, social functioning, and beliefs about others. Reflections about working with this population and this study may be found in Davidson et al., 2010.

Schema Therapy. Schema Therapy is an elaboration of cognitive therapy that has been developed by Young (1994; 1999) specifically for personality disorders, and other difficult individual and couples problems. Schema Therapy involves identifying maladaptive schemas and planning specific strategies and interventions. Four main strategies are cognitive, experiential, behavioral and the therapeutic relationship itself. Cognitive restructuring, modification of maladaptive schemas, is an important cognitive strategy, but is combined with imagery exercises, empathic confrontation, homework assignments and "limited reparenting," i.e., a form of corrective emotional experience (Young, 1999).

Maladaptive schemas typically associated with Antisocial Personality Disorder are: *mistrust/abuse*, i.e., the belief that others will abuse, humiliate, cheat, lie, manipulate, or take advantage; *entitlement*, i.e., the belief that one is superior to others and not bound by the rules and norms that govern normal social interaction; *insufficient self-control*, i.e., the belief that one is incapable of self-control and frustration tolerance; *defectiveness*: i.e., the belief that one is defective, bad, unwanted, or inferior in important respects; *emotional deprivation*, i.e., the belief that one's desire for emotional support will not be met by others; *abandonment*, i.e., the belief that significant others will not or cannot provide reliable and stable support; and *social isolation*, i.e., the belief that one is alienated, different from others, or not part of any group (Bernstein, 2002).

Interpersonal Approach

For Benjamin (2003) psychotherapeutic interventions with Antisocial Personality Disordered individuals can be planned and evaluated in terms of whether they enhance collaboration, facilitate learning about maladaptive patterns and their roots, block these patterns, enhance the will to change, and effectively encourage new patterns.

Benjamin notes that antisocial individuals do not respond well to individual psychotherapy alone. She echoes the sentiments of others by cautioning that the kind and attentive therapist, as well as those who mistakenly believe they are firmly in control, may be "taken for a ride" by these individuals. Conversely, Benjamin notes that the opposite approach of being harsh and unsympathetic will only serve to reconfirm the antisocial individual's belief that they cannot trust those who claim to care. This pattern of "hostile autonomy" guarantees that these individuals are denied benevolent contact with those around them. The therapist's challenge is to break through this barrier and develop a bond with these deeply alienated clients. While individual therapy may be problematic, when combined with other modalities, such as milieu therapy, positive treatment outcome may be possible. The goal of the collaborative phase of treatment is to establish a bonding and some degree of interdependence. Since collaboration in individual psychotherapy cannot be coerced and is seldom chosen by antisocial individuals, Benjamin suggests joining the individual in his or her initial hostile position and then progressively moving toward collaboration.

Other ways of eliciting collaboration she suggested are utilizing sports heroes as role models. The antisocial individual may respond to a story about an athlete's warmth and benevolent power by internalizing these qualities, particularly in conduct disordered adolescents. Another strategy for cultivating warmth may be to allow the antisocial individual the opportunity to occupy a nurturant position, such as providing kittens to prison inmates or teaching kids to play basketball – all while under supervision, of course. Wilderness survival training is another potential modality. In these instances, nurturance and bonding could be facilitated. Carefully managed group therapy can provide opportunities for bonding and control. Family therapy can likewise lead to positive change, but family collusion in maintaining problem patterns must be considered.

Once bonding and interdependence begin, the preconditions for collaboration have been met. Next, the antisocial individual is helped to recognize and understand the self-destructive features of their exploitive lifestyle and pattern. She believes that these individuals can then begin to develop needed self-management and social skills such as self-care, delay of gratification, and empathy for others. Unfortunately, Benjamin offers little discussion and few suggestions for facilitating change for individuals with this disorder.

Group Therapy

Group therapy for antisocial personality disorder is commonly considered to be more effective than individual therapy because it offers antisocial individuals the ability to connect with the experiences of others in a less direct manner than individual therapy. This modality also enables these patients to see their behavior through the eyes of others. Structured forms of group therapy may be quite effective with Antisocial Personality Disordered individuals. Open, exploratory, and nondirective groups (Yalom, 1985) with heterogeneous composition are easily disrupted by antisocial patients, therefore such groups are not advisable for these patients (Liebowitz et al., 1986).

Three types of group treatment have been utilized with these patients: psychoeducational, psychotherapy, and support groups. (Walker, 1992). Psychoeducational groups combine didactic presentation by the clinician which is then processed by group members. Content and agenda is structured as is patient participation. The group is composed of antisocial patients who meet given criteria for participation and are chosen by the clinician. The groups are time-limited and meet weekly for 90 minutes. Because of the complexity of these patients' interpersonal and other problems, these groups have limited utility for antisocial patients.

Psychotherapy groups have somewhat less structure than psychoeducational groups but make use of cohesive themes relevant to these patients. Group membership is determined by the clinician who is family in charge of both content and process. These groups tend to be long term, meet weekly for 90 minutes, and are limited to nine or ten patients. Because a group of ten antisocial patients can be quite formidable, two clinician group therapists are recommended.

Two group therapists serve to diminish the group's potential for acting out against the group leaders, as one clinician is an easy target for isolation as well as attack or dismissal by group members. Two group leaders also offer patients more opportunity for constructive identification because of difference in the clinician's personality and style. Furthermore, it allows for a "good guy-bad guy" routine and allows "lateral passes" by the leaders who may find themselves unable to handle a particular issue or patient (Walker, 1992).

Support groups for antisocial patients are useful for individuals who have had intensive inpatient or outpatient group psychotherapy (Ogrodniczuk, Uliaszek, Lebow, & Kealy, 2021).

While they are based on a self-help model they are led by a clinician. The main focus of these on-going groups with open membership is relapse prevention and the development of peer support.

Walker (1992) described some useful guidelines for setting up these three different types of groups. He also described a number of rules and specific procedures for doing group work with antisocial patients.

Meloy & Yakeley (2010) describe the group process for antisocial personality disorder from a psychodynamic perspective. They note that the therapy group acts as a container for the antisocial individual's projections, as well as a collective auxiliary ego that can reflect on behalf of him or her. This gradually moves the patient to healthier ego functioning.

Therapeutic Community. An extension of group treatment in an inpatient or residential setting in which the milieu is a medium of change is the therapeutic community. Recent research indicates that drug addicted individuals with Antisocial Personality Disorder can benefit significantly from therapeutic community treatment provided they complete the treatment program and continue with aftercare in the community. Treatment completion was found to be the most important factor in reducing recent drug use and post-discharge arrests (Messina et al., 2002).

Marital and Family Therapy

There are a considerable number of studies on the family dynamics and treatment of the antisocial patient mostly involving delinquent youths (Glueck & Glueck, 1950; Minnuchin et al., 1967). A few studies suggest that short term family therapy can also be effective with delinquent adolescents (Alexander & Parsons, 1973; Parsons & Alexander, 1973). Harbir (1981) notes that antisocial patients are seldom motivated to engage in family therapy, but to the extent that the clinician is able to engage the patient's parents or spouse, the more likely therapeutic change is possible. Since the antisocial patient tends to precipitously leave outpatient treatment when difficult and anxiety-provoking issues are faced, it is incumbent on the clinician to maximize therapeutic leverage. Specifically, this means establishing a consistent therapeutic alliance and involving the family at the outset, usually at the beginning of hospital treatment, as a part of a court stipulation or as required adjunct to residential treatment.

A major treatment goal is to help family members, or the spouse in couple's therapy, set limits on the patient (Ogrodniczuk, Uliaszek, Lebow, & Kealy, 2021). Typically, family members and spouses have minimized, ignored, or acted inconsistently in the face of the patient's antisocial behavior. As the family or spouse consistently sets and enforces limits, the patient's pathological behavior reduces, and sometimes treatment amenable symptoms, like depression emerge. This suggests the patient is beginning to change and is more motivated to stop destructive behaviors. As family treatment proceeds, changes in destructive communication patterns can be achieved systematically (Parsons & Alexander, 1973).

Nichols, W. (1996) describes the marital interactional patterns and symptomatology of individuals with Antisocial Personality Disorders and Histrionic Personality Disorders in close interpersonal relationships as well as a suggested treatment plan protocol and strategies for dealing with such couples in a therapeutic context.

Medication

Currently, there are no psychotropic medications specifically indicated for treating individuals with this disorder (Nelson & Tsheringld, 2021). However, there is some evidence that those with this disorder have responded to SSRIs (Silk & Feurino, 2012). For this reason, these medications are used that target specific troubling symptoms, particularly anxiety. Generally, these medications are used as an adjunct to psychotherapy and skills training. Because troubling symptoms often respond to medications sooner than most psychological interventions, medications are usually prescribed at the onset of treatment (Sperry, 1995b). Unfortunately, there is limited research evidence to provide guidelines for the use of SSRIs for other indications or for the use of other medications (Silk & Feurino, 2012).

Combined and Integrative Treatment Approaches

Despite widespread pessimism about the treatability of this disorder there is reason for cautious optimism provided that treatment is combined or multimodal and tailored to the particular needs and circumstances of the individual (Winkeller & Schlesinger, 2021).

There is clear evidence that time itself is the most effective treatment modality. In other words, the intensity of antisocial behaviors tends to dissipate with age (Regier et al., 1988). Purportedly that is due to the cumulative effects of personal, social, legal, and financial repercussions of antisocial behavior. The next most effective is specialized treatment, therapeutic communities or wilderness program that provides firm limits and structure, group work with peers and a structured work program (Woody et al., 1985). To the extent that sufficient therapeutic leverage is present in outpatient settings, treatment outcomes for antisocial patients can be at least guardedly optimistic.

As with borderline personality disorder, most agree that pharmacotherapy should not be the only treatment for Antisocial Personality Disorder (Gunderson, 1986). Kellner (1986) suggests that treatment often begins with a psychotherapeutic modality, after which a trial of medication may be considered for a specific target symptom such as impulsivity, aggressivity, explosiveness, and violence. Treatment, in many cases, will be long because of the patient's unwillingness or inability to persevere. It may consist of a few sessions interspersed with long intervals without any therapeutic work, or for medication monitoring only. In any case, the clinician must attempt to establish a therapeutic while maintaining firm limits. Psychoeducation, whether in an individual or group format, is usually necessary. Kellner

(1986) notes that data supports the use of sustained treatment which invariable involves psychotherapies—individual, group, and family, behavior therapy, and psychoeducation—aimed at teaching self-control and postponement of gratification as well as the use of medication. Though such interventions are exceedingly complex and difficult, Kellner believes they can make a substantial difference in the life and adjustment of these patients.

Many of the studies about combined treatment focus on the treatment of co-occurring antisocial personality disorder and substance use disorders. Ogloff, Talevski, Lemphers, Wood, & Simmons (2015) investigated the relationship between mental illness, substance use disorders, antisocial personality disorder, and offending in a sample of 130 males in a forensic mental health service facility in Australia. They found that the majority of these individuals met the criteria for multiple disorders, highlighting the need for an integrative treatment approach. Havens, Cornelius, Ricketts, Larkin, Bishai, Lloyd, Huettner, & Strathdee (2007) investigated a case management intervention on admission to substance abuse treatment for injection drug users with and without antisocial personality disorder. They found that injection drug users with ASPD were 3.51 times more likely to enter substance abuse treatment after spending time with a case manager. Messina, Farabee, & Rawson (2003) examined the effectiveness of four different types of treatment for cocaine-dependent patients with antisocial personality disorder. These were: cognitive-behavioral therapy (CBT); contingency management (CM); combined CBT and CM; and methadone maintenance. They found that patients with ASPD were more likely to abstain from cocaine use during treatment than those without this disorder, an effect that was significantly related to the contingency management condition.

Chapter 5

Avoidant Personality Disorder

Individuals with avoidant personalities tend to be shy, lonely, hypersensitive individuals with low self-esteem. Although they are desperate for interpersonal involvement, they avoid personal contact with others because of their heightened fear of social disapproval and rejection sensitivity (Sanislow, da Cruz, Gianoli, & Reagan, 2012; Skodol, Bender, & Oldham, 2019; American Psychiatric Association, 2022). While treatment of such individuals involves a number of unique therapeutic challenges, it can be highly effective and successful.

This chapter describes a framework for the assessment and effective treatment of this disorder. It includes sections on diagnosis, psychological assessment, case conceptualization, and treatment interventions. It begins with background information on the disorder as well as a DSM-5-TR description, prototypic description, associated features, and the Alternative Model of Personality Disorders description of this disorder. The section on case conceptualization provides five common clinical formulations of this disorder: psychodynamic, biosocial, cognitive-behavioral, interpersonal, and an integrative conceptualization of this disorder. Several treatment approaches, modalities, and intervention strategies are also described. These includes individual psychotherapy, group therapy, marital and family therapy, medication, and integrative and combined treatment.

Description of the Avoidant Personality Disorder

The Avoidant Personality Disorder can be recognized by the following descriptors or characteristics: styles vs. disorders, triggering event, behavioral styles, interpersonal styles, cognitive styles, affective styles, attachment style, and optimal criterion.

Style vs. Disorder. The avoidant personality can be thought of as spanning a continuum from healthy to pathological, with the avoidant personality style on the healthy and the Avoidant Personality Disorder on the pathological end. Table 5.1 compares and contrasts differences between the avoidant style and disorder.

Triggering Event(s). The typical situation, circumstance or event that triggers or activates the characteristic maladaptive response of the Avoidant Personality Disorder (Othmer & Othmer, 2002), as noted in behavioral, interpersonal, cognitive, and feeling styles, is: "demands for close interpersonal relating and/or social and public appearances."

Behavioral Style. The behavioral style of avoidant personalities is characterized by chronic tenseness and self-consciousness. Their behavior and speech are controlled, and they

Table 5.1 A Comparison of Avoidant Personality Style vs. Disorder

Personality Style	Personality Disorder
Comfortable with habit, repetition and routine. Prefer the known to the unknown	Exaggerates the potential difficulties, physical dangers or risks involved in doing something ordinary but outside his or her usual routine
Close allegiance with family and/or a few close friends; tend to be homebodies	Has no close friends or confidants—or confidants—or only one—other than first degree relatives; avoids activities that involve significant interpersonal contact
Sensitive and concerned about what others Think of them. tend to be self-conscious	Unwilling to get involved with people unless certain of being liked; easily hurt and worriers
Very discrete and deliberate in dealing with others	Fears being embarrassed by blushing, crying or showing signs of anxiety in front of other people
Tend to maintain a reserved, self-restrained demeanor around others	Reticent in social situations because of a fear of saying something inappropriate or foolish, or of being unable to answer a question
Tend to be curious and can focus considerable attention on hobbies, and avocations; however, a few engage in counterphobic coping behaviors	Tend to be underachievers, and find it difficult to focus on job tasks or hobbies

appear apprehensive and awkward. They also tend to be self-critical and devalue their achievements.

Interpersonal Style. Interpersonally, they are rejection sensitive. Even though they desire acceptance by others, they keep distance from others and require unconditional approval before being willing to "open up." They guardedly "test" others to determine who can be trusted to like them.

Cognitive Style. The cognitive style of such individuals can be described as hypervigilant, meaning that they scan the environment looking for clues of potential threat or acceptance. Their thoughts are often distracted by their hypersensitivity. Not surprisingly, they have low self-esteem because of their devaluation of their own achievements and their overemphasis of their own shortcomings.

Affective Style. Their emotional or affective style is marked by a shy and apprehensive quality. Because they are seldom able to attain unconditional approval from others, they routinely experience sadness, loneliness, and tenseness. At times of increased distress, they will describe feelings of emptiness and depersonalization.

Attachment Style. Individuals with a self-view that is negative and world view that vacillates between positive and negative exhibit a composite preoccupied and fearful style of attachment. Their avoidance is based on the desire to be liked and accepted by others, while at the same time fearing rejection and abandonment. The Preoccupied–Fearful Attachment Style adult attachment style is common in individuals with Avoidant Personality Disorder (Lyddon & Sherry, 2001).

Optimal Diagnostic Criterion. Of the various criteria for the Avoidant Personality Disorder, one has been found to be the most useful in diagnosing this disorder. The belief is that by beginning with this criterion, the clinician can test for the presence or absence of the criterion and quickly diagnose the personality disorder (Allnutt and Links, 1996). The "optimal criterion" for this disorder is: "avoids occupational activities that involve significant interpersonal contact fearing criticism, disapproval or rejection."

The following two case examples illustrate the differences between the avoidant personality style (Dr. Q) and the Avoidant Personality Disorder (Ms. A).

Case Study: Avoidant Personality Style

Peter Q. is a 31-year-old eye surgeon who had recently been hired by a large HMO hospital and clinic. He had recently completed residency training, and being new, good looking and single was quickly noticed by the female staff. His specialty was laser surgery for which he was exquisitely skilled and respected by his patients. Although courteous, he was somewhat emotionally distant and shy. Dr. Q seldom participated in staff parties, and if he did make an appearance, he would politely excuse himself after his beeper sounded—which seemed all the time—and he wouldn't return. His social life seemed to be a mystery, and he had little contact after hours with his male colleagues, except for one. Dr. S. had run into Peter at a civil war convention in another city, and to his surprise learned of Peter's long standing hobby and collection of civil war books and memorabilia. In time the two became very good friends, spending considerable time together. Although he had his own apartment, Peter spent much of his free time at home with his parents. Dr. S. soon became a regular guest at the Q. home and was initially was at how warm, cordial and comfortable Peter was in this small setting as compared to the hospital.

Case Study: Avoidant Personality Disorder

Ms. A. is a 27-year-old female student who contacted the University Counseling Center for help with "difficulty concentrating." She indicated that the problem started when Ms. A's roommate of two years precipitously moved out to live with her boyfriend. Ms. A. described herself as being "blown away and hurt" by this. She noted that she had no close friends and described herself as being shy and having had only one date since high school. Since then, she avoided attempts by men to date her because of being rejected when she was a freshman by a guy who had dated her for a month and never contacted her again. On examination, she had poor eye contact with the admissions counselor and appeared very shy and self-conscious.

DSM-5-TR Description

DSM-5-TR emphasizes specific behaviors for this disorders. Individuals who meet criteria for this diagnosis are characterized by an unremitting pattern of being socially inhibited, feeling inadequate, and overly sensitive to the negative evaluations of others. This is typically because they view themselves as socially inept, unappealing, or inferior to others. They consistently avoid work activities that require close interpersonal contact for fear of being criticized or rejected. They will not get involved with others unless they are certain of being accepted. Fearing they will be shamed or ridiculed, they are uncomfortable and act with restraint in intimate relationships. In anticipation of shame or ridicule, they are uncomfortable and are hesitant in intimate relationships. Similarly, they experience feelings of inadequacy and inhibition in new interpersonal situations. Not surprising, they refuse to take personal risks or engage in activities that may prove embarrassing (American Psychiatric Association, 2022).

Prototypic Description

A prototype is a brief description that captures the essence of how a particular disorder commonly presents. Prototypic descriptions are useful and convenient, and clinicians commonly rely on them rather than lists of behavioral criteria or core beliefs (Westen, 2012). Here is a common prototypic description of the Avoidant Personality Disorder: These individuals are frightened and interpersonally awkward. They are also extremely sensitive to criticism and rejection. Just the idea of meeting someone new engenders fear of being humiliated or embarrassed. So, it is much easier to avoid any new work or social relationship that could threaten their personal sense of security and safety. Still, they crave connection with others that they have come to trust. Accordingly, they may have a friend or a relative with whom they can relax and feel safe (Francis, 2013).

Associated Features

Prevalence. AVPD has been identified in 2.7 percent of the general population. It has been diagnosed in 24.6 percent in clinical practice making it one of the most common (Torgersen, 2021).

Differential Diagnosis. Social anxiety disorder (SAD) overlaps with AVPD. They differ in metacognitive abilities, i.e., recognition of others' thoughts and beliefs, wherein those with AVPD tend to misread neutral and positive reactions as negative which only heightens their sensitivity to avoidance and rejection (Moroni et al., 2016; Sperry, 2021).

Development and Course. Avoidant behaviors of shyness, isolation, and fear of new people and situations can be observed in infants and children. While shyness is a precursor of this disorder, it tends to dissipate with age. Those that develop this disorder tend to become shyer and more isolative during the teen and early adult year. In subsequent years this disorder can remit or become less evident so that by age 65 the prevalence is only 0.8 percent (American Psychiatric Association, 2022).

Culture, Sex, and Gender. Some cultures and ethnic groups consider avoidant behaviors appropriate. It may be the result of difficulties in acculturation. Marked avoidance may follow social embarrassment or the failure to achieve major life goals rather than a shy temperament. In such social contexts deliberate avoidance serves to preserve harmony and prevent offending others. While some cultures expect females to be more avoidant and subservient than males, generally this avoidant pattern is equally observed in males and females (American Psychiatric Association, 2022).

Table 5.2 Characteristics of Avoidant Personality Disorder

Triggering Event(s)	Demands for close interpersonal relating and/or social and public appearances
Behavioral Style	Chronically tense and self-conscious
	Aloof, controlled and underactive behavior
	Self-critical and devalue their achievements
Interpersonal Style	Avoids interpersonal contacts fearing rejection
	Cautious to get involved with others
	Restrained intimacy for fear of ridicule
	Preoccupied with social criticism or rejection
	Inhibited in new interpersonal situations
	Reluctant to take social risks
Cognitive Style	Hypervigilant
	Thinking is easily distracted by their hypersensitivity
Feeling Style	Shy and apprehensive
	Feelings of emptiness and depersonalization
Attachment Style	Preoccupied and fearful
Temperament	Irritable
Parental Injunction	"We don't accept you, and probably nobody else will either"
Self View	"I'm inadequate and frightened of rejection"
World View	"Life is unfair, people reject and criticize me, but I want someone to like me. Therefore, be vigilant, demand reassurance, and, if all else fails, fantasize and daydream"
Maladaptive Schemas	Defectiveness; Social Isolation; Approval-Seeking, Self-Sacrifice
Optimal Diagnostic Criteria	Avoids occupational activities that involve significant interpersonal contact fearing criticism, disapproval or rejection

Alternative Model of Avoidant Personality Disorder

The Alternative Model of Personality Disorders (AMPD) offers a clinically useful description of the Avoidant Personality Disorder in terms of typical features and trait facets. Typical features are avoidance of social situations and inhibition in interpersonal relationships related to feelings of ineptitude and inadequacy, anxious preoccupation with negative evaluation and rejection, and fears of ridicule or embarrassment (American Psychiatric Association, 2022). Trait facet criteria include Anxiousness, Withdrawal, Anhedonia, and Intimacy avoidance (Skodol, 2021).

Table 5.2 summarizes these characteristics.

Conceptualizations of the Avoidant Personality Disorder

Psychodynamic Case Conceptualization

Shyness, shame, and avoidant behaviors are conceptualized as defenses against embarrassment, humiliation, rejection, and failure (Gabbard, 1990). Shame and fear of exposure of the self to others are interconnected. Individuals with avoidant personalities tend to feel ashamed about their self-perceptions as weak, unable to compete, physically or mentally defective or disgusting, and unable to control bodily function (Wurmser, 1981). Shame evolves from many different developmental experiences throughout the early childhood years. These developmental experiences, plus a constitutional predisposition to avoid stressful situations, tends to be reactivated in the avoidant patient upon exposure to individuals who matter a great deal to the patient (Gabbard, 1994). Psychodynamic theorists conceptualize the behavior of those with avoidant personality as being motivated by shame for not living up to their ego ideal (Eskedal & Demetri, 2006). This poor self-image results in numerous behaviors intended to protect avoidant individuals, including misreading others' neutral and positive reactions as negative and restricting social experiences to avoid situations where their perceived inadequacies may be revealed.

Biosocial Case Conceptualization

Millon (1981), Millon and Everly (1985) and Millon and Davis (1996; 2000) and believe that the etiology and development of this personality disorder represents an interactive constellation of biogenic environmental factors. They hypothesize that the vigilance characterizing this personality reflects functional dominance of the sympathetic nervous system with a lowered autonomic arousal threshold. This could allow irrelevant impulses to intrude on logical association, diminish control and direction of thought and memory processes resulting in marked interface with normal cognitive processes. Research cited by Kogan et al. (1988) suggests that the trait of shyness is of genetic-constitutional origin, which requires specific environmental experiences to develop into a full-blown pattern of timidity and avoidance.

Parental and peer group rejection are two critical and prevalent environmental influences. The amount of parental rejection appears to be particularly intense and/or frequent. When peer group rejection reinforces parental rejection the child sense of self-worth and self-competence tend to be severely eroded, and result in self-critical attitudes. As a result these individuals restrict their social experiences, are hypersensitive to rejection and become excessively introspective. By restricting their social environment, they subsequently fail to develop social competence which tends to evoke the ridicule of others for their asocial behavior. Because of their hypersensitivity and hypervigilance, they are prone to interpret minor rebuffs as principal indicators of rejection, where no rejection was intended. Finally, because of their excessive introspective, they are forced to examine the painful condition they have created for themselves. Not surprisingly, they conclude that they do not deserve to be accepted by others.

Cognitive-Behavioral Case Conceptualizations

According to Beck (2015), individuals with avoidant personality are fearful of initiating relationships as well as fearful of responding to other's attempts to relate to them because of their overriding belief that they will be rejected. For them, such rejection is unbearable so they engage in social avoidance. Furthermore, they engage in cognitive and emotional avoidance by not thinking about things which could cause them to feel dysphoric. Because of their low tolerance for dysphoria, the further distract themselves from their negative cognitions. Underlying these avoidance patterns are maladaptive schemas or long standing dysfunctional beliefs about self and others. They tend to view themselves as inept socially and incompetent academically and vocationally. They typically view others as critical, demeaning, and uninterested in them. Schemas about self-include themes of being different, inadequate, defective, and unlikable. Schemas about others involve themes of uncaring and rejection.

These individuals are likely to predict and interpret the rejection as caused solely by their personal deficiencies. This prediction of rejection results in dysphoria. Finally, avoidant individuals do not have internal criteria to judge themselves in a positive manner. Thus, they must rely on their perception. They tend to misread a neutral or positive reaction as negative which further compounds their rejection-sensitivity and social emotional and cognitive avoidance. In short, they hold negative schemas which lead them to avoid solutions where they could interact with others. They also avoid tasks which could engender uncomfortable feelings and avoid thinking about matters which produce dysphoria. Because of their low tolerance for discomfort they utilize distractions, excuse making and rationalizations when they begin to feel sad or anxious (Padesky & Beck, 2015).

Turkat (1990) describes this disorder as primarily anxiety-based, and characterized by timidity and anxiety concerning evaluation, rejection, and/or humiliation. He notes that the disorder is very responsive to behavioral interventions, particularly anxiety management desensitization methods, where the hierarchy is based on fear of rejection, criticism, and/or evaluation.

Interpersonal Case Conceptualization

According to Benjamin (2003) persons diagnosed with Avoidant Personality Disorder tended to begin their development sequence with appropriate nurturance and social bonding. As a result, they continued to desire social contact and nurturance. Unfortunately, these individuals were subject to relentless parental control with regard to creating an impressive social image. Visible flaws were cause of great embarrassment and humiliation, particularly for the family. Besides exhortations to be admirable, they experienced degrading mockery for failures, personal imperfections or shortcomings. The adult consequence is that avoidant individuals are socialized to perform adequately and manage an appropriate impression while avoiding occasions for embarrassment or humiliation. Typically, this humiliation was associated with exclusion, banishment, or rejection. As a result, they anticipate rejection and thus socially isolate themselves. Because they are well bonded, they crave relationships and social contact but are absolutely convinced there is little or no risk of rejection or dejection.

Furthermore, although they experienced rejection and ridicule from their families, they also internalized the belief that family is their source of support. Thus, they have intense family loyalty, while harboring equally intense fears of outsiders. In short, avoidant individuals exhibit intense fear of humiliation and rejection. To avoid this, they socially withdraw and restrain themselves, while prying for love and acceptance. They can become very intimate with a select few who pass their highly stringent safety test. Occasionally, they can lose control and explode with rageful indignation.

Integrative Case Conceptualizations

The following integrative formulation provides a biopsychosocial explanation for how this personality is likely to have developed and how it is maintained. Biologically, these individuals commonly were hyperirritable and fearful as infants, and they most likely exhibited the "slow to warm" temperament (Thomas & Chess, 1977). Individuals with this personality pattern are also likely to have experienced various maturational irregularities as children. There irregularities and their hyperirritable pattern are attributed to low around of their autonomic nervous system (Millon & Everly, 1985).

Psychologically, those with Avoidant Personalities typically view themselves as "See, I am inadequate and frightened of rejection." They are likely to view the world as some variant of the theme: "Life is unfair—people reject and criticize me—but, I still want someone to like me." As such, they are likely to conclude: "Therefore, be vigilant, demand reassurance, and if all else fails, fantasize and daydream about the way life could be." A common defense mechanism of the avoidant personality is fantasy. Thus, it is not surprising that Avoidant Personalities are major consumers of romance novels and soap operas.

Socially, predictable patterns of parenting and environmental factors can be noted for the avoidant personality disorder. The avoidant personality is likely to have experienced parental rejection and/or ridicule. Later, siblings and peers will likely continue this pattern of rejection and ridicule. The parental injunction is likely to have been: "We don't accept you, and probably no one else will either." They may have had parents with high standards and worried that they may not have or would not meet these standards and therefore would not be accepted.

This avoidant pattern is confirmed, reinforced and perpetuated by the following individual and systems factors: a sense of personal inadequacy and a fear of rejection leads to hypervigilance which leads to restricted social experiences. These experiences, plus catastrophic thinking, lead to increased hypervigilance and hypersensitivity; leading to self-pity, anxiety, and depression; which leads to further confirmation of avoidant beliefs and styles (Sperry, 2015).

Assessment of Avoidant Personality Disorder

Several sources of information are useful in establishing a diagnosis and treatment plan for personality disorders. Observation, collateral information, and psychological testing are important adjuncts to the patient's self-report in the clinical interview. This section briefly describes some characteristic observations that the clinician makes and the nature of the rapport likely to develop in initial encounters with specific personality disordered individuals. Characteristic response patterns on various objective (i.e., MMPI-II and MCMI-III) and projective tests (i.e., Rorschach and TAT) are also described.

Interview Behavior and Rapport

In the initial interview, Avoidant Personality Disordered individuals tend to be monosyllabic, circumstantial, and guarded. Some may even appear suspicious or quite anxious, but all are hypersensitive to rejection and criticism. Reluctance and guardedness should be approached with empathy and reassurance. The clinician does well to avoid confrontation which likely will be interpreted as criticism. Instead, use empathic responses which encourage sharing of past pain and anticipatory fears. When these individuals feel that the clinician understands their hypersensitivity and will be protective of them, they are willing to trust and cooperate with treatment. After feeling safe and accepted, the character of the interview can change dramatically. Rapport has been achieved, and they feel relieved when they can describe their fears of being embarrassed and criticized, and sensitivity to being misunderstood. They may experience these fears of being embarrassed as silly and express it. If the clinician identifies with position, they are likely to feel ridiculed and withdraw again (Othmer & Othmer, 2002).

Psychological Testing Data

The Minnesota Multiphase Personality Inventory (MMPI-2), the Million Clinical Multiaxial Inventory (MCMI-IV), and the Rorschach Psychodiagnostic Test can be useful in diagnosing the Avoidant Personality Disorder as well as the Avoidant Personality Style or trait (Groth-Marnat, 2009).

On the MMPI-2 a 2-7/7-2 (Depression-Psychasthenia) profile is typical. This profile reflects depression about assumed rejection, as well as apprehension and self-doubt about relating to others (Graham, 2011). When social withdrawal is also present, a high score on O (Social Introversion) is likely, as well as a lowered 9 (Hypomania) scale. When social withdrawal and self-rejection lead to decreased functioning; an elevation on scale 8 (Schizophrenia) may occur (Meyer, 1995).

On the MCMI-IV, an elevation of 85 or above on scale 2B (Avoidant) along with low scores on 4 (Histrionic) and 7 (Compulsive) are likely. Moderate elevators on scales 8B (Masochistic—Self-Defeating) and C (Borderline) may also be present (Millon, Millon, Grossman, Boice, & Sinsabaugh, 2016). The higher S (Schizotypal) is elevated, the more likely decompensation has occurred (Choca & Denburg, 1997).

On the Rorschach, blocked or relatively inactive M (Human Movement) response are likely. A high number of P (Popular) responses occurs, and C (Contrast) often involves passive animals such as deer and rabbits—sometimes being maimed or killed—or passive interactions in the M responses (Meyer, 1995). The new Rorschach Performance Assessment System (R-PAS) is an improved method for scoring and interpreting the Rorschach Inkblot Test. Besides being evidence-based and internationally normed, it increases clinical utility and is easier to use than Exner's Comprehensive System (Mihura & Meyer, 2018).

Treatment Approaches and Interventions

Treatment Considerations

Basically, the overall goals of treatment with avoidant personality-disordered individuals are to increase their capacity to tolerate feedback from others and become more selectively trusting of others (Skodol, 2021a). This means that instead of automatically assuming that others intend to criticize, reject, or humiliate them, or reflexively "testing" the trustworthiness of others, avoidant individuals will be able to take some measured risks in relating to others. This might mean assertively communicating their needs and wants, or it might mean taking the risk of requesting some feedback from others who previously have been supportive of them.

Avoidant individuals already know how to relate to a small and select number of individuals, often relatives. If the clinician simply becomes one of them, the individual's basic pattern of avoidance may remain unchanged. It is only when these individuals learn to recognize the impact of their pattern on others and take risks in new relationships that they can change.

Although individual therapy can help avoidant individuals recognize and analyze their pattern of avoidance and withdrawal, couples therapy and group therapy permit both clinician and individual to observe the impact of this pattern on others, and for the individual to risk new behaviors. If the individual is married or in a long-term relationship, triangular patterns are often present. For instance, the avoidant individual may be married to a spouse who travels extensively and makes few if any emotional demands on their avoidant partner, providing the avoidant partner the opportunity for a secret extramarital affair. This triangular pattern provides some degree of intimacy as well as protection from public humiliation, while also insuring interpersonal distance (Sperry & Sperry, 2016).

Individual Psychotherapies

Psychodynamic Psychotherapy Approaches

Both expressive and supportive aspects of psychodynamic psychotherapy can be most effective in the treatment of the Avoidant Personality Disordered individual (Gabbard, 1994; Yeomans, Clarkin, & Levy, 2021). The supportive aspect involves an empathic appreciation of the humiliation and embarrassment associated with exposure to fearful interpersonal circumstances and the pain connected with rejection. The supportive aspect also involves the clinician's prescription of exposure to the feared situation. Needless to say, firm encouragement must accompany this prescription. More of their fantasies and anxieties will be activated in the actual situation of exposure rather than in their defensive posture of withdrawal. Explaining this fact will further encourage avoidant patients to seek out fearful situations.

The expressive aspect of therapy focuses on exploring the underlying causes of shame as related to past developmental experiences. To the extent the patient is willing to risk confronting the feared circumstance, the expressive aspect of therapy is greatly enhancing. Initial exploratory efforts can be frustrating in that avoidant individuals may be somewhat uncertain about who it is they fear. They tend to provide vague and global explanations such as "rejection" and "shyness" rather than specific fantasies. Thus, the clinician does well to explore specific fantasies within the context of the transference.

These individuals tend to have a considerable degree of anxiety about the psychotherapeutic requirement to openly share thoughts and feelings. Accordingly, when they nonverbally react, i.e., blush, about something that has been verbalized, the clinician might ask them to share their embarrassment and what they imagine the clinician could be thinking and feeling. By pursuing the details of specific situations, these patients can develop a greater awareness of the correlates of the shame affect (Gabbard, 1994).

Interpretive techniques are also useful as either the primary intervention or as adjunctive to behavioral and interpersonal approaches. The basic strategy involves interpretive unconscious fantasies that their fear or impulses will become uncontrollable and harmful to self and others. Not surprisingly, their avoidant behavior maintains a denial of unconscious wishes or impulses (Mackinnon & Michels, 1971). Furthermore, these patients tend to have harsh superegos and subsequently project their own unrealistic expectations of themselves onto others. In doing, they evade expected criticism and embarrassment by avoiding relationships with others. A complete interpretation of them, identifies the unconscious impulse and the fear, and traces the resulting avoidant defensive pattern in early life experiences, in outside relationships, and in the transference (Fenichel, 1945).

Compared to other personality disorders, there has been relatively little formal study of the effectiveness of long-term psychodynamic treatment for avoidant personality disorder. Svartberg, Stiles, & Seltzer (2004) conducted a randomized trial of 40 sessions of cognitive therapy versus psychodynamic therapy with 50 participants who met the criteria for Cluster C personality disorders. Of these 31 qualified for a diagnosis of avoidant personality disorder. Results indicated that both forms of therapy led to significant positive changes; however, only the psychodynamic therapy group showed significant decreases in symptom distress at the end of treatment. Porcerelli, Dauphin, Ablon, Leirman & Bambery (2007) conducted a five-year case study of a 50-year-old male computer technician who received psychoanalysis four times per week. Later sessions after year 2 included elements of cognitive-behavioral and interpersonal therapies. Results indicated that long-term psychoanalysis resulted in clinically significant reductions in symptom severity and relational pathology, with gains being maintained at the 1-year follow up.

Cognitive Behavioral Therapy Approaches

Beck, Freeman, and Associates (2015) provide an in-depth discussion of the Cognitive Therapy approach with Avoidant Personality Disordered individuals. Avoidant individuals are often difficult to engage in treatment given their basic strategy of avoidance and their hypersensitivity to perceived criticism. The therapist must work diligently yet carefully at building trust. Trust tests are common in the early stage of treatment and can include a pattern of cancelling appointments or having difficulty scheduling regular appointments. It is important not to prematurely challenge automatic thoughts, as such challenges can be viewed as personal criticism. Only after these individuals are solidly engaged in treatment should the therapist use cognitive interactions to test their expectancies in social situations. To the extent the therapist utilizes collaboration rather than confrontation and guided discovery rather than direct disputation, these individuals are more likely to view therapy as constructive and are likely to remain in treatment (Fowler, Orme, & Hart, 2021).

Since these individuals often experience high levels of interpersonal anxiety, it is useful to employ anxiety management interventions early in the course of treatment. Because these individuals work at avoiding not only unpleasant affects but also avoid thinking about matters that elicit unpleasant feelings, it is useful to work in increasing emotional tolerance with desensitization methods and reframing. Furthermore, since these individuals may not have learned the basics of social interaction, structured social skills training may need to be incorporated.

Later in therapy, when these individuals have achieved some of their short-term treatment goals and developed sufficient trust in the therapist, efforts to challenge automatic thoughts and restructure maladaptive schemas are appropriate. Issues involving risk of developing close relationship and intimacy are central. Typically, it is necessary to decatastrophize disapproval and rejection. To the extent these individuals have developed sufficient self-efficacy and have experienced enough success on a variety of levels of relationships, they are more receptive to entertaining the notion that disapproval in a close relationship does not equal rejection or devastation. Adding group therapy has a place in the treatment of this disorder, so that they can learn new attitudes and practice new skills in a socially benign and accepting environment. Padesky & Beck (2015) suggest three primary treatment goals: Target emotional avoidance in and between sessions to help the patient become aware of how this pattern contributes to problems; build self-reflection and interpersonal skills such as self-expression, assertion, and conflict negotiation; and develop alternative cognitions that allow for both intimacy and assertiveness in relationships.

In summary, the Cognitive Therapy approach to this disorder recognizes the significant challenge of engaging the avoidant individual in treatment and utilize several efforts to build trust, reduce social anxiety and cognitive and emotional avoidance. It then proceeds to correcting social skills deficits with behavioral methods before turning to cognitive analysis and disputation of automatic thoughts and schemas and provides a safe environment to try out socially proactive behavior.

From a behavioral perspective, management of the avoidant pattern is relatively straightforward (Turkat, 1990). Anxiety-management procedures, assertiveness and social skills training through role playing, direct instruction, and modelling are effective in developing confident social behavior. However, graded exposure is the single most effective behavioral intervention strategy for extinguishing avoidant behavior and anxiety intolerance (Greist & Jefferson, 1992).

Paradoxical intention may also prove useful, particularly with avoidant patients who are also oppositional. With this strategy, the patient seeks rejection in a way that is both predictable, and under the patient's control. For instance, a single male with a fear of dating agrees to an experiment requiring that he be rejected for dates by two women in the coming week. If one of the women approached accepted his offer, he could go out with her, on the condition that he had asked out an additional woman who rejected him. In other words, being rejected becomes a treatment goal. This intervention reduces rejection sensitivity. Use of such a paradoxical intervention may work with the appositionally avoidant patient by accentuating the patient's need to defeat the clinician by doing the opposite of what is suggested or prescribed (Weeks and L'Abate, 1982; Haley, 1978).

Regarding treatment involving comorbid Avoidant Personality Disorder and Social Phobia, Brown, et al. (1997) found that individuals with both generalized and nongeneralized social phobia treated with cognitive behavior therapy improved similarly to those with the more generalized form of social phobia but remained more impaired after treatment. Curiously, the presence of Avoidant Personality Disorder was not predictive of treatment outcome, however, several individuals who met criteria for this diagnosis before treatment, no longer met criteria after treatment. Similarly, Osterbaan et al. (2002) found that individuals with social phobia and comorbid Avoidant Personality Disorder had a poorer response to treatment and remained more impaired in the short term compared to those with the comorbidity. Nevertheless, after 15 months, those with comorbid Avoidant Personality Disorder showed similar progress in the long term.

Schema Therapy. Schema Therapy is an elaboration of cognitive therapy that has been developed by Young (Young, Klosko, & Weishaar, 2003) specifically for personality disorders, and other difficult individual and couples problems. Schema Therapy involves identifying maladaptive schemas and planning specific strategies and interventions. Four main strategies are cognitive, experiential, behavioral and the therapeutic relationship itself. Cognitive restructuring, modification of maladaptive schemas, is an important cognitive strategy, but is combined with imagery exercises, empathic confrontation, homework assignments and "limited reparenting," i.e., a form of corrective emotional experience (Young et al., 2003).

Maladaptive schemas typically associated with Avoidant Personality Disorder include: *defectiveness*: i.e., the belief that one is defective, bad, unwanted, or inferior in important respects; *social Isolation*, i.e., the belief that one is alienated, different from others, or not part of any group; *self-sacrifice*, i.e., the belief that one must meet the needs of others at the expense of one's own gratification; and *approval-seeking*, i.e., the belief that one must constantly seek to belong and be accepted at the expense of developing a true sense of self (Bernstein, 2002).

Interpersonal Approach

For Benjamin (2003), psychotherapeutic interventions with Avoidant Personality Disordered individuals can be planned and evaluated in terms of whether they enhance collaboration, facilitate learning about maladaptive patterns and their roots, block these patterns, enhance the will to change, and effectively encourage new patterns.

Fortunately, avoidant individuals already know how to relate to a select few individuals and thus a supportive therapist can easily provide a safe haven for them. Avoidant individuals respond favorably to accurate empathy and warm support. Gradually, as they share intimacies and feelings of inadequacy, guilt, or shame, they begin to increase self-acceptance. Only then can they realistically begin exploring maladaptive patterns. Since they are exquisitely sensitive to criticism, premature confrontation must be avoided.

General reconstructive changes will occur only if these individuals understand and appreciate the impact of their maladaptive patterns in a way that helps them decide to change. Benjamin advocates couples therapy for avoidant individuals in marriages of long term relationships. Typically, these relationships are characterized by intimacy that assures interpersonal distance and safety for the avoidant partner. Such a pattern of hiding on the margins of relationships is often rooted in unconscious loyalty to the family mandate that avoidant individual remain isolated and safe. In couple's therapy, the clinician would block attempts of partners to humiliate or thrash each other which previously justified what avoidant individual's withdrawal. The most difficult therapeutic task for avoidant individuals is deciding to sacrifice the benefits of their maladaptive patterns and accept the risk of developing new ones. Insight into their humiliation and loyalty to abusive parents or siblings is insufficient. However, Benjamin believes that steady reassurance in a context of competent, protective instruction fosters this change.

Fiore, Dimaggio, Nicolo, Semerari, & Carcione (2008) reported a case study using Metacognitive Interpersonal therapy to treat a 48-year-old male computer manager with obsessive-compulsive personality disorder and avoidant personality disorder. He completed both individual and group therapy to accomplish goals of modulating perfectionism, reducing avoidance behaviors, and acknowledging suppressed desires. Following one year of treatment, this individual no longer met the full criteria for any personality disorder. Gilbert and Gordon (2012) likewise reported the case of a 24-year-old female graduate student being treated with interpersonal therapy for avoidant personality disorder and depression. Following two years of twice-monthly IPT and skills training (a total of 44 sessions), the participant experienced improvements in the areas of self-confidence, somatic complaints, worry, anxiety, and depression.

Group Therapy

Avoidant Personality Disordered patients typically fear group therapy in the same way they fear other new and socially demanding situations. It is for this very reason that group therapy may be specifically and especially effective for the avoidant patients who can be persuaded, and role induced to undertake the exposure (Yalom, 1975). Empathetic group therapy can assist these individuals in overcoming social anxieties and developing interpersonal trust and rapport. Group therapy presents avoidant individuals an opportunity to belong and feel wanted, which challenges their previously held negative beliefs about themselves(Ogrodniczuk, Uliaszek, Lebow, & Kealy, 2021).

Other group members may provide positive feedback about behavior in group that counteracts the avoidant individual's self-image, and the therapist can reinforce this feedback in individual therapy (Fiore, Dimaggio, Nicolo, Semerari, & Carcione, 2008). Benjamin (2003) maintains that safe group therapy, in which the therapist blocks negative or abusive behavior ("trashing") from other members, can have enormous benefits in the areas of self-acceptance and social skills development.

A combination of cognitive therapy and social skills training appear effective. Alden (1989) included aspects of cognitive therapy in the group process. These were: 1) identifying underlying fears; 2) increasing awareness of the anxiety related to fears; and 3) shifting attentional focus from fear related thinking to behavioral action. Didactic information, modeling and the practice of role-playing were basic techniques incorporated into the sessions. Stravynski Grey and Elie (1987) found that a briefer course of group therapy centered on social skills training can be highly effective in ameliorating social skills deficits that exacerbate anxiety about social relatedness.

This type of individual tends to avoid activities that involve significant interpersonal contact for fear of being exposed or ridiculed. Therefore, it takes them longer to adapt to a group-setting and begin to actively participate in treatment. The group therapist's role in pacing the avoidant patient's disclosure and engagement within the group can be very important (Cramer & Azima, 1983). Rennenberg found clients with this disorder so extremely anxious and avoidant that processing directly to social skills training and behavioral rehearsal was unproductive. Stravinsky et al. (1987) suggests beginning with progressive relaxation training and systematic desensitization. Behavioral reversal was used in the group for exposure, itself an effective treatment for social phobia (Stravinsky, Marks, & Yule, 1982). Turner used communication and social skills training during behavioral rehearsal as well.

Structured activities will help the avoidant individuals organize how they think and act so they are more efficient in therapy. Alden (1989) established specific goals for patients to accomplish between sessions in order to enhance generalization from treatment sessions to daily life. The patients selected several social tasks to try, beginning with easier situations and progressing to more difficult ones. In the group setting, she also introduced interpersonal skills training. The process of friendship formation was presented, and clients were encouraged to incorporate these skills into their weekly social tasks. Four sets of behavioral skills that facilitate relating to others were described, modeled by therapists, and discussed and practiced by group members. They included listening/attending skills, empathic sensitivity, appropriate self-disclosure, and respectful assertiveness.

Rennenberg et al. (1990) found that treatment gains through group intervention were stable over one year, however, most patients continued with individual therapy after completing group treatment. It is quite possible that the continued therapy served to reinforce and maintain gains made during the group treatment program. Clinically important changes were reported by patients themselves or their individual therapists. Treated subjects reported decreases in their social reticence, less interference as a result of social anxiety at work and in social situations, fewer symptoms of social anxiety, and greater satisfaction with social activities (Alden, 1989). Wilberg, Karterud, Urnes, Pederson, & Friis (1999) measured the effectiveness of cognitive behavioral therapy groups for individuals with personality disorders, most of whom were classified as avoidant. They found significant improvements for those who participated in the groups compared to those who did not. Harper (2004) found that avoidant individuals who completed a ten-week behavioral group program showed greater improvement in a number of areas than did the control group.

Marital and Family Therapy

Although avoidant individuals need to recognize how their current dysfunctional patterns were developed, they need to focus on their current interpersonal experiences with significant others in their life. As Avoidant Personality Disorders generally provide clinicians with vague descriptions of their interpersonal experiences, others may be helpful in filling in the important gaps of information. Couple and family treatments may be indicated in order to establish a family structure that allows more room for interpersonal exploration outside the tightly closed family circle (Gurman & Kniskern, 1991). Benjamin (2003) advocates couples therapy for avoidant individuals in marriages or long term relationships as typically these are characterized by intimacy that assures interpersonal distance and safety for the avoidant partner. She also notes that those with avoidant personality disorder may likely feel disloyal discussing any humiliation or abuses experienced in the family of origin, which may create an obstacle to family participation in therapy. If they do agree to participate, family members may make matters worse by mocking the therapist, the treatment, or the individual's desire for change (Ogrodniczuk, Uliaszek, Lebow, & Kealy, 2021).

Medication

Currently, there are no psychotropic medications specifically indicated for treating the Avoidant Personality Disorder (Silk & Feurino, 2012). Nevertheless, medications are used that target specific troubling symptoms associated with the disorder, such as depression, anxiety, or sleep problems. Generally, these medications are used as an adjunct to psychotherapy and skills training (Nelson & Tsheringld, 2021).

Because troubling symptoms often respond to medications sooner than most psychological interventions, medications are usually prescribed at the onset of treatment. Unfortunately, there is little research evidence to provide guidelines for the use of such medications. However, because of the comorbidity of this disorder to Social Anxiety Disorder, it was speculated that this personality disorder might respond well to medications with anxiety reducing effects such as selective serotonergic reuptake inhibitors (SSRIs). There is now evidence from a randomized controlled trial that individuals with avoidant personality disorder do respond to low doses of sertraline (Zoloft), an SSRI medication (Silk & Feurino, 2012).

Combined and Integrated Treatment Approach

Clinical experience reveals that many Avoidant Personality Disordered individuals are often unable to focus on the patient-clinician relationship to the extent necessary to work with a purely dynamic therapy. Millon & Davis (2000) suggest an overall poor prognosis for avoidant personality disorder precisely because the problem features of this disorder are the antithesis of what makes psychotherapy successful, such as an open, trusting relationship. Similarly, many have difficulty fully utilizing cognitive-behavioral interventions in the interpersonal context of therapy. Thus, an integrative treatment strategy may be required. Alden (1992) describes an integration of the cognitive and the psychodynamic-interpersonal approaches. The cognitive is, of course, based on Beck and Freeman (1990) and the psychodynamic-interpersonal is based on the Time-Limited Dynamic Psychotherapy approach developed by Strupp and Binder (1984).

The cognitive-interpersonal patterns that characterize the avoidant personality are dysfunctional beliefs of being different or biologically defective as well as beliefs that these defects and feelings are visible to others who will react with disgust, disapproval, or dismissal. These individuals tend to protect themselves by looking to the clinician to provide direction and by understating or even withholding feelings and reactions of what they fear the clinician will disapprove. Thus, the clinician's primary task is to work collaboratively with the patient to modify their cognitive-interpersonal style. Alden (1992) describes four steps in the integrative approach. The first step is recognition of treatment process issues. The clinician must quickly recognize that these patients tend to withhold or understate information that is clinically relevant. Clinicians should expect these patients to respond to direct questions with "I'm not sure" or "I don't know." Such evasive and avoidant responses characterizes the thought process and prevent these patients from encoding details about social encounters.

Unfortunately, clinicians may find themselves interpreting "resistance" or focusing on global and vague interpersonal beliefs and behavior as treatment targets. In either instance, both clinician and patient will experience discouragement and treatment outcomes will be limited. Furthermore, clinicians must recognize the avoidant patient's infectious "hopelessness" and depression, owing largely to their inability to process positive information, lack of attentiveness, and their firmly established negative beliefs and schemas.

The second step is increased awareness of cognitive-interpersonal patterns. Patients need to be encouraged to observe their interpersonal encounters outside sessions by means of self-monitoring and diary-keeping. Alden notes four components of the interpersonal pattern: their beliefs and expectancy of the other person; the behavior that arises from these beliefs; the other's reaction to them; and the conclusion they draw from the experience. As this process of self-observation and analysis proceeds, these patients come to realize their mutual understanding of their interpersonal problem is incomplete and a common pattern emerges. The clinician's role is to draw attention to the beliefs that underlie self-perception that leads to self-protective behaviors.

Step three focuses on alternative strategies. As patients recognize and understand these cognitive-interpersonal pattern and style, the clinician can increase their motivation to try new behavior by helping them recognize that old and new views of self are in conflict, and that this conflict can be reconciled. Helping patients integrate their current beliefs with their earlier interpersonal experiences helps them understand that their social fears and expectations resulted in part from their temperament and parenting. As the patient continues to identify and understand their cognitive-interpersonal patterns they begin to try new strategies, either on their own or at the clinician's prompting.

Step four involves behavioral experimentation and cognitive evaluation. These therapeutic strategies are discussed in detail by Beck and Freeman (1990) to which the reader is referred. Friendship formation and assertive communication are the two basic interpersonal skills that avoidant patients must increase. Role playing and directed assignments are particularly useful in this regard. I've found that the section of Zimbardo's (1977) social skills has been extremely useful as a handout for avoidant patients. Patients are gently guided through exercises to develop assertive communication skills. As a matter of fact, the entire book is an invaluable adjunct in the treatment of the avoidant personality.

Combined Treatment Approach

The basic premise of this book is that a single treatment modality like psychotherapy may well be effective for the highest functioning personality-disordered individual, but less effective for moderate functioning, and largely ineffective for more severely dysfunctional individuals. These lower functioning patients tend to be more responsive to combined treatment modalities. Combined modalities include integrative psychotherapeutic intervention with medication and/or group treatment such as group therapy or support groups. As noted in the section on group treatments, avoidant patients have considerable difficulty with any kind of group. Ideally, lower functioning avoidant patients should be involved in both individual and group therapy concurrently. When this is not possible, time-limited skill-oriented group training sessions or a support group may be sufficient. Aware that their pattern of avoidance and social inhibition makes entry into and continuation with therapeutic groups distressing individual sessions should be focused on transitioning the patient into the group. Medication is often necessary in the early stages of treatment and can be particularly useful in reducing distress and self-protective behavior during the transition into concurrent group treatment (Winkeller & Schlesinger, 2021).

The co-occurrence between personality disorders and substance use disorders is very common, with some estimating that a personality disorder is present in 90 percent of those being treated for polyvalent addiction (Rentrop, Zilker, Lederle, Birkhofer, & Horz, 2014). Dimaggio, D'Urzo, Pasinetti, Salvatoe, Lysaker, Catania, & Popolo (2015) conducted a case study of a 43-year-old male musician with comorbid avoidant personality disorder and substance use disorder (heroin). Treatment progressed according to stages, as follows: drug therapy to manage the symptoms of abstinence from heroin; form a therapeutic bond; foster awareness of emotions and triggers; exploring maladaptive interpersonal schemas; understanding the link between interpersonal events and substance use; acquiring distance from maladaptive schemas; and using adaptive coping skills instead of resorting to substance use.

To overcome the difficulty of treating those with antisocial personality as a result of their social, emotional, and cognitive avoidance, some novel treatments have been explored. Eikenaes, Gude and Hoffart (2006) reported on a quasi-experimental study integrating traditional inpatient treatment with a wilderness program, with positive results.

Chapter 6

Borderline Personality Disorder

Individuals with borderline personality tend to lack a sense of self as a result of which they experience fears of abandonment and feelings of emptiness. They are also likely to experience intense but unstable relationships, emotional instability, outbursts of anger and violence, and impulsivity. Suicidal threats and acts of self-harm are also common (Skodol, Bender, & Oldham, 2019; American Psychiatric Association, 2022).

Of all the personality disorders, the Borderline Personality Disorder is of most concern for clinicians. Specifically, many clinicians believe that this disorder is untreatable, and this belief persists despite research evidence to the contrary. In fact, more research has been published on this disorder than any other personality disorder, and increasingly it indicates that this disorder is quite treatable. For example, Zanarini and colleagues (Zanarini, Frankenburg, Reich, & Fitzmaurice, 2010) followed nearly 300 individuals prospectively over a ten-year period. They found that one half these individuals achieved total recovery. That meant that they no longer met diagnostic criteria for this disorder and also attained reasonable social and occupational functioning. The good news of this important prospective study is that for individuals with this disorder, treatment can be quite successful.

This chapter describes a framework for the assessment and effective treatment of this disorder. It includes sections on diagnosis, psychological assessment, case conceptualization, and treatment interventions. It begins with background information on the disorder as well as a DSM-5-TR description, prototypic description, associated features, and the Alternative Model of Personality Disorders description of this disorder. The section on case conceptualization provides five common clinical formulations of this disorder: psychodynamic, biosocial, cognitive-behavioral, interpersonal, and an integrative conceptualization of this disorder. Several treatment approaches, modalities, and intervention strategies are also described. These include individual psychotherapy, group therapy, marital and family therapy, medication, and integrative and combined treatment.

Description of the Borderline Personality Disorder

The Borderline Personality Disorder can be recognized by the following descriptors and characteristics: styles vs. disorders, triggering event, behavioral styles, interpersonal styles, cognitive styles, affective styles, attachment style, and optimal criterion.

Style vs. Disorder. The borderline personality can be thought of as spanning a continuum from healthy to pathological, wherein the borderline personality style is on the healthy end, and the Borderline Personality Disorder is on the pathological end. Table 6.1 compares and contrasts the antisocial personality style and disorder.

DOI: 10.4324/9781032617930-6

Table 6.1 Comparison of the Borderline Personality Style And Disorder

Personality Style	Personality Disorder
Maintenance of stable interpersonal relationships in which negative and positive perceptions of another are integrated rather than polarized	Pattern of intense and unstable relationships marked by alternating between devaluation and overidealization
Low levels of impulsivity that fall within the normal range of culturally approved indulgence and do not cause devastation to self or others	Impulsive behavior that can be self-damaging, such as spending, sex, substance abuse, shoplifting, reckless driving, or binge eating
Affective stability with tolerable levels of negative emotions	Affective instability marked shifts from baseline mood to depression, irritability or anxiety usually lasting a few hours and only rarely more than a few days
Ability to manage and diffuse anger in ways appropriate to the context in which they occur	Inappropriate and intense anger or lack of control of anger, e.g., frequent displays of temper, constant anger, recurrent physical fights
Sense of connection to self, body and place in the world	Persistent feelings of boredom or emptiness
Possessing an accurate sense of self that is consistent over time without being overly inflexible or overly malleable	Marked and persistent identity disturbance with uncertainty about at least two of the following: self-image, sexual orientation, long term goals or career choice, type of friends desired, preferred values
Ability to tolerate and manage experiences of loss; capacity to realistically assess abandonment/loss	Frantic efforts to avoid imagined or actual experiences of abandonment.
Absence of suicidal behavior, gestures and threats (excludes suicidal ideation) Absence of self-mutilating behavior	Repeated suicidal gestures, behavior, threats, or self-mutilating behavior
Capacity to manage stressful situations and stay cognitively and physically present	Brief, stress-related paranoid ideation or severe dissociative symptoms

The following case examples further illustrate the differences between the Borderline Personality Disorder—Mr. J—and the borderline personality style—Ms. B.

Case Study: Borderline Personality Disorder

Mr. J is a 31-year-old unemployed male who was referred to the hospital emergency room by his therapist at a community mental health center after two days of sustained suicidal gestures. He appeared to function adequately until his senior year in high school, when he became preoccupied with Transcendental Meditation. He had considerable difficulty concentrating during his first semester of college and seemed to focus most of his energies on finding a spiritual guru. At times, massive anxiety and feelings of emptiness swept over him, which he found would suddenly vanish if he lightly cut his wrist enough to draw blood. He had been in treatment with his current therapist for 18 months and became increasingly hostile and demanding as a patient, whereas earlier he had been quite captivated with his therapist's empathy and intuitive sense. Lately, his life seemed to center on these twice- weekly therapy sessions. Mr. J's most recent suicidal thoughts followed the therapist's disclosure that he was moving out of the area.

Case Study: Borderline Personality Style

Janice P is a 29 year old graduate student in Oriental Literature. She had completed her undergraduate degree at the university in business and management with honors and had planned on starting her M.B.A. that fall. A summer tour of Japan and China dramatically changed her life. She fell in love with the Orient: the people, the food, the customs, the ambiance, but especially a literature professor at a Tokyo university she met. She feel madly in love with him the first time at a change meeting, and spent the next two weeks before her flight back to the states totally engrossed with is poetry, his stories and his life. Although he was married, his wife was on a holiday alone. Janice was conflicted about returning home even though he broke off the relationship and entreated him to leave his wife. Ms. B. was crushed that he would not. Nevertheless, she returned to the university with an ardent desire to immerse herself in the study of oriental literature. Because fantasies of returning to Tokyo as a visiting professor and working alongside the love of her life, with he goal of eventually having him all to herself. Yet, even though she was doing well in her classes she occasionally got in touch with the anger and hurt she had experienced that summer. Midway in her first semester in grad school she met a stunning oriental graduate student whom she instantly fell in love with.

Triggering Event. The typical situation, circumstance or event that most likely triggers or activates the characteristic maladaptive response of the Borderline Personality Disorder Personality Disorder (Othmer & Othmer, 2002), as noted in behavioral, interpersonal, cognitive, and feeling styles, is: "frantic efforts to avoid real or imagined abandonment."

Behavioral Style. Behaviorally, borderlines are characterized by physically self-damaging acts such as suicide gestures, self-mutilation, or the provocation of fights. Their social and occupational accomplishments are often less than their intelligence and ability warrant. Of all the personality disorders, they are more likely to have irregularities of circadian rhythms, especially of the sleep–wake cycle. Thus, chronic insomnia is a common complaint.

Interpersonal Style. Interpersonally, borderlines are characterized by their paradoxical instability. That is, they fluctuate quickly between idealizing and clinging to another individual to devaluing and opposing that individual. They are exquisitely rejection-sensitive, and experience abandonment depression following the slightest of stressors. Millon and Davis (1996) consider separation anxiety as a primary motivator of this personality disorder. Interpersonal relationships develop rather quickly and intensely, yet their social adaptiveness is rather superficial. They are extraordinarily intolerant of being alone and they go to great lengths to seek out the company of others whether in indiscriminate sexual affairs, late night phone calls to relatives and recent acquaintances, or late night visits to hospital emergency rooms with a host of vague medical and/or psychiatric complaints.

Cognitive Style. Their cognitive style is described as inflexible and impulsive (Millon, 1981). Inflexibility of their style is characterized by rigid abstractions that easily lead to grandiose, idealized perceptions of others, not as real people, but as personifications of "all good" or "all bad" individuals. They reason by analogy from past experience and thus have difficulty reasoning logically and learning from past experiences and relationships. Because they have an external locus of control, the borderlines usually blame others when things go wrong. By accepting responsibility for their own incompetence, borderlines believe they would feel even more powerless to change circumstances. Accordingly, their emotions fluctuate between hope and despair because they believe that external circumstances are well beyond their control (Shulman, 1982). Their cognitive style is also marked by impulsivity, and just as they vacillate between idealization and devaluation of others, their thoughts shift from one extreme to another: "I like people, no I don't like them"; "Having goals is good, no it's not"; "I need to get my life together, no I can't, it's hopeless." This inflexibility and impulsivity complicate the process of identity formation. Their uncertainty about self-image, gender identity, goals, values, and career choice reflects this impulsive and flexible stance. Gerald Adler (1985) suggested that borderlines have an underdeveloped evocative memory, such that they have difficulty recalling images and feeling states which could structure and soothe them in times of turmoil. Their inflexibility and impulsivity are further noted in their tendency toward "splitting." Splitting is the inability to synthesize contradictory qualities, such that the individual views others as all good or all bad and utilizes "projective identification," that is attributing his or her own negative or dangerous feelings to others. Their cognitive style is further characterized by an inability to tolerate frustration. Finally, micropsychotic episodes can be noted when these individuals are under a great deal of stress. These are ill-defined, strange thought processes especially noted in response to unstructured rather than structured situations and may take the form of derealization, depersonalization, intense rage reactions, unusual reactions to drugs, and intense brief paranoid episodes. Because of difficulty in focusing attention and subsequent loss of relevant data, borderlines also have a diminished capacity to process information.

Affective Style. The emotional style of individuals with this disorder is characterized by marked mood shifts from a normal or euthymic mood to a dysphoric mood. In addition, inappropriate and intense anger and rage may easily be triggered. On the other extreme are feelings of emptiness, a deep "void," or boredom.

Attachment Style. Individuals with a vacillating views of both self and others exhibit the disorganized attachment style. "Disorganized attachment develops from repeated experiences in which the caregiver appears frightened or frightening to the child" (Siegel, 1999, p. 117). This style is associated with dissociative symptomatology which increases their proneness to posttraumatic stress disorder. The Borderline Personality Disorder is characterized by unstable personality structure that seems to shift among the various insecure attachment styles creating a disorganized profile, called the Disorganized Attachment Style (Lyddon & Sherry, 2001).

Optimal Diagnostic Criterion. Of all the criteria for the Borderline Personality Disorder, one has been found to be the most useful in its diagnosis. The belief is that by beginning with this criterion, the clinician can test for the presence or absence of the criterion and quickly diagnose this disorder. The optimal criterion for this disorder is: frantic efforts to avoid real or imagined abandonment (Allnutt & Links, 1996)

Childhood Abuse and Etiology. There is increasing research evidence that a history of early abuse or neglect is common in adults with personality disorders, particularly Borderline Personality Disorder (Herman, Perry, & van der Kolk, 1989; Zanarini et al., 2000; Bernstein (2002) indicates that childhood histories of *severe* emotional abuse is noted in adults diagnosed with Borderline Personality Disorders. Data on sexual abuse among individuals with this disorder are troubling, in that the odds of such an individual attempting suicide in adulthood is over ten times that of those who were never sexually abused (Soloff, Lynch, & Kelly, 2002).

Many clinicians have come to assume that this disorders is cause by such childhood abuse. Research largely supports this presumption. Nevertheless, it does not suggests that abuse is the primary causes of all cases of Borderline Personality Disorder. But exactly how prevalent is such trauma in those presenting for treatment? A recent meta-analytics study (Fossatti, Madeddu, & Maffei, 1999), indicate that in individuals diagnosed with Borderline Personality Disorder the prevalence rates of abuse are in the range of 60–80 percent. This means that 20–40 percent of these individuals do *not* report such histories. Presumably, such individuals are more likely to be the so called "higher functioning" borderlines. In other words, while there are traumatic pathways in the development of personality disorders, there are also non-traumatic pathways. An important treatment implication is that such clients, who were not traumatized but rather may have been otherwise wounded as children in their efforts to meet emotional needs, may be responsive to a broader range of therapeutic interventions than more focused approaches such as Dialectical Behavior Therapy. These other interventions might include exploratory, uncovering, and abreactive interventions which are less likely to be regressive or iatrogenic than they would be with clients with trauma histories (Graybar & Boutilier, 2002).

DSM-5-TR Description

Individuals with this personality disorder are characterized by an unremitting pattern of unstable relationships, emotional reactions, identity, and impulsivity. They engage in frantic efforts to avoid abandonment, whether it is real or imagined. Their interpersonal relationships are intense, unstable, and alternate between the extremes of idealization and devaluation. They have chronic identity issues and an unstable sense of self. Their impulsivity can result in self-damaging actions such as reckless driving or drug use, binge eating, or high-risk sex. These individuals engage in recurrent suicidal threats, gestures, acting out or self-mutilating behavior. They can exhibit markedly reactive moods, chronic feelings of emptiness, emotional outbursts, and difficulty controlling their anger. They may also experience brief, stress-related paranoid thinking or severe episodes of dissociation (American Psychiatric Association, 2022).

Prototypic Description

These individuals have intense and frustrating relationships which begin with high hopes but predictably degenerate into conflict and disappointments. Because they are terrified of being abandoned, they drive others away with unrealistic demands, relentless anger, and self-fulfilling expectations of abandonment. Real or imagined losses can lead to suicide attempts or self-mutilation. The result is repeated destructive relationships and a fragile sense of self. They may engage in impulsive sexual and aggressive behaviors. Suicide rates are high for such individuals. However, those who survive may find some sense of balance and serenity in midlife (Francis, 2013).

Associated Features

Prevalence. BPD has been identified in 2.7 percent of the general population. with about 6 percent in primary care settings, about 10 percent in outpatient mental health clinics, and 20 percent in psychiatric inpatient settings (American Psychiatric Association, 2022).

Differential Diagnosis. Impulsive and antisocial behaviors in those with BPD are associated with increased risk for suicide. Nevertheless, while recurrent suicidal behavior is a defining feature of the disorder, a ten-year study found that suicide attempts declined from 79 percent to 13 percent over time. Depressive or bipolar disorders commonly co-occur with BPD. Accordingly, if criteria are met, it is essential that both disorders should be diagnosed and treated (American Psychiatric Association, 2022).

Development and Course. BPD has been diagnosed in 12- and 13-year-old adolescences, but adult onset is more common. While BPD was considered to have a poor symptomatic course, studies show that stable remissions of between one and eight years are common. Impulsivity lessens, while emotional reactivity does not, without effective therapy. Lack of recovery is related to receiving disability benefits and experiencing poor physical health (American Psychiatric Association, 2022).

Culture, Sex, and Gender. The BPD pattern has been identified across cultures. Varying social contexts and demands can foster specific borderline features or be confused with BPD. Accordingly, a valid diagnosis of BPD must be evaluated in light of cultural norms. While community studies find the rate of BPD is the same in men and women, BPD is more common in women in clinical settings, presumably because of a higher degree of help-seeking (American Psychiatric Association, 2022).

Alternative Model of Borderline Personality Disorder

The Alternative Model of Personality Disorders (AMPD) offers a clinically useful description of the Borderline Personality Disorder in terms of typical features and trait facets. Typical features are instability of self-image, personal goals, interpersonal relationships, and affects, accompanied by impulsivity, risk taking, and/or hostility Trait facet criteria include Emotional lability, Anxiousness, Separation insecurity, Depressivity, Impulsivity, Risk taking, and Hostility. Four or more are required including at least one of following: Impulsivity, Risk Taking, or Hostility (American Psychiatric Association, 2022).

Conceptualizations of the Borderline Personality Disorder

Psychodynamic Case Conceptualization

Kernberg (1975) targets the rapprochement sub-phase of Mahler's separation-individuation developmental theory as the point of fixation for borderline pathology. At the phase children lacks object constancy and thus cannot integrate the good an bad and aspects of themselves or their mothers. Neither can they separate from the mother since they have yet to internalize a whole, soothing internalized usage of her that sustain them during her physical absence. Kernberg points out that a disturbance in the mother's emotional availability during the rapprochement sub-phase can result in an excess of aggression in the child, maternal problems with parenting, or both.

Masterson (1976) and Masterson and Klein (1990) implicate the rapprochement sub-phase but emphasize the mother's behavior rather than the child's aggression. Typically a borderline herself the mother is deeply conflicted about their children growing up and becoming their own person. Thus, these children receives the message that if they grow up something awful will happen to them and/or to their mothers, and that remaining dependent is the only way of maintaining the maternal bond. This prospect of separation and individuation thus provokes "abandonment depression" in borderlines. No integration between a rewarding object unit and a withdrawing object unit is possible at this rapprochement sub-phase accounting for the symptom of the borderline syndrome.

Adler's (1985) understanding of borderline pathology is influenced by Kohut (1971, 1977) and Fraiberg (1969) and is based on a deficit rather than a conflict model as with Kernberg. Inconsistency in maternal behavior and availability results in the borderline's failure to develop a "holding-nothing" internalized object. This accounts for feelings of emptiness, depressive tendencies, and oral rage. Furthermore, the borderline individual has difficulty summoning up internal images of the natural nurturing figure in stressful situations. This cognitive deficit of evocative memory suggests a regression to developmental age between eight and 18 months. These inadequate resources leave the borderline prone to fragmentation of the self which is accompanied by profound emptiness called "annihilation panic."

Mentalization Approach. Bateman & Fonagy's (2007) mentalization approach to Borderline Personality Disorder is rooted in object relations and attachment theory. Sometimes referred to as "mentalizing," this is the process by which individuals interpret their own subjective cognitions, behaviors, and emotions, as well as those of others. The ability to mentalize is believed to arise as a function of childhood development by age four. Rather than an automatic consequence of maturation, it is dependent on the quality of an individual's early object relationships. Interactions with the primary caregiver, usually the mother, act as the foundation from which individuals make sense of their mental states and interpersonal interactions. To fully develop this capacity, infants must have a stable, affectionate, safe, and attentive adult to mirror their experiences. Bateman & Fonagy suggest that those with borderline personality lack the ability to interpret mental states and accurately understand their relationships, as a result of psychological trauma in early or late childhood. Neglect, abuse, and incongruent emotional mirroring all lead to insecure/hypersensitive attachments and poor self-regulation.

Transference-Focused Psychotherapy Approach. Clarkin, Yeomans, & Kernberg (2015) subscribe to a similar etiology for Borderline Personality Disorder in their approach, called Transference-Focused Psychotherapy (TFP). Grounded in object relations theory, Clarkin et al. theorize that the specific symptoms of BPD result from a lack of identity integration and incoherence between an individual's experience and understanding of self and others. This unintegrated psychological state is called identity diffusion. Those with Borderline Personality Disorder rely on defensive strategies that distort reality, such as dissociation and splitting. The result of these cognitive distortions is that negative or aggressive affects are not seen as coming from within but from outside the self, leading to feelings of helplessness, anger, and insecurity. Transference-Focused Psychotherapy conceptualizes psychological structure as the product of early interactions with caregivers, which are internalized as the individual develops. In the case of BPD, this process is interrupted by traumatic and/or inconsistent relationships with caregivers. The absence of an integrated self leads to chronic distress and feelings of emptiness for which borderline individuals impulsively act out in an attempt to relieve their discomfort.

Biosocial Case Conceptualization

Millon and Davis (1996) views the borderline's lack of a clear, coherent sense of identity as central to the pathogenesis of this disorder. He believes that identity confusion and/or diffusion is the result of biopsychosocial factors that combine to impair a coherent sense of identity. Because of this central deficit, poor coordinated actions, over-modulated affects, poorly controlled impulses and a failure of consistent effort result. Thus, the borderline individual dependents on others for protection and reassurance, and are hypersensitive to loss or separation of these supports. Based on this research, Millon (1981) and Millon and Everly (1985) contend that the borderline syndrome is essentially more severe and regressed variants of the dependent, histrionic or passive aggressive personality disorders. They describe three subtypes of this disorder.

Borderline-dependent individuals tend to exhibit a passive infantile pattern and possess family histories of low energy levels. This pattern evokes parental warmth and overprotection, and they subsequently form strong attachments and dependency to a single caregiver, which ultimately restricts their opportunity to learn the necessary skills of social independence and self-efficacy. This sets the stage for rejection by those on whom they have come to rely.

Borderline-histrionic individuals more often possess family histories characterized by high autonomic reactivity, and they exhibit hyperresponsiveness as a result of exposure to high levels of stimulation. Parental control tends to be exercised by contingent reinforcement patterns for which these children feel competent and accepted only if their behavior is explicitly approved by others, and thus they "perform" to secure support, attention, and nurturance.

Borderline-passive aggressive individuals tend to have exhibited "difficult child" (Thomas & Chess, 1977) temperaments. As irritable, difficult to soothe infants they likely received inconsistent responses from their caregivers, caring at times, harried and frustrated at others, and even withdraw. They might have been products of broken homes, and likely had a parent who modelled the erratic, vacillating, passive-aggressive behavior they display as adults.

Cognitive-Behavioral Case Conceptualization

Three common cognitive behavioral case conceptualizations have been described. They are Cognitive Therapy, Schema Therapy, and Dialectical Behavior Therapy.

Cognitive Therapy. According to Beck (1990, 2015) three basic assumptions are noted in those with this personality disorders: "I am powerless and vulnerable"; "I am inherently unacceptable" and "the world is dangerous and malevolent"(Pretzer, 1990; Arntz, 2015). Because of their inherent belief they are helpless in a hostile world without a source of security they vacillate between autonomy and dependence with being able to rely on either. In addition, borderlines tend to display "dichotomous thinking", the tendency to evaluate experiences in mutual exclusive categories, all good or all bad, success or failure, trustworthy or deceitful. The combination of dichotomous thinking and basic assumptions are the basis of borderline emotion and behavior, including acting out, self-destructive behaviors.

Schema Therapy. Young (1990; Young, Klosko, & Weishaar, 2003) describe a schema-focused conceptualization of this disorder. The basic premise is that "early maladaptive schemas" develop during childhood and result in maladaptive behavior patterns which reinforce these schemas. These schemas include the abandonment/loss schema: "I'll be alone forever. No one would live me or want to be close to me if they really got to know me"; and the emotional deprivation schema: "No one is ever there to meet my needs, to be strong for me, to care for me."

Dialectical Behavior Therapy. Linehan (1987; 2013) describes a behavioral conceptualization of this disorder. The basic premise is that inadequate emotional regulation and an invalidating environment predispose an individual to this disorder. In addition, there is an invalidating environment "in which communication of private experience is met by erratic, inappropriate, and extreme responses. In other words, the expression of private experience is not validated; instead, it is often punished, and/or trivialized" (Linehan, 1993a, p. 49). Linehan (1993a) contends that a poor fit between a difficult child and an invalidating environment fosters the development of this disorder. The borderline pattern is believed to be physiologically based and reinforced by experiences with significant others who discount their emotional experiences. Subsequently, borderline individuals develop little or no skill in emotion regulation. In short, the combination of intense emotional responses, inadequate emotional regulation skills, and an invalidating environment predispose an individual to unrelenting crisis for which these individuals are unable to effectively cope.

Interpersonal Case Conceptualization

Structural Analysis of Social Behavior Approach. Benjamin's (1996, 2003a) approach to case conceptualization Structural Analysis of Social Behavior. It posits that individual with Borderline Personality Disorder typically grew up in a family marked by a chaotic, soap-opera lifestyle. Without these dilemmas, life was experienced as hollow, boring, and empty. Whether these chaotic dramas were blatant or sequestered from public view, the borderline-to-be played a central role resulting in the impulsivity, mood instability, and unpredictably characteristic of life without constancy. The developmental histories of these individuals often included traumatic abandonment experiences, the isolation of which was typically marked by physical and/or sexual abuse. This abuse-laden aloneness became inexorably linked with the notion that the borderline-to-be was a bad person. These abuse experiences "taught" the individual to shift from idealization to devaluation. And to the extent that sexual abuse experiences were painful, they set the stage for self-mutilation, as pleasure became confused with pain during such episodes. Family norms dictated that autonomy was bad while dependency and sympathetic misery with the family were good. As such movement toward independence, competence or happiness elicited self-sabotage. Furthermore, young borderline individuals learned from their families that misery, sickness, and debilitation draw forth love and concern from others. The adult consequences is the borderline disordered individuals believe that caregivers and lovers secretly love misery. In short, there is a morbid fear of abandonment and a wish for protective nurturance particularly from a lover or caregiver. Initially, friendly dependency on the nurturer gives way to hostile control when the caregiver or lover fails to deliver enough. Borderline individuals believes that significant others secretly like dependency and neediness and a vicious introject attacks the self in the face of any signs of success or happiness. Treatment based on this model is called Interpersonal Reconstructive Therapy (Benjamin, 2003b; 2007).

Interpersonal Psychotherapy Approach. A related interpersonal conceptualization of this disorder is an adaptation of Interpersonal Psychotherapy which was originally developed for treatment of chronic depression or Dysthymic Disorder, called Persistent Depressive Disorder in DSM-5-TR (Weissman, Markowitz, & Klerman, 2000; 2007). In this adaptation, Borderline Personality Disorder is characterized as a mode-inflected condition similar to chronic depression but punctuated by sporadic, ineffective outburst of anger and impulsivity (Markowitz, Bleiberg, Pessin, & Skodol, 2007).

Integrative Case Conceptualization

The following integrative formulation provides a biopsychosocial explanation for how this personality is likely to have developed and how it is maintained. Biologically, borderlines can be understood in terms of the three main subtypes: borderline-dependent, borderline-histrionic, and borderline-passive aggressive. The temperamental style of the borderline-dependent type is that of the passive infantile pattern (Millon, 1981). Millon hypothesized that low autonomic nervous system reactivity plus an overprotective parenting style facilitates restrictive interpersonal skills and a clinging relational style. On the other hand, the histrionic subtype was more likely to have a hyperresponsive infantile pattern. Thus, because of high autonomic nervous system reactivity and increased parental stimulation and expectations for performance, the borderline-histrionic pattern was likely to result. Finally, the temperamental style of the passive-aggressive borderline was likely to have been the "difficult child" type noted by Thomas and Chess (1977). This pattern plus parental inconsistency marks the affective irritability of the borderline-passive aggressive personality.

Psychologically, borderlines tend to view themselves, others, the world, and life's purpose in terms of the following themes. They view themselves by some variant of the theme: "I don't know who I am or where I'm going." In short, their identity problems involve gender, career, loyalties, and values while their self- esteem fluctuates with each thought or feeling about their self- identity. Borderlines tend to view their world with some variant of the theme: "People are great, no they are not"; "Having goals is good, no it's not"; or, "If life doesn't go my way, I can't tolerate it." As such they are likely to conclude "Therefore keep all options open. Don't commit to anything. Reverse roles and vacillate thinking and feelings when under attack." The five defensive operations utilized by the Borderline Personality Disordered individuals are denial, splitting, primitive idealization, projective identification, omnipotence, and devaluation (Shulman, 1982).

Socially, predictable patterns of parenting and environmental factors can be noted for the Borderline Personality Disorder. Parenting style differs depending on the subtype. For example, in the dependent subtype overprotectiveness characterizes parenting, whereas in the histrionic subtype a demanding parenting style is more evident, while an inconsistent parenting style is more noted in the passive-aggressive subtype. But because the borderline personality is a syndromal elaboration and deterioration of the less severe Dependent, Histrionic, or Passive Aggressive Personality Disorders, the family of origin in the borderline subtypes of these disorders is likely to be much more dysfunctional, increasing the likelihood the child will have learned various self-defeating coping strategies. The parental injunction is likely to have been, "If you grow up and leave me, bad things will happen to me (parent)."

This borderline pattern is confirmed, reinforced, and perpetuated by the following individual and systems factors: Diffuse identity, impulsive vacillation, and self-defeating coping strategies lead to aggressive acting out, which leads to more chaos, which leads to the experience of depersonalization, increased dysphoria, and/or self-mutilation to achieve some relief. This leads to further reconfirmation of their beliefs about self and the world as well as reinforcement of the behavioral and interpersonal patterns (Sperry, 2015).

Table 6.2 summarizes the characteristic features of this disorder.

Table 6.2 Characteristics of Borderline Personality Disorder

Triggering Event(s)	Expectation of meeting personal goals and/or maintaining close relationships
Behavioral Style:	Impulsivity
	Acting out behaviors
	Helpless, empty "void"
Interpersonal Style:	Fear of abandonment
	Unstable, intense relationships
	Alternates between extremes of idealization and devaluation
Cognitive Style:	Inflexible, rigid thinking
	Failure to learn from experience
	External loss of control
Emotional Style:	Emotionally reactive and dysregulated
	Inappropriate, intense anger
	Extreme liability of mood and affect
Attachment Style	Disorganized
Temperament:	*Dependent type:* passive infantile pattern—low autonomic nervous system reactivity
	Histrionic type: hyperresponsive infantile pattern—high autonomic reactivity
	Passive Aggressive type: "difficult" infantile pattern—affect irritability
Parental Injunction:	"If you grow up, bad things will happen to me (parent)."
	Overprotective or demanding or inconsistent parenting
Self-View:	"I don't know who I am or where I'm going." Identity problems involving gender, career, loyalties, and values. Self-esteem fluctuates with current emotion.
World View:	"People are great, no they're not. Having goals is good, no it's not. If life doesn't go my way, I can't tolerate it. Don't commit to anything."
Maladaptive Schemas	Abandonment; Defectiveness; Abuse/Mistrust; Emotional Deprivation; Social Isolation; Insufficient Self-Control
Optimal Criteria	Frantic efforts to avoid real or imagined abandonment

Assessment of Borderline Personality Disorder

Several sources of information are useful in establishing a diagnosis and treatment plan for personality disorders. Observation, collateral information, and psychological testing are important adjuncts to the patient's self-report in the clinical interview. This section briefly describes some characteristic observations that the clinician makes and the nature of the rapport likely to develop in initial encounters with specific personality-disordered individuals. Characteristic response patterns on various objective (i.e., MMPI-2 and MCMI-IV) and projective tests (i.e., Rorschach and TAT) are also described.

Interview Behavior and Rapport. Interviewing Borderline Personality Disordered individuals presents a special challenge because of their instability and ambivalence. Instability or liability is noted in their moods, goals, and rapport with the clinician. Instability regarding rapport is handled by empathically focusing on it. This is done by directing the discussion, keeping the discussion on track, and curbing diversions and outbursts. Asking open ended questions is preferable to seeking precise answers to closed-ended pointed questions (Ackley, Mack, Beyer, & Erdberg, 2011). Instability is also processed by separating it as a pathological part that needs to be explored. Since it also affects rapport, the clinician must continually acknowledge its presence and effect. The result is that these patients become less defensive and more willing to disclose, thus furthering rapport.

Dealing with ambivalence requires confronting their contradictions while at the same time exhibiting and understanding of their ambivalent feelings. Therapeutic confrontation illustrates their splitting and projective identification and moderates overidealized or devaluation. It further helps these individuals realize that their ambivalence results from perceived lack of support and understanding of mother which they allow to profound influence their sense of well-being (Othmer & Othmer, 2002).

Psychological Testing Data The Minnesota Multiphasic Personality Inventory (MMPI-2), the Millon Clinical Multiaxial Inventory (MCMI-IV), the Rorschach Psychodiagnostic Test, and the Thematic Apperception Test (TAT) can be useful in diagnosing the Borderline Personality Disorder as well as the borderline personality style (Groth-Marnat, 2009).

On the MMPI-2 elevations on scales 2 (Depression), 4 (Psychopathic Deviate), 8 (Schizophrenia) are common (Graham, 2011). Scales O (Social Introversion) and K (Correction) tend to be high, F (Frequency) is typically low. If emotional dysregulation—particularly of anger—is prominent, scale 6 (Paranoia) will be high. Although relatively rare, 2–6 (Depression-Paranoia) 6–2 profile is associated with Borderline pathology (Meyers, 1995).

On the MCMI-IV, elevation on scale C (Borderline) is most likely and concurrent elevation on scale 8A (Negativistic—passive aggressive) is also likely (Millon, Millon, Grossman, Boice, & Sinsabaugh, 2016). Elevations on such clinical scales as A (Generalized anxiety disorder), H (Somatic symptom disorder), N (Bipolar I disorder), and/or D (Dysthymia Disorder) can be expected (Choca & Denburg, 1997).

On the Rorschach illogical and confabulated combinations (i.e., "A horse's head with two sea horses growing out of his ears" for Card 10) are common (Singer & Larsen, 1981; Swiercinsky, 1985). Such responses are most likely on cards 10 and 2. The new Rorschach Performance Assessment System (R-PAS) is an improved method for scoring and interpreting the Rorschach

Inkblot Test. Besides being evidence-based and internationally normed, it increases clinical utility and is easier to use than Exner's Comprehensive System (Mihura & Meyer, 2018).

On the TAT, "primitive splitting" may be noted in characters that are judged as all bad, (i.e., devils), in characters wherein only one side of the personality is admitted to or portrayed, or when good-bad characteristics are juxtaposed incongruously. Separation anxiety themes, extreme portrayals of affect, and acting out rather than delayed gratification themes are not uncommon (Bellak, 1997).

Treatment Approaches and Interventions

Treatment Considerations

The Borderline Personality Disorder is one of the more common presentations seen in both the public sector and in private practice. It can be among the most difficult and frustrating conditions to treat. Clinical experience suggests that it is important to assess the individual for overall level of functioning and treatment readiness in making decisions about treatment approaches, modalities, and strategies.

The Borderline Personality Disorder is the most researched of all the personality disorders. To date, several randomized controlled treatment studies have been published. An evaluation of seven controlled trials of DBT concluded that DBT met the criteria for a well-established treatment according to the American Psychological Association's Division 12 Task Force for empirically supported therapies (Lynch, Trost, Salsman, & Linehan, 2007).

Individual Psychotherapy

Many consider individual psychotherapy to be the cornerstone of treatment for the Borderline Personality Disorder. Although these are widely divergent opinions on the appropriateness or efficacy of the various individual psychotherapeutic approaches, there is consensus on some general principles. Waldinger (1986) describes five points of consensus on treating the borderline personality. First, the therapist must be active in identifying, confronting, and directing the patient's behaviors during sessions. Second, a stable treatment environment must be afforded in terms of setting and maintaining limits and boundaries, scheduling, payment of fees, and role expectations of patient and clinician. Third, connection between the patient's actions and feelings on the present need to be established. Fourth, self-destructive behavior must be made ungratifying. And fifth, careful attention must be paid to countertransference feelings.

Regardless of the specific psychotherapeutic approach utilized, the literature indicates that treatment of the borderline patient is difficult, countertransference problems are common, and the results are uneven (Gunderson, 1989). Some borderline patients experience negative therapeutic reaction and others untoward effects of individual psychotherapy. In some instance these patients should not be afforded individual treatment. Francis, Clarkin, and Perry (1984) offer the "no treatment option" and offer specific criteria for its use. Nevertheless, when treatment is indicated, attention to the patient's needs and expectations for treatment and efforts to match and tailor treatment are essential in maximizing treatment outcomes.

This section describes various psychodynamic, cognitive-behavioral, and interpersonal approaches.

Psychodynamic Psychotherapy Approaches

Given the stereotypes of psychoanalysis, many find it surprising that mentalization therapy and transference focused psychotherapy are particularly effective in the treatment of Borderline Personality Disorder. Still, there are other psychodynamically oriented forms of treatment that can also be useful. These include psychoanalytic psychotherapy, supportive psychotherapy, and short-term dynamic psychotherapy (Yeomans, Clarkin, & Levy, 2021). Each of these is described in this section.

Psychoanalytic Psychotherapy. There are basically two psychoanalytic opinions regarding the treatment of the borderline patients based on the role of early interpretation and the management of negative transference. One view is that confrontation must occur early in the course of treatment and that interpretation of primitive transference be made in here-and-now situations. The other view is that the early interpretations of aggressive theme is ineffective and possibly disruptive. Kernberg (1984) and Masterson (1976) among others, espouse the first view, while Chessick (1982) and Buie and Adler (1982) and others advocate the second. Nevertheless, both views agree that personality reconstruction is the goal of treatment, requiring three or more sessions a week for a minimum of four years.

Masterson (1976) and Masterson and Klein (1989) have elegantly described the psychotherapeutic process with borderline patients. Supportive psychotherapy is differentiated from reconstructive psychotherapy. The goal of reconstructive psychotherapy is to work through the abandonment depression—feelings of depression, anger and rage, fear, guilt, passivity and helplessness, emptiness and void that follow a recent experience of separation and loss—associated with the original separation-individuation phase. This leads to the achievement of ego autonomy and the transformation of split object relations into whole object relations and the split ego into a whole ego. Three stages of psychotherapy are noted by Masterson: the testing phase in which confrontation in which the clinician utilizes communicative matching to support the patient's emerging individuation, is the principal technique, the working through phase and the separation phase.

The expected outcome of such treatment is not only reduction in impulsive behavior and other regressive reactions to stressors, but also improved stability in interpersonal relationships. Such personality reconstruction allows the individual to function normally or on a neurotic level (Gunderson, 1989).

Mentalization Based Treatment. Based on the work of Bateman & Fonagy (2007, 2010), Mentalization Based Treatment (MBT) is intended to help borderline patients develop the capacity to accurately identify and respond to the subjective mental states of themselves and others. This includes helping patients maintain a stable sense of self and appropriate level of arousal. The originators of this treatment maintain that MBT is not a unique therapy model, but rather a therapeutic stance intended to achieve a specific goal. As such, MBT permits the use of many different techniques which may be found in other treatments.

Two important aspects of Mentalization Based Treatment are the therapeutic stance and mentalizing the transference between the patient and therapist. The therapeutic stance encompasses a number of factors, including therapist humility derived from "not knowing"; patience in understanding differences in perspective between therapist and patient; validating and accepting different perspectives; actively seeking to understand the patient's experience by asking questions, not searching for explanations; and clarifying when something is unclear.

In this method of treatment, the primary vehicle for change is the relationship between therapist and patient. Bateman and Fonagy do not focus on transference interpretation to increase the patient's insight, as is common in other psychodynamic therapy approaches. They assert that the ability to benefit from interpretation requires a level of mentalizing capacity that borderline patients typically do not possess. Rather, MBT uses the transference relationship to encourage patients to focus their attention on another individual's mind and examine their own perceptions. Mentalizing the transference is accomplished in six steps: validation of the patient's transference with the therapist; exploration of events which generated the transference; accepting enactment on the part of the therapist; collaborating with the patient to develop an interpretation; offering an alternative perspective; and monitoring the patient's reaction to the process. A randomly controlled trial comparing outpatient mentalizing-based treatment and structured clinical management for borderline personality disorder found that borderline patients in the MBT group experienced a steeper reduction in problems such as suicide attempts and hospitalizations (Bateman & Fonagy, 2009).

Transference-Focused Psychotherapy. Clarkin et al. (2015) developed Transference Focused Psychotherapy (TFP) with the goals of improving behavioral control, increasing self-reflection, and cultivating affect regulation skills in borderline patients. This is accomplished through the relationship between the therapist and patient, as in Mentalization Based Treatment. Transference Focused Psychotherapy is a highly structured, manualized, evidence-based approach to the treatment of Borderline Personality Disorder. Therapy sessions are 45-minites long and are held two times a week. During the first year of treatment, the primary goal is to contain parasuicidal behaviors and other forms of self-destructive acting out. The ultimate goal of TFP is identity integration.

Techniques include contracting and limit-setting along with exploring the patient's inner world in the here-and-now transference relationship. The treatment contract is especially important for this type of treatment, as this structure provides a safe context in which the patient's patterns may manifest as gives the therapist a way to explore the meaning behind deviations from the contract. In Transference Focused psychotherapy, interpretation is seen as the means by which integration occurs.

Supportive Psychotherapy. From a dynamic perspective supportive psychotherapy is less intensive and regressive than psychoanalytic psychotherapy or psychoanalysis. The goals of supportive therapy with borderline individuals are principally to improve their adaptation to daily life and reduce their self-destructive responses to interpersonal stressors (Kernberg, 1984).

The basic techniques of supportive psychotherapy consists of exploring the patients' primitive defenses in the here-and-now for the purpose of helping them achieve control by nonanalytic means and fostering a better adaptation to reality by helping them become more aware of the disorganizing affect of their defensive operations. Manifest and suppressed transferences—rather than unconscious and repressed transferences—are explored and utilized for classification of related interpersonal problems the patient faces (Kernberg, 1984).

Such supportive psychotherapy is utilized commonly with moderate and lower functioning borderline outpatients. Typically, sessions are scheduled weekly and may continue for several years. The result of the Menninger Outcome Study suggest that supportive treatment is able to bring about the basic personality change that were expected only from reconstructive dynamic psychotherapy (Wallerstein, 1986). So, despite Kernberg's (1984) characteristic of supportive psychotherapy as "a treatment of last resort," supportive psychotherapy is a potent intervention.

Klein (1989a) describes two types of supportive treatment for lower functioning borderlines. In the first, confrontive psychotherapy, the treatment process involves confronting resistances that maintain maladaptive behaviors until they become ego dystonic. A therapeutic alliance takes the place of transference acting out. Treatment also involves the implementation of adaptive modes of dealing with underlying affects, such of new patterns replacing previous self-destructive behaviors and defenses. Unlike reconstructive psychotherapy, this approach does not facilitate the patient working through abandonment depression. The goals of this therapy are limited to increasing the patient's capacity to work to achieve some consistency in interpersonal relationships.

Klein (1989a) also describes an approach to "counseling" with very low functioning borderline patients. This approach is the treatment of choice for patients with a history of repeated early abuse, neglect or separation trauma, or repeated, severe psychiatric regressive episodes, or a history of repeating life threatening suicidal or homicidal actions. The goal of this treatment is to reduce anger, anxiety, and depressive affects that persistently interfere with the patient's capacity to function adaptively. The counselor serves as an auxiliary ego for the patient and utilizes a combination of such techniques as reality testing, encouragement, direction, problem-solving, and medication.

Short-Term Dynamic Psychotherapy. While it was previously assumed that borderline patients were unfit for short-term dynamic psychotherapy, it now appears that short-term and time-limited approaches have some utility with selective patients. In as few as ten to 20 sessions, treatment can be focused on specific relational or situational problems. And, because such a specific focus the likelihood of a regressive transference developing is limited. This approach may be suitable for borderline patients who present with concerns about being engulfed, overwhelmed or too dependent. It may also be useful for those who have a history of terminating more regressive treatment. Furthermore, it may serve as a springboard for moving into long-term therapy.

Klein (1989b) describes a short-term treatment protocol for borderline patients. The goals are containment, i.e., they come to recognize, control, and contain their propensity to act out; learning, i.e., that emerging affects that covered their defenses can and must be verbalized rather than acted out; and adaptation, i.e., they channel their energies associated with these affects into adaptive and sublimated behavior and expressions. This short-term approach follows Masterson's model except that the frequency of sessions is limited, and confrontation is the principal technique utilized, although clarification, interpretation and communicative matching are sometimes needed. Sessions are scheduled once or twice a week for a year or less, and day-to-day problems of adaptation and healthy defenses are the focus of treatment.

Research Support for Psychodynamic Interventions. There are now some empirical studies supporting the clinical value and utility of dynamically oriented therapy with Borderline Personality Disorder. In one study, individuals treated with an approach based on self-psychology and who remained in treatment for two years appeared to have profited from therapy (Stevenson & Meares, 1992; Meares, Stevenson, & Comerford, 1999). Because it was a post-hoc, naturalistic study with a waiting list control group for comparison, it cannot be certain that the results can be attributed to this dynamic approach.

A random controlled study of a psychoanalytically oriented approach to treatment in a partial hospitalization study has also been reported (Bateman & Fonagy, 1999; 2001). The treatment was intensive and extensive and consisted of: weekly psychoanalytic psychotherapy, thrice-weekly group analytic psychotherapy, weekly psychodrama and expressive therapy, and a weekly community meeting, along with mediation management. Whether positive treatment outcomes could be attributed to the specific structure and milieu of the partial hospitalization program itself or to the psychodynamic approach utilized by therapists in the program is unclear.

A structured, manualized approach, specifically designed for treating Borderline Personality Disorder and called "Transference Focused Psychotherapy" appears promising. This approach focuses on affect-laden themes in the current patient-therapist relationship. These include containment of self-destructive and suicidal behaviors, various ways of sabotaging treatment, and the identification and recapitulation of significant object relations patterns. This uncontrolled trial showed markedly decreased hospitalizations, day hospital treatment, and very low drop out rate (Clarkin et al., 2001).

Cognitive Behavioral Therapy Approaches

Cognitive Therapy. According the Beck, Freeman, and Associates (1990), the Cognitive Therapy approach has significant advantages over other approaches in the treatment of Borderline Personality Disordered individuals. Basically, completion of Cognitive Therapy is possible in one-and-a-half to two-and-a-half years (Freeman et al., 1990) as compared to psychoanalytical oriented therapies which typically require five to seven years (Masterson, 1981).

Establishing a collaborative working relationship is often a particularly challenging first step in the treatment process. Since trust and intimacy are major issues for these individuals, taking a collaborative, strategic approach based on guided discovery is suggested. Explicitly acknowledging and accepting the individual's difficulty in trusting the therapist, communicating clearly, assertively, and honestly, following through on agreements, and behaving in a consistently trustworthy manner provides the individual with evidence on which trust can be based. Furthermore, setting limits including specifying a treatment contract is advised. An initial focus in concrete behavioral goals is useful in reducing the impact of the borderline individual's difficulty with intimacy and trust. Many of these individuals find it less threatening to work on issues for which little introspection is required, and where the focus on behavior rather than on feelings or thoughts. Not surprisingly, a major focus in Cognitive Therapy is changing maladaptive schema. Borderline individuals here believe that the world is a dangerous place, that they are helpless, and that they are inherently flawed in a way that inevitably leads to rejection and abandonment by others. It is suggested that these beliefs must be gradually challenged by "chipping away" at them, by testing expectancies against previous experience, by developing behavioral experiences to test expectancies, and developing new competencies and coping skills. These individuals must learn to challenge dichotomous thinking both during and between sessions, as decreased dichotomous thinking often results in decreased mood liability and impulsivity. Behavioral interventions, such as self-instructional training (Meichenbaum, 1977) may be useful in further reducing self-destructive impulsive behaviors.

Non-compliance with treatment is not an uncommon problem with personality-disordered individuals, and often the reason is fear of change (Fowler, Orme, & Hart, 2021).

Since they assume the world is dangerous and they have a low tolerance for ambiguity, they find change, including growth in the course of treatment threatening. Addressing change openly, examining risks and benefits, planning changes as a series of small steps, and not pressing for change to quickly are recommended. Fears about termination of treatment evoke abandonment and rejection issues which must be carefully addressed. In summary, the Cognitive Therapy of Borderline Personality Disordered individuals begin by developing a collaborative working relationship of trust and then focuses on modulating moods, impulses and behavior with cognitive-behavioral methods, setting the stage so that basic schemas such as abandonment, defectiveness, incompetence, and mistrust can be modified and changed.

In line with Turkat's (1990) formulation that the basic issue for borderlines is problem-solving deficiencies, Turkat proposes a treatment methodology involving several strategies. They are basic problem-solving training, concept formation training, categorization management, and processing speed management.

Dialectical Behavior Therapy. The defining feature of this treatment approach is its emphasis on dialectics, the reconciliation of opposites. The basic dialectic for therapists working with DBT is accepting the client's behaviors, thoughts and affects in the moment while simultaneously encouraging them to change (Stanley, Brodsky, & Gratch, 2021).

Accordingly, DBT treatment requires "moment to moment changes in the use of supportive acceptance versus confrontation and change strategies. This emphasis on acceptance as a balance to change flows directly from the integrative of a perspective drawn from Eastern (Zen) practice with Western Psychological practice" (Linehan, 1993, p. 19).

Linehan (1993; 2015) specified four primary modes of treatment in DBT: individual therapy; group-based skills training, telephone contact, and therapist consultation. Group therapy and other modes of treatment may be added at the discretion of the therapist.

The individual therapist is the primary therapist, and the main work of therapy is carried out in the individual therapy sessions. Individual therapy is conceptualized as having three stages: beginning, middle, and end (Marra, 2005). Essential components of individual therapy from a DBT perspective include: dialectical analysis and coaching clients to think dialectically about their own situation; validation of the client's feelings, thoughts and experiences; balancing emotion-focused and solution-focused coping; prompting improved shifting of attention from internal to external cues; teaching new psychological coping skills, and non-pejorative interpretation of the client's behavior and affect.

Skills training is usually carried out in a group context, ideally by someone other than the individual therapist. In the skills training groups clients are taught skills considered relevant to the particular problems of personality-disordered individuals. There are four groups of skills: core mindfulness skills, interpersonal effectiveness skills, emotion modulation skills, and distress tolerance skills. Each of these skills targets key style/temperament over modulations. However, it is possible to accomplish skill training in the context of individual therapy with select clients (Marra, 2005).

Telephone contact with the therapist after hours is offered not as psychotherapy but rather to help and support in clients to find alternatives to self-injury and for relationship repair when the client believes she damaged her relationship with her therapist and wants to rectify it prior to the next session.

DBT therapists are encouraged to participate regularly in therapist consultation groups. These groups provide both emotional support for therapists dealing with difficult clients as well as for ongoing training in DBT methods.

Following an initial period of pre-treatment involving assessment, commitment and orientation to therapy, DBT consists of three stages of treatment.

1 This stage focuses on reducing parasuicidal and suicidal behaviors, therapy interfering behaviors and behaviors that comprise quality of life. It also focuses on developing the necessary skills to resolve these problems. Skills training is usually carried out in a group context, ideally by someone other than the individual therapist. In the skills training groups clients are taught skills considered relevant to the particular problems of personality-disordered individuals. There are four groups of skills: core mindfulness skills, interpersonal effectiveness skills, emotion modulation skills, and distress tolerance skills.
2 This stage deals primarily with difficult problems of living, including treatment of post-traumatic stress related issues when present. Much of this work is done in individual sessions.
3 The focus of this stage is on self-esteem and individual treatment goals. The targeted behaviors of each stage are brought under control before moving on to the next phase. In particular, post-traumatic stress related problems, such as those related to childhood sexual abuse, are not dealt with directly until stage 1 has been successfully completed. Therapy at each stage is focused on the specific targets for that stage which are arranged in a definite hierarchy of relative importance. These include: decreasing suicidal behaviors, decreasing therapy interfering behaviors, decreasing behaviors that interfere with the quality of life, increasing behavioral skills, decreasing behaviors related to post-traumatic stress, improving self-esteem, and individual targets negotiated with the client.

The core strategies in DBT are 'validation' and 'problem-solving'. Attempts to facilitate change are surrounded by interventions that validate clients' behavior and responses in relation to the client's current life situation, and that demonstrate an understanding of their difficulties and suffering. Problem-solving focuses on the establishment of necessary skills. Other treatment modalities include contingency management, cognitive therapy exposure-based therapies, and medication. Because parasuicidal, suicidal and other forms of acting-out behaviors are common with BPD individuals, contingency management is commonly employed in each stage of treatment.

The provision of DBT therapy is easier to accomplish in an inpatient, partial hospitalization or residential treatment setting than in private practice. The reason is that as described by Linehan (1993a), DBT is bet implemented with a treatment team in which one therapist provides psychosocial skill training, another provides individual therapy, others can provide a consultation function, and the therapists have access to a therapist consultation group for support.

Marra (2005) has offered suggestions for the adapting DBT treatment in private practice settings. While he recommends that skills training be provided by another therapist, he offers guidelines when that is not possible. Nevertheless, he encourages therapists in private practice who want to use DBT to have regular contact with a psychotherapy consultant as a substitute for involvement in a therapist consultation group. The purpose of such consultation is to clarify diagnosis, treatment plans and specific interventions with another professional who can offer a fresh perspective, confront the therapist's interpretation of data and situations, and warn of potential boundary violations.

Cognitive Coping Therapy. This is an active, directive, didactic and structured cognitive behavioral approach for treating personality-disordered individuals (Sharoff, 2002). It is a complete and self-contained approach to treatment which begins with assessing an individual's coping skills—in terms of skill chains, subskills and microskills—and then increasing skill competence in targeted areas as needed. Five key skill areas with representative treatment modalities include: *cognitive skills*—problem-solving, self-instruction training, and self-management; *emotion skills*—emotional containment and compartmentalization; *perceptual skills*—perspective taking, thought stopping, and psychological distance taking; *physiological skills*—meditation and relaxation training, and *behavior skills*—communication and assertiveness training. Sharoff (2002) describes a detailed protocol—and case example—for using this structured approach with Borderline Personality Disorder.

Schema Therapy. Schema Therapy is an elaboration of cognitive therapy that has been developed by Young (1994; 1999; Young, Klosko, & Weishaar, 2003) specifically for personality disorders, and other difficult individual and couples problems. Schema Therapy involves identifying maladaptive schemas and planning specific strategies and interventions. Four main strategies are cognitive, experiential, behavioral and the therapeutic relationship itself. Cognitive restructuring, modification of maladaptive schemas, is an important cognitive strategy, but is combined with imagery exercises, empathic confrontation, homework assignments and "limited reparenting," i.e., a form of corrective emotional experience (Young, 1999; Young et al., 2003).

Maladaptive schemas typically associated with Borderline Personality Disorder are: *abandonment,* i.e., the belief that significant others will not or cannot provide reliable and stable support; *defectiveness*: i.e., the belief that one is defective, bad, unwanted, or inferior in important respects; *mistrust/abuse*, i.e., the belief that others will abuse, humiliate, cheat, lie, manipulate, or take advantage; *emotional deprivation, i.e.,* the belief that one's desire for emotional support will not be met by others; *social Isolation*, i.e., the belief that one is alienated, different from others, or not part of any group; and *insufficient self-control*, i.e., the belief that one is incapable of self-control and frustration tolerance(Bernstein, 2002). Young et al. (2003) provides a detailed treatment protocol for utilizing the schema-focused approach with Borderline Personality Disorder.

Other Cognitive-Behavioral Interventions. Smucker (1999) describes a cognitive behavioral approach that incorporates guided imagery to focus directly on images and affects associated with early childhood abuse in borderline individuals. This approach developed out of Smucker's experience in working with severe traumatized borderline individuals who often met criteria for Post-Traumatic Stress Disorder and had failed in previous treatments.

Interpersonal Approach

Benjamin (1996; 2003a; 2007) has written extensively about this approach. In her view, psychotherapeutic interventions with borderline personality-disordered individuals are best planned and evaluated in terms of whether they enhance collaboration, facilitate learning about maladaptive patterns and their roots, block these patterns, enhance the will to change, or effectively encourage new patterns.

Benjamin offers a number of observations on facilitating collaboration. She insists that therapists offer these individuals a contrast in a strength building rather than in enabling regression. A collaboration based on strength building must emphasize in sessions as well as in phone calls or in the clinic lobby that the mutual goal is to build on strengths so these individuals can pull themselves back together. The collaboration must be against "it", their destructive pattern(s). Healthy collaboration further requires that transference and countertransference disasters be avoided through firm physical and verbal boundaries. Benjamin cautions that the treatment approach she advocates is not appropriate for individuals who are unable to agree to a contract in strength building.

Borderline individuals need to learn to recognize that perceived abandonment sets off a chain of self-destructive patterns. These individuals are likely to relinquish self-mutilation, self-sabotage, and homicidal or suicidal acting out if they can 'divorce' their internalized abusive attachment figures. Essentially, they must give up the desire to be affirmed by these internalized representations. This occurs by developing a dislike of those figures, or by developing a superseding attachment to someone more constructive, such as the clinician. Once these tasks are achieved, the focus of treatment shifts to facilitating new learning. The basic goal is learning how to give and take autonomy while remaining friendly.

Interpersonal Reconstructive Therapy (IRT). IRT was developed by Benjamin (2003b; 2007) for the treatment of this disorder. Like many other treatments for Borderline Personality Disorder, IRT conceptualizes the problem as one of inadequate attachment to caregivers in early development. Problem patterns are categorized according to the Structural Analysis of Social Behavior (SASB), a method developed by Benjamin. Behaviors are described according to the focus (on other, self, or self as if by other), affiliation (placed on a love-hate axis), and interdependence (placed on an emancipate-control axis). The borderline patient's behavior towards the therapist is classified in the IRT system as either "Regressive Loyalist," or "Red," when the patient is engaging in old, destructive patterns, and "Growth Collaborator," or "Green," when the patient responds to the therapist in new, effective ways. Red and Green remain in conflict throughout the course of treatment until finally the Growth Collaborator becomes dominant in the patient's mind. There are five stages in Interpersonal Reconstructive Therapy: Establishing collaboration between therapist and patient; learning about old patterns of behavior, such as where they originate and what purpose they serve; blocking destructive patterns; increasing the will to change; and learning new patterns. As with other treatments with personality reconstruction as the goal, IRT is a long-term form of therapy that may span multiple years.

Group Therapy

Data on the efficacy of group therapy for the treatment of personality disorders is rather "soft." There are many case reports and even a few controlled studies, but no randomized clinical trials, except for the Borderline Personality Disorder. There are numerous case reports and clinical trials, and even one randomized clinical trial reported on group treatment with Borderline Personality Disordered individuals. What's more, there is general consensus that group therapy, under specified conditions, has enormously therapeutic efficacy (Ogrodniczuk, Uliaszek, Lebow, & Kealy, 2021).

This section will review both dynamic and behavioral group approaches as well as highlight some representative research studies.

The psychodynamic group literature on borderline personality begins in the 1950's. There is general consensus that group dynamic therapy can be a useful adjunct to individual dynamic-therapy, but that it cannot be the only treatment (Hulse, 1958; Slavson, 1964; Day & Semrad, 1971; Horowitz, 1980). Horowitz (1980) cautions that borderline patients require individual psychotherapy to support them throughout group engendered stress and to integrate the affects the groups provokes in them. Furthermore, without individual psychotherapy premature termination from group therapy is likely. On the other hand, Pines (1975) contends that concurrent dynamic individual psychotherapy is not necessary because the group process itself is a potent holding environment capable of containing primitive impulses and projections. Horowitz (1977) also contends that he individual psychotherapist does not function as group therapist in order to reduce the possibility of jealousy and fantasies of favoritism among other group members.

Most writing on dynamic group therapy for borderline prefer heterogeneous to homogenous groups. They insist that borderline patients are more effectively treated in groups consisting of higher functioning individuals with neuroses and other personality disorders (Day & Semrad, 1971; Horowitz, 1977; Stone & Weissman, 1984). There is, however, outcome research that supports the use of homogenous groups wherein all patients have Borderline Personality Disorder diagnoses (O'Leary et al., 1991; Finn, 1990; Linehan et al., 1991).

The advantages of dynamic group therapy include "dilution of intense transference" (Horowitz, 1980) which results from the presence of multiple transferential objects, instead of the single all-encompassing individual clinician. Rage is instead diluted and directed toward other group members. Borderline patients also find it easier to accept feedback and confrontation from group peers than from a therapist. Groups also provides many opportunities to understand and master such borderline defenses as splitting and projective identification.

There are some disadvantages and difficulties with group treatment of borderline patients. First, these patients may be easily scapegoated because of their primitive manner of expression. Second, they may feel deprived amidst the competition of other group members for the group leader's nurturance. And they may maintain a certain distance in the group because of their privacy attachment to their individual psychotherapist (Gabbard, 2014).

Dynamically oriented groups with borderlines tend to span the continuum from ego psychology (O'Leary et al., 1991; Finn, 1990) to self-psychology (Harwood, 1992).

Behavioral group therapies for borderline patients focus less on underlying and explanations from the symptomatic behavior, and more helping these patients acquire the specific skills necessary to control their affects, reduce their cognitive distortions, and projective identifications, and find alternatives to self-destructive behaviors. Linehan (1985, 1988, 1993, 2015) provides a manual-guided strategy for the treatment of self-destructive behavior and impulsivity called "dialectical behavior therapy." Although geared primarily to chronically parasuicidal borderline females, the treatment strategies and interventions have applicability to higher functioning individuals. The group session employs didactic, shell training, and behavioral rehearsal techniques directed at dependency and other interpersonal patterns, as well as improving affect tolerance. These twice weekly sessions for one year are complemented with weekly individual counseling.

There is some noteworthy research with borderlines in group treatment that will be briefly highlighted. Nehls (1991, 1992) reports process and outcome data on group therapy of borderline patients in homogenous treatment format. The group format was highly structured, through group members defined their own treatment goals. Patient outcomes included decreased depression and hostility which was associated largely with two interventions: providing and seeking information. Dick and Wolfe (1986) reported data on a time-limited dynamic group therapy with heterogeneous groups containing a number of borderline patients. The group met daily for twelve weeks. One year past group follow-up showed an 82 percent reduction in the use of psychiatric services compared to a control group of untreated patients. Three year follow-up showed the gains had been maintained. Finally, Linehan et al. (1991) examined parasuicidal female borderline patients randomly assigned to dialectical behavior therapy groups or to traditional community treatment for a one year period. Those in behavioral groups had fewer incidents of parasuicide, were more likely to remain in individual therapy, and had fewer inpatient psychiatric days as compared to those in traditional treatment. Follow up measures two years after this initial study, as well as subsequent studies, indicated that DBT was an effective treatment and gains were maintained over time (Linehan et al., 1993, 2006). Another randomly controlled trial in which DBT was compared to general psychiatric management found that both forms of treatment were equally effective in treating borderline personality disorder (McMain et al., 2009).

A manual-guided approach called Relationship Management Psychotherapy is a time-limited group approach. This form of therapy allows borderline patients to choose their own treatment and requires those who threaten self-harm or act in aggressive ways to be expelled from the inpatient program for 24 hours. It has been compared with open-ended individual dynamic psychotherapy in a randomized clinical trial (Clarkin, Marzaliali, & Monroe-Blum, 1991). Hoch, O'Reilly, and Carscadden (2006) compared the mean annual outcome rates for 27 patients consecutively enrolled in a relationship management therapy program from 1998 to 2000. They found significant reductions in the use of restraint, staff observation, self-harm, and days of inpatient treatment.

Marital and Family Therapy

Families of borderline patients often exhibit severe pathology, which may be of etiological significance. Parents of borderline patients have high incidence of affective disorders, alcoholism, antisocial personality disorder, and Borderline Personality Disorder or traits. The parental relationship is usually characterized by neglect and overprotectiveness. Family therapy can be useful, and in some instances necessary, in maintaining borderline patients in outpatient psychotherapy. This is particularly the case when borderline patients remain financially and/or emotionally dependent on their parents.

Family therapy with borderlines has been developed along at least three theoretical lines. The first is the psychodynamic, particularly in terms of object relations and systems theory. Everett et al. (1989) have the most complete discussion of this approach in there book *Treating the Borderline Family: A Systemic Approach*. They specify five treatment goals: increasing the family's ability to reduce the systemic splitting process; increasing family members' capacities for owning split-off objects and moving toward interacting with others as a "whole person"; reducing oppositional and stereotypic behavior of all family members; "resetting" external boundary for both unclear and intergenerational systems; and "resetting" internal boundary for spousal, parent-child, and sibling subtypes; and permitting a clearer alliance between the parents and limiting reciprocal intrusiveness of children and parents. Five treatment strategies for accomplishing these goals in an outpatient family treatment setting are: developing and maintaining a therapeutic structure; reality testing in the family; interactional disengagement; intervening in the intergenerational system; and solidification of the marital alliance and sibling subsystem (Ogrodniczuk, Uliaszek, Lebow, & Kealy, 2021).

Another treatment orientation is the structural family approach developed by Minnuchin (1975). Schone and Kovel (1988) describe severe borderline pathology in terms of spouse subsystem is internally over-involvement and contemporarily distant and disengaged from the hold subsystem. In effect, borderline females have a systems equivalent of object splitting wherein family subsystems are organized around dichotomous extremes: collusion and sabotage; loyalty and scapegoating; inclusion and rejection; nurturance and neglect; and symbiosis and abandonment. It is this structural pattern of family interaction that is the focus of systemic change. Lachkar (1992) provides an extensive discussion of an integrated object relations and self-psychology approach to the marital treatment of the borderline patient. She provides a detailed treatment protocol and several case reports illustrating this method.

A third option is the Relationship Enhancement Therapy approach for borderline families and couples. Relationship Enhancement was developed by Guerney (1977) which integrate social skills training, psychodynamic principles, and interpersonal therapy techniques. Since borderline patients have major deficits in self-differentiation and communication, the Relationship Enhancement's focus on skill building in some areas seems promising with couple and family settings, particularly for mild to moderately dysfunctional borderline patients (Waldo and Harman, 1993; Harman & Waldo, 2001). The clinician functions largely as a coach to develop the necessary relational skills, usually in two hour sessions. Waldo and Harmon (1993) report a case of time-limited intervention that was successful. A 12-month follow-up showed that the changes had been maintained. These authors also describe and illustrate the use of two therapists working conjointly with couples in which one partner presents with Borderline Personality Disorder (Waldo & Harman, 1998). The fundamental principles of relationship enhancement therapy are further discussed in Accordino, Keat, and Guerney (2003), as well as a case study of an adolescent with serious mental illness and substance dependence.

Lachkar (1999) offers additional insight into the treatment of couples in which one partner has a borderline personality structure while the other partner presents with a narcissistic pattern. Solomon (1999) also addresses the treatment of the borderline-narcissistic couple from a somewhat different psychoanalytic perspective.

Medication

Medication is commonly used in the treatment of this and other personality disorders (Nelson & Tsheringld, 2021). Usually, the treatment targets are affective instability, interpersonal sensitivity, impulsivity, aggressivity, transient psychotic episodes, and self-harming behavior. Lithium and carbamazepine have targeted affective instability, while serotonergic agents have been effective with impulsivity and aggressivity. Serotonergic agents, like fluoxetine and sertraline, are effective for reducing the interpersonal sensitivity and reactivity (Reich, 2002). For those with rejection sensitivity, and a history of good treatment compliance, a trial of an MAOI can be considered if all other approaches have failed. Serotonergic agents have some efficacy in lower functioning histrionic individuals who exhibit impulsivity and affective instability (Reich, 2002). Transient psychotic episodes, including mild thought disorders and dissociation, are best addressed with atypical antipsychotics instead of traditional neuroleptics which have the risk of tardive dyskinesia. Finally, for self-harming behavior, trials of SSRIs have been helpful. If not, an adjunctive trial of naltrexone can be considered, if necessary (Reich, 2005).

In recent year, quetiapine (Seroquel) has become the most commonly prescribed medication for borderline personality disorder probably because it reduces various symptoms such as anxiety presumably because it has a sedating effect. It is an antipsychotic medication that is generally well tolerated. That means it has few adverse effects and specifically has low potential for extrapyramidal (tremor and stiffness) symptoms. However, it can cause weight gain (Diamond, 2009). Very well-designed research has been reported that confirms what clinicians have known for some time. In a randomized controlled trial, it was found that low dose quetiapine (150 mg/day) was effective in reducing the overall severity of symptoms in those with borderline personality disorder. Most improvement was noted in verbal and physical aggression but less on impulsivity and depression (Black, Zanarini, Romine, Shaw, Allen, & Schulz, 2014).

There are some potential complications or disadvantages with pharmacotherapy in the treatment of borderline individuals. First, is the matter of noncompliance either related to side effects or to secondary gain. Medications can serve as leverage to control the prescribing clinician or other caregivers. Demands for frequent changes in dosage or type of medication, overdosing, and failure to take the medication prescribed are all means of transference acting out. Second, borderline individuals may appear to others to have improved from medication but report they feel worse, or vice versa. Gunderson (1989) suggested that this apparent paradox may ensue to the extent the individual believes that symptomatic improvement will result in undesirable consequences, such as loss or abandonment of dependent gratifications.

Combined and Integrated Treatment Approaches

There is considerable consensus that combined treatment is essential, or at least preferable, for borderline pathology given its severity and apparent treatment resistance. Clearly, differences exist between the prognosis and treatability of the high functioning borderline (i.e., Global Assessment of Functioning, [GAF] over 65) and the low functioning borderline (i.e., GAF below 45). Reports of treatment success using only traditional individual psychoanalytic psychotherapy may be possible with the highest functioning borderline individual but are not likely with lower functioning borderline individuals. In line with the basic premise of this book, the lower the patient's functioning and motivation and readiness for treatment, the more treatment must be integrated and combined.

The most common recommendations for combined treatment is to prescribe both individual therapy and group therapy (Winkeller & Schlesinger, 2021). There is currently no consensus on which theoretical approaches to combine or whether both should be combined or sequenced. The earliest recommendations of combined treatment was by Tacbacnik (1965) who advocated concurrent dynamic individual psychotherapy and dynamic group therapy. On the other hand, Horowitz (1977; 1980) advocates sequencing dynamic group and individual therapy in which the group experience prepares the patient to productively utilize individual therapy. Clarkin et al. (1991) also recommend combined individual and group modalities but favors individual behavior treatment with long term manual-guided group treatment.

Others recommend combining individual therapy and family therapy. These include Kernberg (1984) who describes the indications for concurrent as well as sequential utilization of these modalities.

Berger (1987) recommends combined psychotherapy and pharmacotherapy because these individuals are difficult to treat with only one modality. He notes that combined treatment can be complicated by the borderline's tendency to idealize one treatment and negate the other. Koenigsberg (1993) offers a very thoughtful review of combining medications and psychotherapy, highlighting the indications and contraindications for this treatment decision. He also describes the complications inherent in combined treatment strategy but believes these can be addressed by special structuring of treatment, attention to countertransference issues, and vigilance for splitting. Koenigsberg contends that combining medication and psychotherapy has considerable value for seriously symptomatic patients, those prone to treatment noncompliance, or likely to intractable affective storms and psychotic regression. Bellino, Rinaldi, and Bogetto (2010) found that combined therapy with antidepressants and interpersonal psychotherapy was more effective than single pharmacotherapy alone in the treatment of borderline patients. Further examination by these researchers revealed that patients with more severe psychopathology had a better chance to improve with this combined treatment (Bellino, Bozzatello, & Bogetto 2015).

Lazarus (1985) the developer of Multimodal Therapy endorses the combined use of several modalities, concurrently or sequential, for a variety of difficult patients, including borderline individuals. Vaccani (1989) describes treating the alcohol-abusing Borderline Personality Disorder with psychotherapy, family therapy, group therapy, and Alcoholics Anonymous meetings. Nehls and Diamond (1993) describes the modalities for lower functioning borderlines in a community-based setting. The modalities that are coordinated and continuous include: individual therapy, group therapy, medication, drug and alcohol services, psychosocial rehabilitation, crisis intervention, and crisis houses.

It is now generally accepted that an integrated treatment model is best suited to address personality disorders (Livesley, 2012; Clarkin, Cain, & Livesley, 2015). While there exist some significant differences between the various treatment models developed for borderline personality disorder, certain elements common to all of them that contribute to treatment success have been identified. Perhaps the most important of these is the cultivation and maintenance of a positive therapeutic relationship between therapist and patient. This is comprised of five main elements regardless of orientation or model: cultivating emotional awareness; structuring treatment; being responsive; supervision or team involvement and support; and exploring ruptures in the relationship (McMain, Boritz, & Leybman, 2015).

Chapter 7

Dependent Personality Disorder

Individuals with dependent personalities present with a pervasive pattern of dependency and submissiveness. They tend to be excessively passive, insecure, self-sacrificing, and non-assertive individuals who become overly dependent on one or more persons for guidance and support (Bornstein, 2012; Skodol, Bender, & Oldham, 2019; American Psychiatric Association, 2022).

Despite the fact that it is one of the least studied personality disorders (Simon, 2009), treatment of the Dependent Personality Disorder can be highly effective and successful.

This chapter describes a framework for the assessment and effective treatment of this disorder. It includes sections on diagnosis, psychological assessment, case conceptualization, and treatment interventions. It begins with background information on the disorder as well as the DSM-5-TR description, prototypic description, associated features, and the Alternative Model of Personality Disorders description of this disorder. The section on case conceptualization provides five common clinical formulations of this disorder: psychodynamic, biosocial, cognitive-behavioral, interpersonal, and an integrative conceptualization of this disorder. Several treatment approaches, modalities, and intervention strategies are also described. These includes individual psychotherapy, group therapy, marital and family therapy, medication, and integrative and combined treatment.

Description of the Dependent Personality Disorder

The Dependent Personality Disorder can be recognized by the following descriptors and characteristics: styles vs. disorders; triggering event; behavioral styles; interpersonal styles; cognitive styles; affective styles; attachment style, and optimal criterion.

Style vs. Disorder. The dependent personality can be thought of as spanning a continuum from healthy to pathological, with the dependent personality style at the healthy end and the Dependent Personality Disorder at the pathological end. Table 7.1 compares and contrasts differences between the dependent style and the disorder.

The following two case examples further illustrate differences between the Dependent Personality Disorder (Mr. C.) and the dependent personality style (Ms. B.).

> **Case Study: Dependent Personality Disorder**
>
> Ms. C. is a 38-year-old, single woman with panic symptoms that had begun approximately three years earlier. Once the panic attacks began, Ms. C. moved back into her parents' home and has become nearly totally housebound, fearing that "panic could strike any time." She described both of her parents as caring, concerned, and "my best friends," on whom she is overly reliant. She looks to them to support her financially and emotionally, and to make decisions for her. Ms. C. has also become progressively habituated to the Valium that she was prescribed for panic symptoms.

> **Case Study: Dependent Personality Style**
>
> Mr. B. has been a social worker at a foster-care agency for the past seven years. He finds his job fulfilling and is well liked by the other staff members, as well as the children and prospective parents with whom he works. He is a very concerned, caring, and gentle person. A year earlier, he had begun dating Sandra L., one of the pediatricians who consults for the agency. Their relationship has been happy and fulfilling for both of them, probably because of Mr. B.'s efforts. He cannot get over the fact that a doctor would be interested in being with him, and he expresses his appreciation in numerous ways. He can not spend enough time with her or do enough things for her. He idealizes her, makes every effort to make her feel comfortable and secure, and regularly seeks her opinions and advice. Yet he insists that he has a mind of his own; after much deliberation and soul searching, he bought an expensive sports car even though Sandra thought it was extravagant.

Triggering Event. The typical situation, circumstance or event that most likely triggers or activates the characteristic maladaptive response of the Dependent Personality Disorder (Othmer & Othmer, 2002), as noted in behavioral, interpersonal, cognitive, and feeling styles, is: "expectations of self-reliance and/or being alone."

Behavioral Style. The behavioral style of dependent personalities are characterized by docility, passivity, and non-assertiveness.

Interpersonal Style. In interpersonal relations, they tend to be pleasing, self-sacrificing, and clinging, and constantly require the assurance of others. Their compliance and reliance on others lead to a subtle demand that others assume responsibility for major areas of their lives.

Table 7.1 Comparison of Dependent Personality Style and Disorder

Personality Style	Personality Disorder
When making decisions *they* are comfortable seeking out the opinions and advice of others; but ultimately make their own decisions	Unable to make everyday decisions without an excessive amount of advice or reassurance from others; allows others to make the most of their important decision
Carefully promote harmony with important persons in their life through being polite, agreeable and tactful	Agrees with people even when they believe they are wrong, because of fear of being rejected
Although they respect authority and prefer the role of team member, they can initiate and complete tasks on their own	Has difficulty initiating projects or doing things on their own
Thoughtful and good at pleasing others. Occasionally, they will endure personal discomfort in accomplishing a good deed for the key people in their lives	Volunteer to do things that are unpleasant or demeaning in order to get other people to like them
Tend to prefer to company of one or more individuals to being alone	Feels uncomfortable or helpless when alone, or go to great lengths to avoid being alone
Tend to be strongly committed to relationships and work hard to sustain them	Feels devastated or helpless when close relationships end; and frequently preoccupied with fears of being abandoned
Can take corrective action in response to criticism	Easily hurt by criticism or disapproval

Cognitive Style. The cognitive style of dependent personalities is characterized by suggestibility. They easily adopt a Pollyannaish attitude toward life. Furthermore, they tend to minimize difficulties, and because of their naiveté, are readily persuadable and others easily take advantage of them. In short, this style of thinking is uncritical and unperceptive.

Emotional Style. Their emotional or affective style is characterized by insecurity and anxiousness. Because they lack self-confidence, they experience considerable discomfort at being alone. They tend to be preoccupied with the fear of abandonment and of the disapproval of others. Their mood tends to be one of anxiety or fearfulness, as well as having a somber or sad quality.

Attachment Style. The preoccupied attachment dimension is characterized by a sense of personal unworthiness and a positive evaluation of others. These individuals tend to be very externally oriented in their self-definitions. This Preoccupied Attachment Style is common in individuals with Dependent Personality Disorder (Lyddon & Sherry, 2001).

Optimal Diagnostic Criterion. Of all the diagnostic criteria for the Dependent Personality Disorder, one has been found to be the most useful in diagnosing this disorder. The belief is that by beginning with this criterion, the clinician can test for the presence or absence of the criterion and more quickly diagnose the personality disorder (Allnutt & Links, 1996). The optimal criterion for this disorder is: needs others to assume responsibility for most major areas of his or her life.

DSM-5-TR Description

Individuals with this personality disorder are characterized by an excessive and unremitting need to be cared for and cling to others because of their fear of separation. They constantly seek the advice and reassurance of others when making decisions. More than anything, they want others to take responsibility for most major areas of their lives. Not surprisingly, they seldom express disagreement with others for fear they will lose their support and approval. Because they lack confidence in their own judgment and ability, they have difficulty starting projects and doing things on their own. These individuals will even engage in actions that are difficult and unpleasant in order to receive support and caring from others. Because of unrealistic fears of being unable to take care of themselves, they feel helpless or uncomfortable when faced with being alone. When a close relationship is about to end, they immediately seek out another caring and supportive relationship. Finally, they become preoccupied with fears of being left to take care of themselves (American Psychiatric Association, 2022).

Prototypic Description

A prototype is a brief description that captures the essence of how a particular disorder commonly presents. Prototypic descriptions are useful and convenient, and clinicians commonly rely on them rather than lists of behavioral criteria or core beliefs (Westen, 2012). Here is a common prototypic description of the Dependent Personality Disorder: These individuals feel inadequate, weak, and needy. They don't take very good care of themselves. They find it nearly impossible to make their own decisions, and they don't feel good about being alone. Their neediness makes them submissive and subservient. So they are more than willing to put others' needs and views above their own. Basically, they will do whatever it takes to get others to care for them, to give them affection, and give direction to their lives (Francis, 2013).

Associated Features

Prevalence. DPD has been identified in 1.0 percent of the general population and 15.0 percent in clinical practice (Torgersen, 2021).

Differential Diagnosis. Dependency is a feature shared by various anxiety disorders, i.e., separation anxiety disorders in adults, panic disorder, and agoraphobia, as well as depressive disorders. It is also common in borderline and histrionic personality disorders (American Psychiatric Association, 2022).

Development and Course. While the development of DPD remains unclear, there are some common features among those who meet criteria for this disorder. These include child abuse or neglect, a life-threatening illness during childhood, a family member who has DPD or another anxiety disorder, or a history of abusive relationships (American Psychiatric Association, 2022).

Culture, Sex, and Gender. Dependent behavior is characteristic of DPD only when it is in excess of the individual's cultural norms or reflets unrealistic concerns. While cultural norms or religious practices that emphasize reliance on authority may foster DPD, neither passivity, deferential. In clinical settings DPD is more common in females than males (American Psychiatric Association, 2022).

Alternative Model of Dependent Personality Disorder

The Alternative Model of Personality Disorders offers a clinically useful description of the Dependent Personality Disorder in terms of typical features and trait facets. Typical features are a pervasive and excessive need to be taken care of that leads to submissive and clinging behavior and fears of separation (American Psychiatric Association, 2022). Trait facet criteria include submissiveness, anxiousness, and separation insecurity (Skodol, 2021).

Conceptualizations of the Dependent Personality Disorder

Psychodynamic Case Conceptualizations

Early psychoanalytic writers posited that dependent personalities were formed in the oral phase of psychosexual development. Contemporary formulations view the development of dependency as a function of parental—particularly maternal—overinvolvement and intrusiveness throughout all phases of development. These individuals often present histories of parental reward for maintaining loyalty, and subtle parental rejection whenever they attempted separation and independence. They would react with crying and clinging behavior, while being immobilized by fear and dread of abandonment. Their submissive stance is the result of multiply determined unconscious factors. Gabbard (1990) notes that dependent personalities typically seek to be cared for by others because of their underlying anxiety, which often masks aggression. Dependency thus may be viewed as a compromise formation defending against hostility. Furthermore, dependent behavior can also be used to avoid reactivation of past traumatic experiences.

Biosocial Case Conceptualization

Millon and Everly (1985) speculate that dependent personalities exhibited fearful, withdrawing, or sad temperaments as infants. Accordingly, such behaviors were likely to elicit overly protective behavior from caretakers. Millon (1981) notes that these dependent individuals tend to have ectomorphic—thin and frail—or endomorphic—heavy and cumbersome—body types, which contribute to low energy thresholds and a lack of physical vigor.

Environmental factors such as parental overprotection, competitive deficits, and social-role programming appear to interact with these biological predispositions, resulting in the dependent personality pattern. Parental overprotection often precludes the development of autonomous coping behavior, such as assertiveness, problem solving, and decision making. Hend, Baker, and Williamson (1991) report that families of individuals with Dependent Personality Disorders are characterized by low expressiveness and high control, as compared with families in clinical and normal control groups, which is indicative of the pervasive reinforcement of dependent behavior. Outside the parental relationship, these children often experience social humiliation and doubts about their efficacy in interpersonal situations. Through such repeated experiences, they learned, particularly as adolescents, that it is better to remain submissive than to strive to be competitive. Furthermore, cultural and social norms seem to reinforce passive dependent behavior patterns among women and endomorphically and ectomorphically built men. Finally, dependent personality patterns are self-perpetuating through reinforcement of dependent behaviors; avoidance of growth-promoting activities, that is, those that might be challenging, threatening, or anxiety producing; and self-detraction, by which they not only convince others that they are inferior, defective, and incapable of independence, but also themselves (Millon & Davis, 1996).

Cognitive-Behavioral Case Conceptualizations

According to Beck (2015), the dependent personality is rooted in basic assumptions about the self and the world. Typically, they view themselves as inadequate, weak, helpless, incompetent, and needy. They view others as strong, nurturing, supportive, and able to care for them. Related beliefs include needing the assistance of strong and caring individuals in order for them to survive and to make decisions for them. They also are convinced that must remain close to and not displease such individuals. Not surprisingly, such beliefs are reflected in their main strategy or pattern of subordinating themselves and pleasing others (Beck, 2015; Brauer & Reinecke, 2015).

Therefore, these individuals are likely to conclude that they must rely on someone else who is stronger and more adequate to take care of and protect them. For this security they pay a considerable price: First, they must relinquish responsibility and subordinate their own needs. Second, they must relinquish opportunities to learn such skills as assertiveness, decision making, and problem solving. Finally, they must contend with fears of rejection and abandonment if their clinging relationship ends. The main cognitive distortion of such dependent individuals is dichotomous thinking with respect to independence (Brauer & Reinecke, 2015). For example, they believe that they are both totally connected to another and dependent or totally alone and independent, with no gradation between. Also, they believe that things are either "right" or "wrong," and that there is either "absolute success" or "absolute failure." Another cognitive distortion observed among dependent personalities is "catastrophizing," particularly regarding relationships. Common cognitive distortions are: "I never would be able to do that," "I can't," and "I'm too dumb to do that."

Turkat (1990) suggests a behavioral formulation for this disorder that centers on a pervasive fear of decision making and an inability to act assertively. Since these individuals have not previously learned either of these skills, these become basic therapeutic tasks, after their overwhelming anxiety is effectively managed.

Interpersonal Case Conceptualizations

According to Benjamin (2003), persons with Dependent Personality Disorder experienced sufficient caring and attention as infants to enable them to bond with others. They also learned to rely on others and expect that others will be there to meet their needs. However, the parents of potential dependent-disordered individuals did not wean this level of nurturing when it was developmentally appropriate to do so. Subsequently, these individuals learned compliant dependent behavior, as well as to avoid autonomy at all costs. As a result, they developed poor self-concepts by default, and as adults continue to view themselves as inadequate and overly tolerant of the blaming of others. Because they have not learned to take care of self and life's demands, they must depend on others. Since they have limited coping resources, they must tolerate abuse, which is the price of the needed caretaking. Typically, dependent individuals-in-training were mocked by peers and siblings for their incompetence. As a result, their feelings of inadequacy and incompetence were reinforced and reconfirmed. In short, these individuals are characterized by marked submissiveness to a dominant other person, who presumably will provide unending nurturance and guidance. Such a relationship is maintained even if it means tolerating abuse, since dependent-disordered individuals believe themselves to be incompetent and unable to survive without the dominant other.

Integrative Case Conceptualization

The following integrative formulation provides a biopsychosocial explanation for how this personality is likely to have developed and how it is maintained. Biologically, these individuals are characterized by a low energy level. Their temperament is usually described as melancholic. As infants and young children, they were characterized as fearful, sad, or withdrawn.

Psychologically, they can be understood and appreciated in terms of their view of themselves, their world view, and their life goal. The self-view of these individuals tends to be a variant of the theme: "I'm nice, but inadequate (or fragile)." Their view of self is self-effacing, inept, and self-doubting. Their view of the world is some variant of the theme: "Others are here to take care of me, because I can't do it for myself." Their life goal is characterized by some variant of the theme: "Therefore, cling and rely on others at all cost."

The social features of this personality disorder can be described in terms of parental, familial, and environmental factors. The dependent personality is most likely to be raised in a family in which parental overprotection is prominent. It is as if the parental injunction to the child is "I can't trust you to do anything right (or well)." The dependent personality is likely to have been pampered and overprotected as a child. Contact with siblings and peers may engender feelings of unattractiveness, awkwardness, or competitive inadequacy, especially during the preadolescent and adolescent years. These can have a devastating impact on the individual, and further confirm the individual's sense of self-deprecation and doubt.

This personality is reinforced and becomes self-perpetuating by a number of factors: a sense of self-doubt, an avoidance of competitive activity; and particularly by the availability of self-reliant individuals who are willing to take care of and make decisions for the dependent person in exchange for the self-sacrificing and docile friendship of the dependent personality. (Sperry, 2015).

Table 7.2 summarizes the characteristics of this disorder.

Assessment of Dependent Personality Disorder

Several sources of information are useful in establishing a diagnosis and treatment plan for personality disorders. Observation, collateral information, and psychological testing are important adjuncts to the patient's self-report in the clinical interview. This section briefly describes some characteristic observations that the clinician makes and the nature of the rapport likely to develop in initial encounters with specific personality-disordered individuals. Characteristic response patterns on various objective (i.e., MMPI-2 and MCMI-IV) and projective (i.e., Rorschach and TAT) tests are also described.

Table 7.2 Characteristics of Dependent Personality Disorder

Triggering Event(s)	Expectations of self-reliance and/or being alone
Behavioral Style	Docile, passive, insecure, and submissive
	Lacks assertiveness
	Self-doubting and lacks self-confidence
Interpersonal Style	Pleasing, clinging, and compliant
	Requires reassurance to make decisions
	Abdicates responsibility to others
	Avoids disagreements
	Self-abasing to receive the support of others
	Urgently seeks new relationships when one ends
Cognitive Style	Suggestible and pollyannaish
Feeling Style	Pleasant and anxious, timid, or sad when stressed
Temperament	Low energy level; fearful, sad or withdrawn melancholic
Attachment Style	Preoccupied
Parental Injunction	"You can't do it by yourself"
Self-View	"I'm nice, but inadequate (or fragile)"
World View	"Others are here to take care of me, because I can't do it myself"
Maladaptive Schemas	Defectiveness; self-sacrifice; approval-seeking; self-sacrifice
Optimal Diagnostic Criteria	Needs others to assume responsibility for most major areas of his or her life

Interview Behavior and Rapport

In the initial interview, individuals with Dependent Personality Disorders will commonly wait for the clinician to initiate the conversation. After an opening statement by the clinician, these patients can present an adequate description of their current situation, but then will retreat to silence. Predictable comments are: "I don't know what to say. I've never seen a therapist before," or "Ask me questions so I'll know what's important to talk about." When the clinician responds and asks other questions, the cycle may repeat itself. Nonetheless, interviewing these individuals can be enjoyable, and establishing rapport is relatively easy. After some initial anxiety, they will begin to trust the clinician and the therapeutic process. So long as the clinician provides pleasant advice and support, and shows empathy for their indecisiveness and failures, the interview flows smoothly. However, when the clinician attempts to explore the detriments engendered by their submissiveness, they become uncomfortable and want support. If the dependency is not pursued with an empathic ear, they will change therapists. If pursued sympathetically, they will cooperate and meet their clinician's expectations. They answer questions to the point and will clarify and elaborate on demand. They can tolerate abrupt transitions and will allow deep feelings to be probed. But they cannot tolerate confrontation and interpretation of their dependency (Othmer & Othmer, 2002).

Psychological Testing Data

The Minnesota Multiphasic Personality Inventory (MMPI-2), the Millon Clinical Multi-axial Inventory (MCMI-IV), the Rorschach Psychodiagnostic Test, and the Thematic Apperception Test (TAT) can be useful in diagnosing Dependent Personality Disorder, as well as the dependent personality style or trait (Groth-Marnat, 2009).

On the MMPI-2, the most likely profile is the 2-7/7-2 (Depression-Psychasthenia), which characterizes individuals who are passive, dependent, and docile. A high 3 (Hysteria) scale is common, as is a mildly elevated K (Correction) scale (Graham, 2012). Passivity and naiveté are reflected in a high L (Lie) scale, while the F (Frequency) scale is in the average range. Acceptance of the stereotypical female role is reflected by a low scale 5 (Masculinity-Femininity). Lack of resistance to coercion from authority shows in a low 4 (Psychopathic Deviate) scale. A low scale 9 (Hypomania) reflects passivity and lack of initiative (Meyer, 1995).

On the MCMI-IV a high score on scale 3 (Dependent) would be anticipated (Millon et al., 2016). An elevation on scale A (Generalized anxiety disorder) is common, particularly when these individuals feel insecure about placing their welfare in the hands of others (Choca et al., 1992).

With regard to the Rorschach, if dependent personalities feel accepted by the examiner and believe that the examiner expects a high number of responses, they will produce an extensive record. Otherwise, fewer than average responses can be expected. Most common are A (Animal), M (Human Movement), and P (Popular) responses. Finally, C (Color) tends to be used more often than F (Form) in determining responses (Meyer, 1995).

The new Rorschach Performance Assessment System (R-PAS) is an improved method for scoring and interpreting the Rorschach Inkblot Test. Besides being evidence-based and internationally normed, it increases clinical utility and is easier to use than Exner's Comprehensive System (Mihura & Meyer, 2018).

Generally speaking, the TAT responses of dependent personalities are not particularly distinctive. However, themes of dependency and compliance are common on card 2 (Bellak, 1993).

Treatment Approaches and Interventions

Treatment Considerations

The differential diagnoses for this personality disorder include the Histrionic Personality Disorder and the Avoidant Personality Disorder. Common symptom diagnoses that are associated with the Dependent Personality Disorder include the Anxiety Disorders, particularly Simple Phobia and Social Anxiety Disorder, and Panic Disorder. Other common DSM-5-TR disorders include Conversion Disorder, and Somatic Symptom Disorder. The experience of loss of a supportive person or relationship can lead to a number of affective disorders including Persistent Depressive Disorder and Major Depressive episodes. Finally, because Dependent Personality Disorders can have lifelong training in assuming the "sick role" they are especially prone to the Factitious Disorders.

In general, the long-range goal of psychotherapy with a dependent personality is to increase the individual's sense of independence and ability to function interdependently. At other times, the therapist may need to settle for a more modest goal. That is, helping the individual become a "healthier" dependent personality. Treatment strategies typically include challenging the individual's convictions or dysfunctional beliefs about personal inadequacy, and learning ways in which to increase assertiveness. A variety of methods can be used to increase self-reliance. Among these are providing the dependent person directives and opportunities for making decisions, being alone, and taking responsibility for his or her own well-being (Sperry, 2015).

Individual Psychotherapy

For the various individual psychotherapeutic modalities, there are reports of successful treatment for Dependent Personality Disorder. Although no large case series or controlled treatment trials have yet to be published, several case reports suggest that positive treatment outcomes are common. Treatment tends to be shorter and less difficult than for other personality disorders, such as the borderline, narcissistic or antisocial personality disorder.

Psychodynamic Psychotherapy Approaches

A central purpose of psychodynamic psychotherapy is to help patients cope better with previous separations and object losses (Yeomans, Clarkin, & Levy, 2021). Patients enter therapy with the unconscious wish to reinstate earlier relationships and bring them to a more satisfactory resolution. Accordingly, the clinician comes to symbolize the object losses, and therapy succeeds if the clinician becomes a better object than the objects of the patient's childhood. The clinician gratifies certain fundamental wishes that the parent-object did not adequately gratify, as well as provides a more reasonable and benign model for identification. If therapy is a success, the internalization of the objects will be more positive and less laden with anger and guilt, thereby making separation a genuine maturational event (Strupp & Binder, 1984). A major dilemma in the psychotherapy with patients with Dependent Personality Disorders is that they do not readily relinquish the new object and tend to cling tenaciously to the clinician.

In this form of resistance, the patient leans dependently on the clinician as an end in itself, rather than as a means to an end. Thus, as therapy unfolds, these patients may forget what complaint or symptom brought them into treatment, and their only purpose becomes the maintenance of their attachment to the clinician. Dreading termination, they tend to experience a reexacerbation of their initial symptoms. They will endeavor to make the clinician collude in their avoidance of making decisions or asserting themselves in the hope of continuing their dependency. The clinician, however, must frustrate these wishes and prompt independent thoughts and actions in these patients. By conveying that the anxiety produced by this frustration is tolerable and productive, the clinician encourages the patient toward achieving insight and independence (Gabbard, 1994).

In long-term psychodynamic psychotherapy, the emergence of a dependent transference toward the clinician is thus promoted, which is then dealt with in a way to promote emotional growth. Patients are told that extra sessions may be allowed early in therapy, particularly during periods of heightened anxieties. This assurance of readily available support aids in developing a trusting relationship with and transferring dependent wishes onto the clinician. The clinician must encourage patients to express feelings and wishes and to bear the anxiety of making decisions dealing with episodes of anxiety and accepting pleasurable experiences. Furthermore, the clinician will need to clarify and interpret the transference elements, as well as support the patients in finding more self-reliant ways of coping when they plead with the clinician to take a more directive role in their lives.

During the final stage of therapy, the clinician gradually increases the level of expectation for self-initiated behavior and autonomous decision making. The clinician reinforces the patient's increased ability to cope with crises without extra sessions and to self-soothe and self-manage episodes of heightened anxiety. This requires resolution of the patient's wish to be dependent and instead to accept a more self-reliant position in the therapeutic relationship (Hill, 1970). Finally, it should be noted that individuals with Dependent Personality Disorders commonly create countertransference problems in their clinicians related to dependency conflicts. Thus clinicians must anticipate countertransference contempt or disdain toward dependent patients (Gabbard, 1994).

According to Bornstein (2012), Western society's demands to become autonomous and self-sufficient result in a series of implicit rules and restrictions placed on individuals during childhood. Ambivalence about this expectation may result in both conscious and unconscious conflicts about the "unacceptable" desire for dependency. Bronstein suggests that psychoanalytic psychotherapy is particularly well-suited to address this conflict, with the goal being to make individuals consciously aware of it and open to change. Luborsky & Crits-Cristoph (1990) developed the Core Conflictual Relationship Theme (CCRT) method to resolve dependency dynamics and conflicts. The main element of the CCRT method is an in-depth analysis of the patient's relationships. This included wishes, fears, and intentions; the other person's response; and the patient's reaction. The therapist also creates a supportive "holding environment" within the therapeutic relationship to minimize anxiety and defensiveness while working through dependency-related transference and countertransference.

Time-Limited Dynamic Psychotherapy

Kantor (1992) notes that long-term analytic psychotherapy is arduous and time-consuming and should be recommended primarily when patients are highly motivated and the dependency is ego syntonic. Otherwise, the treatment may become interminable because of such resistances as unwillingness to work hard in treatment because this means terminating therapy, which they anticipate will be unbearable. Generally speaking, long-term psychotherapy with motivated patients requires two to four sessions a week over three or more years to work through a dependent transference.

For these and other reasons, time-limited dynamic psychotherapy has been advocated as the treatment of choice for most of these patients (Flegenheimer, 1982; Gunderson, 1989). Knowing at the outset that treatment will end after 12, 16, or 20 sessions means that these patients must confront their deepest anxieties about loss and individuation, as well as their fantasies about unlimited nurturance and timelessness (Mann, 1973). Such time-limited therapies are most likely to succeed when three conditions are present: a circumscribed, dynamic conflict or focus; a patient who can quickly form a therapeutic alliance; and little or no tendency to act out or regress to severe dependency (Strupp & Binder, 1994; Luborsky, 1984). Time-limited therapy is less successful with dependent individuals who have limited ego strengths or greater degrees of separation anxiety (Gabbard, 1994). For such patients, Wallerstein (1986) suggests a supportive treatment approach in which sessions are tapered down to one every few months, provided there is no threat to termination.

Flegenheimer (1982) has critically reviewed six different brief dynamic psychotherapy approaches—those of Sifneos, Alexander, Mann, Malan, Davanloo, and Wolberg. He believes that Mann's, Alexander's, and Wolberg's approaches are tailor-made for the many dependent personality-disordered individuals. Passive, indecisive patients are likely to feel comfortable with the paternalistic stances of Alexander or Wolberg, where the clinician initially takes charge, gives advice, and makes decisions. The approach enables these patients to try new behaviors because they are "told to." The positive response to new behaviors engenders and reinforces those new patterns of behavior. Likewise, more passive dependent patients tend to do well with Mann's approach, wherein a termination date is set at the first session. The dependency of the patient allows the "golden glow" of Mann's first phase of therapy to develop to the fullest, setting the stage for subsequent disillusionment and preparing for a meaningful separation experience.

Mann's approach (1973 requires little modification of the standard analytically oriented approach and requires the least amount of confrontation of the briefer psychotherapies. Not surprisingly, this rather gentle technique tends not to engender major resistances in dependent patients.

Time-limited approaches are advocated as the starting point for treatment of most dependent patients. For those who have multifocal conflicts or otherwise fail to improve in briefer therapies, longer term dynamic therapies, supportive therapy, or psychoanalysis would be treatment options.

Cognitive Behavioral Therapy Approaches

Beck et al. (2004) provides an extended description of the cognitive therapy approach with individuals with Dependent Personality Disorders. The basic goal of therapy is increased autonomy and self-efficacy. Autonomy is defined as the capability to act independently of others, along with the capability to develop close and intimate relationships. Because dependent individuals are squeamish about the word "independent" and fear that competence will lead to abandonment, achieving these goals must be accomplished with considerable delicacy. Since these individuals often come to treatment anticipating that clinicians will solve their problems and make their decisions, it is necessary to allow some dependence initially in order to engage them. The structured collaborative nature of cognitive therapy encourages the dependent individual to play an active role in the treatment process, beginning with the agenda and goal setting. The use of guided discovery and Socratic questioning early in treatment helps these individuals to begin to face their own solutions and decisions, reducing overreliance on the therapist and others. As therapy proceeds, progress toward goals can be utilized as powerful evidence to challenge the dependent individual's assumptions of personal helplessness.

Challenging the dichotomous belief about independence—that one is both totally dependent and helpless or totally independent and isolated—helps to modify the distorted notion that autonomy is a commitment to total alienation. Besides challenging and disputing automatic beliefs and maladaptive schemas concerning dependency and helplessness, therapists are encouraged to utilize behavioral methods such as assertiveness training and behavioral experiments, as well as to modify the very structure of therapy.

This modification can be accomplished in several ways, such as by gradually changing to a group format or concurrent individual and group therapy, "weaning" sessions by scheduling them less frequently toward the end of the therapy or setting a specific termination date early in treatment and focusing therapy as preparation for termination. Since termination typically evokes rejection and abandonment schemas in these individuals, offering the option of one or two booster sessions—late in the course of treatment—following termination can ease the transition. In short, the cognitive treatment of Dependent Personality Disorders begins with a collaborative relationship in which the therapist allows a measure of dependency, which is gradually replaced with guided discovery, and challenges the dichotomy beliefs of independence. As treatment proceeds, schema reconstruction and modification of the structure of treatment, along with behavioral methods, are utilized to achieve treatment goals (Fowler, Orme, & Hart, 2021).

It is particularly important that the therapist monitor his or her thoughts and feelings toward the dependent patient. Therapists may feel the urge to forego thorough evaluation or make other exceptions for these seemingly "pathetic" individuals. In this case, the therapist's directiveness is covertly aiding the patient's pathological pattern and undermining the goal of autonomy. It may be useful for the therapist to create a Dysfunctional Thought Record to determine whether any deviations from protocol are in the interest of the patient or whether they foster continued dependence. Beck and associates note that dependent patients are more likely than others to report that they have fallen in love with therapists. Therefore, it is of particular importance to avoid "special" treatment.

A more behaviorally oriented approach to this disorder is based on the formulation that the dependent personality is hypersensitive to independent decision making (Turkat, 1990). The corresponding behavioral strategy is bidirectional anxiety management procedures focused on independent decision making. Since individuals with Dependent Personality Disorder are often undersocialized, social skills training may be indicated. Assertive communication and friendship and dating skills are often minimal in lower functioning dependent patients. Fay and Lazarus (1993) offer cognitive-behavioral protocols in assertiveness, friendship, and dating skills. Brauer, L. & Reinecke, M. (2015) recommend that therapists help dependent patients face the sources of their anxiety by developing behavioral skills in a systematic, graduated fashion. This may be accomplished via modeling by the therapist during sessions, *in vivo* practice, and observing others who are more autonomous and assertive.

Cognitive Coping Therapy. Cognitive Coping Therapy is an active, directive, didactic and structured approach for treating personality-disordered individuals (Sharoff, 2002). It is a complete and self-contained approach to treatment which begins with assessing an individual's coping skills–in terms of skill chains, subskills and microskills–and then increasing skill competence in targeted areas as needed. Five key skill areas with representative treatment modalities include: *cognitive skills*–problem solving, self-instruction training and self-management; *emotion skills* – emotional containment and compartmentalization; *perceptual skills* – perspective taking, thought stopping, and psychological distance taking; *physiological skills* –meditation and relaxation training, and *behavior skills*–communication and assertiveness training. Sharoff (2002) describes a detailed protocol—and clinical example—for using this structured approach with a complex and difficult Dependent Personality Disorder case.

Schema Therapy. Schema Therapy is an elaboration of cognitive therapy that has been developed by Young (Young, Klosko, & Weishaar, 2003) specifically for personality disorders, and other difficult individual and couples problems. Schema Therapy involves identifying maladaptive schemas and planning specific strategies and interventions. Four main strategies are cognitive, experiential, behavioral and the therapeutic relationship itself. Cognitive restructuring, modification of maladaptive schemas, is an important cognitive strategy, but is combined with imagery exercises, empathic confrontation, homework assignments and "limited reparenting," i.e., a form of corrective emotional experience (Young et al., 2003).

Maladaptive schemas typically associated with Dependent Personality Disorder are: *defectiveness*: i.e., the belief that one is defective, bad, unwanted, or inferior in important respects; *dependence*, i.e. the belief that one is unable to competently everyday responsibilities without considerable help from others; *approval-seeking*, i.e., the belief that one must constantly seek to belong and be accepted at the expense of developing a true sense of self; and *self-sacrifice, i.e.,* the belief that one must meet the needs of others at the expense of one's own gratification (Bernstein, 2002).

Interpersonal Approach

For Benjamin (2003), psychotherapeutic interventions with persons with Dependent Personality Disorders can be planned and evaluated in terms of whether they enhance collaboration, facilitate learning about maladaptive patterns and their roots, block these patterns, enhance the will to change, and effectively encourage new patterns.

According to Benjamin, those with dependent personality disorder appear to be the ideal patient, at least superficially. They comply with all recommendations and prescriptions, from homework to paperwork and payment. The more authoritative the therapist is, the more the dependent goes along for the ride. However, she notes that the dependent individual's apparent attitude of friendly cooperation actually complicates the development of a collaborative therapeutic alliance and undermines efforts to change. Essentially, eliciting more and better help from clinicians is the agenda for dependent individuals. They see no reason to collaborate with clinicians against their maladaptive pattern of dependency. Therapy may go on forever. The clinician's challenge at the onset of treatment is to engage with the position opposite their usual one: stop submitting, learn about being independent, and separate. Initially, this seems impossible for these individuals because, with their histories of intense enmeshment, they cannot understand what it means to be differentiated. They believe that there are only two options: to control others or to submit to others. Since they believe that controlling represents bossiness, aggressivity, and bullying of others, they reject it in favor of submission. However, if they are helped to understand that separation and competence, rather than control, are the opposite of submission, they can change. Blocking maladaptive patterns in dependent individuals often requires the assistance of their significant others, such as family members. The paradoxical suggestion that others restrict their offers of help at times when dependent individuals are functioning well is a way to reward independent behavior. Such suggestions must be followed with other interventions that change the strong wish to be dependent and strengthen the wish to become more competent and independent.

Essentially, dependent individuals must first recognize their dependent pattern and the high price they pay to maintain it, and then explore alternatives. To the extent that they can collaborate against "it" and face the present-day meaning of this pattern, they may decide to change. As this occurs, the implementation of a new pattern is relatively straightforward. Benjamin points out that standard behavioral techniques such as assertiveness communication and feeling identification and expression can be quite effective.

Group Therapy

Group treatment has been shown to be successful in the treatment of Dependent Personality Disorders. Two considerations are involved in deciding whether group treatment will be an effective format. The first consideration relates to the patient's degree of impairment; where motivation and potential for growth exist, a more interactional psychotherapy group may be indicated (Ogrodniczuk, Uliaszek, Lebow, & Kealy, 2021). Such a context provides a therapeutic milieu for exploring the inappropriateness of passive dependent behavior and for experimenting with greater assertiveness (Yalom, 1985). However, if dependent traits reflect severe personality impairment or the absence of prosocial behavior such as assertive communication, decision making, and negotiation, an ongoing supportive problem-solving group or a social skills training group might be indicated. The second consideration refers to whether referral should be made to a homogeneous group, with treatment targeted at dependency issues shared by all group members, or a heterogeneous group, where group members have different personality styles or disorders. Frances et al. (1984) provide selection criteria for both types of group formats. Clinical lore suggests that dependent patients tend to get "lost" in heterogeneous groups. Yalom (1995) seems to be describing the dependent personality in his discussion of the "silent patient" in groups. Yet time-limited assertiveness-training groups that are homogeneous and have clearly defined goals have been shown to be very effective (Lazarus, 1981).

Two studies involving the treatment of dependent patients have been reported in the literature. Montgomery (1971) utilized homogeneous group formats for dependent patients who were previously being seen in an individual format in a clinical setting. The patients were described as clinging and dependent, and as expecting magical cures and medication. Engagement within the group provided the patients with the opportunity to redirect their attention-seeking behavior from regressive to more socially adaptive purposes. Montgomery reports that all but three of 30 patients eventually discontinued medication. Sadoff and Collins (1968) reported group therapy for dependent patients who also stuttered. Weekly group treatment, which emphasized dynamic interpretation, was shown to be effective. Positive changes in stuttering and dependency were reported.

Marital and Family Therapy

The professional literature on family therapy interventions with the Dependent Personality Disorders is almost nonexistent. Harbir (1981) notes that individuals with Dependent Personality Disorders are usually brought to family therapy by their parents. They are frequently older adolescents or young adults between the ages of 20 and 35 who present with a neurotic or psychotic symptom. Harbir describes a prototypical case of a 29-year-old man with a diagnosis of dependent personality who essentially was totally dependent on his parents for his maintenance. A more functional younger sister had moved out on her own the previous year. Although he did some part-time work at home for his father, he neither made his own meals, cleaned his own room, nor washed his own clothes. He was content to live the rest of his life with his parents, if they would permit it. There was no clear-cut presenting problem, other than the identified patient's unwillingness to work outside the home. Clearly, the son, mother, and father were deeply enmeshed, although the son was much more dependent on the mother than the father, and vice versa. Structural techniques were employed by the clinician to decrease the intensity of the mother-child interaction. Essentially, various tasks were prescribed that encouraged the father and son to form a separate relationship. Tasks that encouraged social activities outside the family also were prescribed. Since the son had developed few peer relationships, these tasks initially were quite difficult for both the son and his parents.

After one year of family treatment, the son was able to emancipate sufficiently and could work and socialize outside the home. Could these results have been accomplished in individual therapy? Perhaps, but it was not likely in that time frame, and without some cooperation from the parents. Changing the enmeshed family relationship tends to be anxiety provoking for all parties, and thus there is considerable resistance from other family members when only one member of the family is in therapy.

Very little has been published on marital therapy for persons with Dependent Personality Disorders. Malinow (1981) notes that dependent patients can function adequately if their marital partners consistently meet their needs, but typically become symptomatic and impaired when that support is withdrawn or withheld. Turkat (1990) believes that it is useful to engage the cooperation of the marital partner in treatment for two reasons: (1) because of the negative impact on the relationship as the dependent individual becomes less anxious and more independent; and (2) because the patient's progress can be facilitated if the partner collaborates in accomplishing the treatment goals. Barlow and Waddell (1985) describe a time-limited couples group for the treatment of agoraphobia. Most of the symptomatic partners exhibited features of the dependent personality. In group, the nonsymptomatic partners took the roles of "coach" and "confidant," collaborating on treatment goals. Taking on these roles meant relinquishing the role in which they reinforced their partner's agoraphobia and dependency. During the course of this ten-session treatment protocol, not only did panic and agoraphobia symptoms remit, but the marital relationship shifted from dependency to more interdependence.

A common marital relational pattern is the dependent/narcissistic couple in which one partner presents with Dependent Personality Disorder and the other partner presents with Narcissistic Personality Disorder. Nurse (1998) provides a detailed rationale and treatment protocol for working with such couples based on Millon's theory of personality disorders (Millon & Davis, 1996).

Links & Stockwell (2004) examined couples therapy for patients with dependent personality disorder and identified two dimensions of dependency that determine whether or not patients benefit from this type of intervention. They provide details surrounding two cases to represent each dimension. The first focuses on interpersonal dependency that results from insecure attachment. Links & Stockwell note that this couple failed to benefit from couples therapy because of an enmeshed relationship. The second dimension involves a lack of assertiveness and self-confidence in the dependent individual. These deficits result in a crisis within the relationship that may successfully be addressed in the context of couple's therapy. The authors maintain that it is imperative to determine which dependence dimension predominates to evaluate the appropriateness of couples therapy.

Beck et al. (2004) explain that treatment geared towards increasing the autonomy and assertiveness of the dependent individual may result in upsetting his or her spouse. Often times, the significant others of those with dependent personality disorder enjoy the unequal balance of the power in the relationship and may see changes to this as a threat. In this case, marital or family therapy can help family members adjust to changes in the identified patient and potentially grow as a unit (Ogrodniczuk, Uliaszek, Lebow, & Kealy, 2021). If, however, significant others are not willing to accept the changes brought about in treatment, the dependent individual must determine whether or not to end the relationship.

Medication

Currently, there are no psychotropic medications specifically indicated for treating individuals with dependent personality disorder (Silk & Feurino, 2012). Nevertheless, medications are used that target specific troubling symptoms associated with the disorder, such as depression, anxiety, or sleep problems. Generally, these medications are used as an adjunct to psychotherapy and skills training (Nelson & Tsheringld, 2021). Because troubling symptoms often respond to medications sooner than most psychological interventions, medications are usually prescribed at the onset of treatment (Sperry, 1995b). Unfortunately, there is little research evidence to provide guidelines for the use of such medications with this disorder (Silk & Feurino, 2012).

Combined and Integrative Treatment Approaches

In many ways, the dependent personality is an "orphan" in the clinical literature, and this certainly is evident in the area of combined and integrative treatment. Another type of combined treatment involves utilizing different modalities simultaneously. Barlow and Waddell's (1985) effort to combine behavior therapy in a group setting with couples was previously described. Not surprisingly, the results of combining modalities are noteworthy. Lazarus (1981, 1985) provides further documentation about the overall efficacy, and cost effectiveness, of multimodal interventions.

Until a few years ago little has been written regarding integrative treatment (Winkeller & Schlesinger, 2021). Nevertheless, clinical practice is replete with efforts to utilize anxiety-reducing strategies in both dynamic and cognitive therapies. For example, Glantz and Goisman (1990) describe a unique integration of relaxation techniques with object-relations psychodynamic psychotherapy with dependent patients. A breath controlling and progressive muscle-relaxation strategy was used to merge split self-representations in the course of exploration psychotherapy. The technique was introduced after signs of split self-representation had been identified. Patients were taught the technique, and it was prescribed as an intersession treatment task. Once they were able to relax adequately in session, they were asked for visual images of first one and then another of the conflicting self-representations. After clear images had been elicited and discussed, they were encouraged to merge the images. Twenty-four of the 27 personality-disordered patients in the study, many of whom were dependent personalities, responded with greater compliance, improved interpersonal relationships, and reduced resistance.

For those with co-morbid dependent personality and substance use disorders, Ekleberry (2014) states that participation in self-help programs such as AA and NA may be helpful; however, she cautions that these individuals may fall prey to aggressive and narcissistic group members.

Chapter 8

Histrionic Personality Disorder

Individuals with histrionic personalities initially appear to be charming, likable, energetic, and seductive, but as time passes, they may be viewed as emotionally unstable, immature, and egocentric. While it is noted in males, this personality pattern predominates in females, and typically presents with a caricature of femininity in dress and manner (Blashfield, Reynolds, & Stennett, 2012; Skodol, Bender, & Oldham, 2019; American Psychiatric Association, 2022).

While treatment of such individuals involves a number of unique therapeutic challenges, it can be highly effective and successful.

This chapter describes a framework for the assessment and effective treatment of this disorder. It includes sections on diagnosis, psychological assessment, case conceptualization, and treatment interventions. It begins with background information on the disorder as well as the DSM-5-TR description, prototypic description, associated features, and the Alternative Model of Personality Disorders description of this disorder. The section on case conceptualization provides five common clinical formulations of this disorder: psychodynamic, biosocial, cognitive-behavioral, interpersonal, and an integrative conceptualization of this disorder. Several treatment approaches, modalities, and intervention strategies are also described. These include individual psychotherapy, group therapy, marital and family therapy, medication, and integrative and combined treatment.

Description of the Histrionic Personality Disorder

The Histrionic Personality Disorder can be recognized by the following descriptors and characteristics: styles vs. disorders, triggering event, behavioral styles, interpersonal styles, cognitive styles, affective styles, attachment style, and optimal criterion.

Style vs. Disorder. This histrionic personality can be thought of as spanning a continuum from healthy to pathological, wherein the histrionic personality style is on the healthy end and the Histrionic Personality Disorder is on the pathological end. Table 8.1 compares and contrasts the histrionic personality style and disorder.

The following two case examples further illustrate differences between the Histrionic Personality Disorder (Ms. P.) and the histrionic personality style (Mr. M.).

Case Study: Histrionic Personality Disorder

Ms. P. is a 20-year-old female undergraduate student who requested psychological counseling at the College Health Services for "boyfriend problems." Actually, she had taken a nonlethal overdose of minor tranquilizers the day before coming to the Health Services. She said she took the overdose in an attempt to kill herself because "life wasn't worth living" after her boyfriend had left the afternoon before. She was an attractive, well-dressed woman adorned with makeup and nail polish, which contrasted sharply with the very casual fashion of most coeds on campus. During the initial interview she was warm and charming, maintained good eye contract, yet was mildly seductive. At two points in the interview she was emotionally labile, shifting from smiling elation to tearful sadness. Her boyfriend had accompanied her to the evaluation session and asked to talk to the clinician. He stated the reason he had left the patient was because she made demands on him which he could not meet, and that he "hadn't been able to satisfy her emotionally or sexually." Also, he noted that he could not afford to "take her out every night and party."

Case Study: Histrionic Personality Style

Mr. M. is a 41 year old literary agent who spent the early years of his career representing non-fiction writers with major publishing houses. He has been quite successful for several years but has also become somewhat disenchanted with is behind the scenes efforts. While he has made several of his clients extraordinarily wealthy and famous he dreamed of the time when he too would be financially independent and in the limelight. When cable T.V. licenses became available, he sensed the opportunity to fulfill his dream. He would become president of his own station and host his own talk show. After all, he had several high-visibility clients whom he could get to be guests on his show. He set out to garner financing for his plan. With his charming manner and alluring vision, he quickly intrigued several backers and got the station launched. The only problem was he hadn't thought much about the production side of the enterprise. He quickly arranged for interviews for an executive producer. William T. was the fourth person he interviewed. Trevor knew as soon as he walked in that he was right for the job. After a ten minute interview William was hired. Mr. M's hunch about both William and the success of the talk show he hosted proved to be right.

Triggering Event. The typical situation, circumstance or event that most likely triggers or activates the characteristic maladaptive response of the Histrionic Personality Disorder Personality Disorder (Othmer & Othmer, 2002), as noted in behavioral, interpersonal, cognitive, and feeling styles, is: "opposite sex relationships."

Behavioral Style. The behavioral style is characterized as charming, dramatic, and expressive, while also being demanding, self-indulgent, and inconsiderate. Persistent attention-seeking, mood lability, capriciousness, and superficiality further characterize their behavior.

Table 8.1 Comparison of Histrionic Personality Style and Disorder

Personality Style	Personality Disorder
Enjoy compliments and praise	Constantly seeks or demands reassurance, approval or praise
Charming, engaging and appropriately seductive in appearance and behavior.	Inappropriately sexually seductive in appearance or behavior
Attentive to their appearance and grooming, enjoying clothes, style and fashion	Overly concerned with physical attractiveness
Lively and fun-loving, often impulsive, but can delay gratification	Expresses emotion with inappropriate exaggeration; self-centered and little tolerance for gratification
Enjoy being the center of attention, and can rise to the occasion when all eyes are on them	Uncomfortable in situations where they cannot be the center of attention
Sensation-oriented, emotionally demonstrative and physically affectionate. React emotionally but appropriately.	Display rapidly shifting and shallow expression of emotion.
Utilize and style of speech which his appropriately global and specific.	Utilize a style of speech that is excessively impressionistic and lacking in detail.

Interpersonal Style. Interpersonally, these individuals tend to be exhibitionistic and flirtatious in their manner, with attention-seeking and manipulativeness being prominent. They also tend to have empathic deficits, just as narcissistic personality-disordered individuals.

Cognitive Style. The cognitive or thinking style of this personality can be characterized as impulsive and thematic, rather than being analytical, precise and field-independent. Their tendency is to be non-analytic, vague, and field-dependent. They are highly suggestible and rely heavily on hunches and intuition. They avoid awareness of their own hidden dependency and other self-knowledge and tend to be "other-directed" with respect to the need for approval from others. Therefore, they can easily dissociate their "real" or inner self from their "public" or outer self.

Emotional Style. Their emotional or feeling style is characterized by exaggerated emotional displays and excitability including irrational outbursts and temper tantrums. Although they are constantly seeking reassurance that they are loved, they respond with only superficial warmth and charm and are generally emotionally shallow. Finally, they are exquisitely rejection sensitive.

Attachment Style. The preoccupied attachment dimension is characterized by a sense of personal unworthiness and a positive evaluation of others. These individuals tend to be rather externally oriented in their self-definitions. The Preoccupied Attachment Style is common in individuals with Histrionic Personality Disorder.

Optimal Diagnostic Criterion. Of all the diagnostic criteria for the Dependent Personality Disorder, one criterion has been found to be the most useful in diagnosing this disorder. The belief is that by beginning with this criterion, the clinician can test for the presence or absence of the criterion and quickly diagnose the personality disorder (Allnutt & Links, 1996). The "optimal criterion" for this disorder is: "uncomfortable in situations in which he or she is not the center of attention."

DSM-5-TR Description

Individuals with this personality disorder are characterized by an unremitting pattern of attention seeking and emotionality. They tend to be uncomfortable in situations where they cannot be the center of attention. Their emotional reactions tend to be shallow and rapidly shifting. Typically, they draw attention to themselves with the way they dress. Their manner of speech tends to be impressionistic with few details. These individuals are easily influenced by others or circumstances. They are likely to perceive relationships as more intimate than they really are. They often engage in provocative and inappropriate seductive sexual behavior. Furthermore, they are dramatic and overly exaggerate their emotional expressions (American Psychiatric Association, 2022).

Prototypic Description

A prototype is a brief description that captures the essence of how a particular disorder commonly presents. Prototypic descriptions are useful and convenient, and clinicians commonly rely on them rather than lists of behavioral criteria or core beliefs (Westen, 2012). Here is a common prototypic description of the Histrionic Personality Disorder: These individuals are the exhibitionists in life. If they are female they use charm, physical appeal, and seductiveness to command attention. There is an intensity to their relationships and emotions, but a shallowness at the same time. If they are male, they are more likely to command attention by bragging about a business deal or investment, or their prowess in sports or sex. Their interests and attitudes are easily influenced by what others think and value. They come on strong and seek intimacy quickly. But such intimacy wears thin quickly which leaves them feeling unappreciated (Francis, 2013).

Associated Features

Prevalence. HPD has been identified in 1.2 percent of the general population and 9.7 percent in clinical practice (Torgersen, 2021).

Differential Diagnosis. HPD is not uncommonly mistaken for Borderline Personality Disorder since both disorders share common traits like attention seeking, manipulation, and rapidly shifting moods. However, BPD is differentiated from HPD by self-destructiveness, chronic feelings of emptiness, and disruptive anger in close relationships. Furthermore, individuals may display histrionic personality traits, but it is only when these traits become inflexible, maladaptive, and impairing that HPD is diagnosable (American Psychiatric Association, 2022).

Development and Course. HPD appears to develop as a result of both genetics and childhood experiences. Children of parents with HPD may exhibit histrionic behavior they learned from a parent or as a way to get attention from their parents Child abuse and neglect, lack of discipline, or positive reinforcement of dramatic behaviors in childhood can be causal. This pattern is usually evident by the age of 15 (Yalch, Ceroni & Dehart, 2023).

Culture, Sex, and Gender. In clinical settings HPD is more frequently diagnosed in females. However, the gender ratio is not significant different from the ratio of females to males within those clinical settings. The presence of HPD should be distinguished from reactive and contextual expression of histrionic traits that arise in response to socialization pressures in competitive peer groups including the need to be liked rather than pervasive and enduring traits consistent with this disorder (American Psychiatric Association, 2022).

Alternative Model of Histrionic Personality Disorder

The Alternative Model of Personality Disorders (AMPD) offers a clinically useful description of the Histrionic Personality Disorder in terms of typical features and trait facets. Typical features are a pervasive pattern of excessive emotionality and attention seeking (American Psychiatric Association, 2022). Trait facet criteria include Emotional lability, Attention seeking, Manipulativeness (Skodol, 2021).

Conceptualizations of the Histrionic Personality Disorder

Psychodynamic Case Conceptualizations

Gabbard (1990) argues that the Histrionic Personality Disorder needs to be distinguished from the Hysterical Personality Disorder. The later has a central place the tradition of psychoanalytic thinking and refers to a higher functioning healthier group of patients, then the group characterized by DSM-5-TR criteria. Histrionic females typically lack maternal nurturance and turn to their fathers for gratification of their dependence needs. They learn that they can gain their father's attention through flirtatious and exhibitionistic displays of emotion. As she matures, she learns she must repress her genital sexuality to remain "daddy's little girl." Similarly, histrionic males will have also experienced maternal deprivation and turned to their fathers for nurturance. If their father is emotionally unavailable, they may develop a passive, effeminate identification or hyper masculine one in reaction to anxiety about effeminacy. He may not become homosexual, but his heterosexual relationships are means of reassuring himself relative to underlying genital inadequacy. These men will be disappointed with all women since they cannot measure up to mother. Some will choose a celibate life style to maintain their loyalty to their mother, while others will indulge in macho behavior such as body building and Don Juanism, i.e., compulsive seduction of women, to reassure themselves they are "real men" (Kellerman & Burry, 1989).

Biosocial Case Conceptualizations

Millon (1981) and Millon and Davis (1996) note that individuals with Histrionic Personality Disorders often display a high degree of emotional lability and responsiveness during infancy and early childhood which they attribute to low excitability thresholds for limbic and posterior hypothalamic nuclear. However, environmental factors seem to play the major role in the development of this pathology. Millon and Everly (1985) list three such factors: parental reinforcement of attention-seeking behavior; histrionic parental role models; and reinforcement of interpersonally manipulative behavior. In effect, as children these individuals learned to employ cuteness, charm, attractiveness, and seduction to secure parental reinforcement. Furthermore, this disorder is self-perpetuated through short-lived relationships, preoccupation with externals and massive repression. Specifically, by sealing off and repressing aspects of their inner worlds, histrionic individuals deny themselves opportunities to develop psychologically.

Cognitive-Behavioral Case Conceptualizations

Beck (2015) describes a cognitive therapy view of the Histrionic Personality Disorder based on specific underlying assumptions and cognitive distortions. Two underlying assumptions are posited: "I am inadequate and unable to handle life by myself" and "I must be loved by everyone to be worthwhile." Believing they are incapable of caring for themselves, histrionic individuals actively seek the attention and approval of others and expect others to take care of them and their needs. Believing they must be loved and approved by others promotes rejection sensitivity. Finally, feeling inadequate and desperate for approval, they are under considerable pressure to seek attention by "performing" for others. These beliefs also give rise to a thinking style characterized as impressionistic, global and unfocused which is not conducive to a differentiated sense of self (Sungar & Gunduz, 2015). Not surprisingly, this global, exaggerated thinking style engenders common cognitive distortions (Beck, 2015), such as dichotomous thinking, overgeneralization and emotional reasoning.

Taking a more behavioral tact, Turkat (1990), differentiates the Histrionic Personality Disorder in two types: the controlling type in which the basic motivation is achieving total control through the use of manipulative and dramatic ploys; and the reactive type in which the basic motivation is seeking reassurance and approval. Turkat does not believe the controlling type is amenable to behavior treatment. Unable to read other's emotions and interventions accurately, these individuals remain shallow, self-centered and uncomfortable when immediate reinforcement is not immediately forthcoming from others. In short, they suffer from a primary deficit in empathy.

Interpersonal Case Conceptualizations

For Benjamin (1996), persons with Histrionic Personality Disorder were likely to be loved for their good looks and entertainment value, rather than for competence or personal strength. They learned that physical appearance and charm could be used to control important others. The household of histrionic personalities tended to be a shifting stage. Unpredictable changes stemmed from parental instability, possibly associated with alcohol or substance use. The chaos in these families was more likely to be dramatic and interesting rather than primitive and life threatening as with borderline personalities. On the other hand, the help seeking histrionic subtypes were likely to be nurtured for being ill. They learned that complaints and disabilities were an effective way to elicit warm concern. Along with encouragement of denial these families rewarded sickness. Finally, they exhibit a strange fear of being ignored, together with a wish to be loved and taken care of by important others, who can be controlled through charm or sickness. In short, a friendly trust is accompanied by a secretly disrespectful agenda of forcing delivery of the desired nurturance and love. Inappropriate seductive behaviors and manipulative suicide attempts exemplify such coercions.

Integrative Case Conceptualization

The following integrative formulation provides a biopsychosocial explanation for how this personality is likely to have developed and how it is maintained. Biologically and temperamentally, the histrionic personality is characterized by a high energy level and emotional and autonomic reactivity. Millon and Everly (1985) noted that histrionic adults tended to display a similarly high degree of emotional lability and responsiveness as they did in infancy and early childhood. Their temperament then can be characterized as hyperresponsive and externally oriented towards gratification.

Psychologically, they can be understood and appreciated in terms of their view of themselves, their world view, and their life goal. The self-view of the histrionic will be some variant of the theme: "I am sensitive, and everyone should admire and approve of me." The world view will be some variant of: "Life makes me nervous so I am entitled to special care and consideration." Life goal is some variant of the theme: "Therefore, play to the audience, and live in the moment."

In addition to biological and psychological factors, social factors such as parenting style and injunction, and family and environmental factors influence the development of the histrionic personality. The parental injunction for the histrionic personality involves reciprocity: "I'll give you attention, if you do X." A parenting style that involves minimal or inconsistent discipline helps insure and reinforce the histrionic pattern. The histrionic child is likely to grow up with at least one manipulative or histrionic parent who reinforces the child's histrionic and attention-seeking behavior. Finally, the following sequence of self and system perpetuants are likely to be seen in the Histrionic Personality Disorder: denial of one's real or inner self; a preoccupation with externals; the need for excitement and attention seeking which leads to a superficial charm and interpersonal presence; and the need for external approval. This, in turn, further reinforces the dissociation and denial of the real or inner self from the public self, and the cycle continues (Sperry, 2016). Table 8.2 summarizes these characteristics.

Table 8.2 Characteristics of Histrionic Personality Disorder

Behavioral Style:	Self-dramatization
	Suggestibility
	Charming and excitement-seeking
Interpersonal Style:	Needs to attract others' attention
	Seductive or provocative interactions
	Exhibitionistic and/or flirtatious
	Misreads intimacy of relationships
Cognitive Style:	Impulsive
	Thematic, field-dependent
	Impressionistic style of speech
Feeling Style:	Rapidly shifting, shallow expression of emotions
	Exaggerated emotional display
Temperament:	Hyperresponsive infantile pattern
	Externally oriented for gratification
Attachment Style	Preoccupied
Parental Injunction:	"I'll give you attention when you do what I want"
Self-View:	"I need to be noticed"
World View:	"Life makes me so nervous, so I'm entitled to special care and consideration"
Maladaptive Schemas	Approval-Seeking; Emotional Deprivation; Defectiveness
Optimal Diagnostic Criteria	Is uncomfortable in situations in which he or she is not the center of attention

Assessment of Histrionic Personality Disorder

Several sources of information are useful in establishing a diagnosis and treatment plan for personality disorders. Observation, collateral information, and psychological testing are important adjuncts to the patient's self-report in the clinical interview. This section briefly describes some characteristic observations that the clinician makes and the nature of the rapport likely to develop in initial encounters with specific personality-disordered individuals. Characteristic response patterns on various objective (i.e., MMPI-2 and MCMI-III) and projective tests (i.e., Rorschach and TAT) are also described.

Interview Behavior and Rapport. Interviewing Histrionic Personality Disordered individuals can be enjoyable but, at the same time, challenging. Initially these individuals may be more interested in admiration and approval than in a therapeutic relationship. Rapport, therefore, may be difficult to establish. Exaggerated emotionality, vagueness, superficiality, and phoniness are common in the first encounter. With a male clinician, histrionic females may be flirtatious and seductive. But, with a female clinician they are more likely to engage in a power struggle. To elicit sufficient information to complete a diagnostic evaluation usually requires the clinician to overcome their vagueness and dramatic exaggerations. Open-ended and unstructured questions are not useful since these individual easily become sidetracked. It is preferable to pursue a main theme such as a work problem or an interpersonal conflict and elicit concrete examples, while curbing rambling and contradictions. Confronting contradictions typically results in anger and loss of rapport. Instead, express empathy and encouragement. It is predictable that when they feel empathy and understanding slipping away, that they will return to dramatization (Othmer & Othmer, 2002).

Psychological Testing Data. The Minnesota Multiphase Personality Inventory (MMPI-2), the Millon Clinical Multiaxial Inventory (MCMI-II), the Rorschach Psychodiagnostic Test, and the Thematic Apperception Test (TAT) can be useful in diagnosing the Histrionic Personality Disorder as well as the Histrionic Personality Style or trait (Groth-Marnat, 2009).

On the MMPI-2 the 2-3/3-2 (Depression-Hysteria) profile is most commonly found. When clinically distressed these individuals are likely to have elevations on 2 greater than 7OT. If not, scale 3 will be more elevated. The 3-4/4-3 (Hysteria-Psychopathic deviant) and 4-9/9-4 (Psychopathic Deviant-Hypermania) patterns are also noted in these individuals Graham, 2012). Scales 4, 7 (Psychasthenia), and 8 (Schizophrenia) may also be moderately elevated, with scale 4 reflecting their tendency to be overdramatic and self-absorbed, while self-doubt and anxiety raise the 7 score, and impulsive emotionality elevating the 8. Scale 5 is also likely to be elevated in males—but quite low in females—reflecting the association of hysteria with traditional feminine role behavior (Meyer, 1995).

On the MCMI-IV, an elevation on scale 4A (Histrionic) is expected (Millon et al., 2016). Because these individuals are attention seekers, scales 1 (Schizoid) and 2 (Avoidant) tend to be very low, while H (Somatic symptom disorder) may be high, since somatization can be used as an attention getting device, as can N (Bipolar I disorder) (Choca et al., 1992).

On the Rorschach, these individuals provide a low number of responses, as well as a low number of W (Whole), M (Human Movement), C (Pure Color), and shading (Y, YF, or T) responses. Occasionally, these individuals will give a "blood" response to a color card (Meyer, 1995). The new Rorschach Performance Assessment System (R-PAS) is an improved method for scoring and interpreting the Rorschach Inkblot Test. Besides being evidence-based and internationally normed, it increases clinical utility and is easier to use than Exner's Comprehensive System (Mihura & Meyer, 2018).

On the TAT, these individuals typically produce stories containing dependency and control themes. Their stories may also become personalized, generating some affective display. Occasionally, blocking occurs on cards with sexual or aggressive percepts. Rarely, primitive splitting may be noted in characters that are all good or all bad on incongruous juxtapositions (Bellak, 1993).

Treatment Approaches and Interventions

Treatment Considerations

The differential diagnosis of the Histrionic Personality Disorder includes the Narcissistic Personality Disorder and the Dependent Personality Disorder. It also includes the Histrionic-Borderline Disorder which is a decompensated version of the Histrionic Personality Disorder. Also, Millon (1981) describes a Histrionic-Antisocial Personality Disorder. Associated symptom diagnoses include: Persistent Depressive Disorder, Social Anxiety Disorder, and Obsessive-Compulsive Personality Disorder. In addition, Major Depression and Bipolar Disorders are common in the decompensated Histrionic Personality Disorder.

The treatment of the Histrionic Personality Disorder may present a considerable challenge for clinicians. For the purposes of this discussion, we will limit ourselves to some general considerations about treatment goals, limits, and medications. General treatment goals include helping the individual integrate gentleness with strength, moderating emotional expression, and encouraging warmth, genuineness, and empathy. Because the histrionic personality can present as dramatic, impulsive, seductive, and manipulative with potential for suicidal gestures, the clinician needs to discuss the matter of limits early in the course of therapy regarding professional boundaries and personal responsibilities. Some histrionic personalities, particularly those that bear some resemblance to "hysteroid dysphoria," may respond to certain antidepressants. Otherwise, unless a concurrent acute psychotic or major depressive episode is present, psychotherapy is the principal mode of treatment (Sperry, 2015).

Individual Psychotherapy

This section will briefly review the major psychotherapeutic approaches for treating the Histrionic Personality Disorder in an individual psychotherapy format. Later sections will describe other treatment formats such as group therapy, couples therapy, and pharmacotherapy. The individual treatment approaches are: psychodynamic psychotherapy, cognitive-behavioral therapy, and interpersonal psychotherapy.

Psychodynamic Psychotherapy Approach

Gabbard (1990) is quite optimistic about the responsiveness of higher functioning individuals with Histrionic Personality Disorder to psychoanalytically oriented psychotherapy. He reports that such individuals readily develop a therapeutic alliance and perceive the therapist as helpful. On the other hand, Gabbard believes that treatment with lower functioning individuals with this personality disorder should employ therapeutic strategies utilized for the borderline personality disorder.

Winer and Pollock (1989) indicate the basic dynamic in all presentations of the Histrionic Personality Disorder is the excessive, unresolved effort to have all of their needs met by someone else. The general goal of dynamically oriented therapies is to examine the origins of the pattern and explore the neurotic strategies: seductiveness, temper tantrums, charm, or logical thinking—these individuals employ in order to fulfill their needs (Yeomans, Clarkin, & Levy, 2021).

The classical psychoanalytic method emphasizes therapist neutrality and requires that the patient have sufficient ego strength to regress in a controlled manner. The transference that develops is analyzed with mutative interpretations, and presumably leads to enduring personality change. Thus, proper handling of transference, particularly erotic transference, is important. Gabbard (1990) notes that mishandling of erotic transference is probably the most frequent cause of treatment failure with these individuals. However, with more disturbed and unstable Histrionic Personality Disordered individuals, transference distortions require that resolving transference distortions by interpretation be undertaken with great caution. In fact, some (Khan, 1975; Havens, 1976) suggest that erotic transference not be allowed to develop too firmly or to be interpreted. Rather, counterprojective techniques are advised. These are direct or subtle, verbal or nonverbal response which communicate to the patient that the therapist is not a transference figure of childhood (Havens, 1976).

Horowitz and Lerner (2010) have more recently identified three phases of the psychodynamic treatment of histrionic personality disorder: therapist interventions to increase state stability and reduce crises; increasing connection with others and eliminating obstacles to personality growth; and increasing self-coherence and developing intimacy with a sense of integrity. Psychodynamic psychotherapy with histrionic patients has also been examined by Fernandez (2010) in a single case study involving a 25-year-old female psychology student. This treatment, consisting of couch analysis four times per week, was deemed to be a failure. While the patient had good capacity for insight and provided rich material to process in sessions, she frequently missed appointments or arrived late. This manner of resistance is common for histrionic patients seeking attention, and ultimately derailed the therapy process. O'Donohue, Fowler, and Lilienfeld (2007) note that the effectiveness of psychodynamic psychotherapy specifically for histrionic personality disorder has not been demonstrated in controlled studies.

Brief Dynamic Psychotherapy

While long-term psychoanalytically oriented psychotherapy is considered the mainstay of dynamic treatment (Quality Assurance Project, 1991) time-limited individual psychotherapy may also be quite useful, particularly with higher functioning histrionic individuals. The approaches of Malan (1972) and Sifneos (1972, 1984) seem quite promising. The short-term-anxiety-provoking psychotherapy (STAPP) approach developed by Sifneos may be a particularly "good fit" for higher functioning histrionic individuals who present with satisfactory impersonal relationships psychological mindedness, the ability to easily engage and interact with a therapist, and a circumscribed presenting complaint. On the other hand, Mann's (1973, 1984) time-limited approach which requires patients to quickly engage and disengage from therapy "without suffering unduly" may pose considerable difficult for these individuals who characteristically develop intense and sticky transference with therapist (Chodoff, 1989). Winston and Pollock (1991) describe Brief Adaptive Psychotherapy (BAP) as particularly effective with histrionic individuals. BAP has an ego psychological orientation which focuses on maladaptive patterns of beliefs and behaviors. The maladaptive pattern is thoroughly assessed as its underlying elements are explored in detail with particular attention on transference and resistance.

Cognitive Analytic Therapy (CAT) (Ryle, 2004) is another time-limited model of psychodynamically-oriented treatment that has been used for personality disorders. It consists of a narrative reformulation and the sequential diagrammatic reformulation (SDR). Patients receive 24 weekly sessions and four follow-up sessions spread out over a six-month period. Following the first three assessment sessions, personality patients are read a letter from the therapist that reformulates the origins of their distress and identifies target problems and procedures. In Kellet's (2007) single-case study with a woman diagnosed with histrionic personality disorder, these were: the need to be noticed; pacing of relationships; focus on physical appearance; and trust issues. The SDR was developed over the next 4 sessions. This is used to create therapeutic "exits" from the problem roles and behaviors identified in the SDR. These included, among others, less self-criticism, interacting with others without wearing make-up or provocative clothes, and learning to tolerate not being the center of attention. Cognitive Analytic Therapy ends with a "goodbye letter" jointly formulated by the patient and therapist to summarize achievements, prepare for future obstacles, and address any feelings of abandonment related to the termination of therapy.

Cognitive Behavioral Therapy Approaches

According the Beck and Associates (2004) Cognitive Therapy is particularly appropriate in treating Histrionic Personality Disordered individuals provided they remain in treatment. Although usually cooperative and motivated for therapy, the histrionic's global, diffuse thinking style is quite different from the systematic, structural nature of Cognitive Therapy. Thus, these individuals initially find treatment difficult and frustrating as they learn to focus attention on a single issue at a time, and then monitor their thoughts and feelings.

There are a number of necessary conditions for successful cognitive treatment of this disorder. Since these individuals are generally dependent and demanding in relationships, they use of collaborative and guided discovery are particularly well suited. Taking an active role and utilizing questioning is quite helpful in stemming the histrionic individual's view of clinicians as rescuers and saviors. Setting limits that are clear and firm, while rewarding assertive requests within these limits and demonstrating caring in other ways is another necessary condition of treatment. The next condition is establishing treatment goals. These goals must be meaningful and perceived as urgent by these individuals and be specific and concrete enough that short term as well as long term benefits can become realities. This counters the histrionic individual's tendency to set broad, vague, noble sounding goals. An important key to keeping these individuals in therapy is achieving one or more of the specific, short term goals that were collaboratively established (Fowler, Orme, & Hart, 2021).

The mainstay of treatment with these individuals involves: challenging automatic thoughts; the self-monitoring of cognition which is helpful in controlling their impulsivity; and the restructuring, modification and interpretation of maladaptive schemas. Challenging their most basic assumption such as "I am inadequate and have to rely on others to survive" is aided by cognitive-behavioral methods such as assertion, problem solving and behavioral experiments which can increase their self-efficacy and help them feel more competent. Another central belief that must be modified is that the loss of a relationship is always disastrous. Fantasizing about the reality of what would happen if a relationship would end, and recalling how they survived before that relationship began, can help these individuals "decatastrophize" their beliefs about rejection. The behavioral approach with the "controlling type" of histrionic personality (Turkat, 1990) has not been shown to be effective (Turkat & Maisto, 1985; Turkat, 1990). The "reactive type" is more amenable to change, specifically with empathy training. Turkat (1990) describes this intervention which consists of social skills training in active listening, paraphrasing and reflection. The goal is to teach these patients to focus increasingly on other's needs and feelings. Role playing with video feedback has been particularly effective. The use of dramatic behavioral experiments and training in problem solving skills are also advocated by Beck and Freeman (1990).

Sungur and Gunduz (2015) outline several treatment goals that may be used, depending on individual patient needs. The first of these affect awareness and regulation skills. This is intended to help histrionic patients improve frustration tolerance and learn new, more adaptive behaviors in order to reduce the frequency of dramatic or aggressive behavior. The second possible treatment goal is to confront fears about rejection and decatastrophize ideas about loss of approval or attention. This can be accomplished by separating the patient's behaviors from the "self," so that any criticisms are not taken as attacks to self-worth that require defensiveness. Sungur and Gunduz also point to the goal of social and communication skills development in the treatment of histrionic personality disorder. This includes building empathy, active listening, and being a good audience member rather than being at the center of the stage. The final goal is increasing self-sufficiency, problem solving skills, and a sense of identity without dependence on others' approval.

In short, effective Cognitive Therapy approach to the Histrionic Personality Disorder will be systematic and structural, including firm limit setting and specific treatment goals, and include cognitive (disputation of automatic thoughts and schemas restructuring of basic maladaptive beliefs and schemas) as well as behavioral methods.

Schema Therapy. Schema Therapy is an elaboration of cognitive therapy that has been developed by Young (Young, Klosko, & Weishaar, 2003) specifically for personality disorders, and other difficult individual and couples problems. Schema Therapy involves identifying maladaptive schemas and planning specific strategies and interventions. Four main strategies are cognitive, experiential, behavioral and the therapeutic relationship itself. Cognitive restructuring, modification of maladaptive schemas, is an important cognitive strategy, but is combined with imagery exercises, empathic confrontation, homework assignments and "limited reparenting," i.e., a form of corrective emotional experience (Young et al., 2003).

Maladaptive schemas typically associated with Histrionic Personality Disorder include: *emotional deprivation*, i.e., the belief that one's desire for emotional support will not be met by others; *defectiveness*: i.e., the belief that one is defective, bad, unwanted, or inferior in important respects; and *approval-seeking*, i.e., the belief that one must constantly seek to belong and be accepted at the expense of developing a true sense of self (Bernstein, 2002).

Interpersonal Approach

For Benjamin (2003), psychotherapeutic interventions with Histrionic Personality Disordered individuals can be planned and evaluated in terms of whether they enhance collaboration, facilitate learning about maladaptive patterns and their roots, block these patterns, enhance the will to change, and effectively encourage new patterns.

Benjamin notes that to establish a therapeutic alliance facilitating collaboration with the histrionic individual based on knowledge of the basic pattern, wishes and fears of that individual. It is essential that the therapist communicate warmth and competent support while not reinforcing the histrionic's dependent, needy position. The working contract is with the individual's observing ego while the "enemy" is the damaging pattern. A major tasks of beginning treatment is transforming the histrionic's view of treatment as making fantasies come true to a place where personal development can be facilitated. Thus, treatment interventions can be evaluated on the basis of whether or not they accomplish this. If an intervention results in more demanding dependency, then it has failed to achieve the aforementioned goals.

Facilitating collaboration with the histrionic patient is no easy task. Gender dynamics can play a particularly important role. For example, female therapists may have difficulty communicating the accepting warmth and support so desired by the female histrionic patient because of the latter's dim view of the therapist's competence. Male therapists will have an easier time establishing the therapeutic contract—at least at first. Regardless of gender, therapists must be clear in their boundaries and intentions for their relationship with the histrionic patient. The therapy relationship is for the needs and learning of the patient, not the therapist. Benjamin notes it should be clear that the therapist's salary or fees are enough to meet his or her needs in this relationship, and that it is not a social relationship. This challenges the marriage fantasy commonly held by histrionic patients.

The task of learning to recognize patterns is complicated in that histrionic individuals have not sufficiently developed an observing ego to help them to recognize and reflect on patterns. In fact, they've come to believe that if they become competent, they would be left alone, and no one would care for them. Establishing stability is tantamount to losing their identity. While the female histrionic can internalize the female clinician's modelling of benign and constructive examination of patterns, the male clinician must help the individual look about her fears that if she becomes competent the clinician will decide she is unattractive and stop treatment.

Next, the clinician focuses the histrionic individual's attention on potentially destructive patterns of acting out based on underlying fears and wishes. By providing gentle challenges, the clinician protects these individuals from their own past. The goal is to expand options and enhance awareness in light of what is being learned about patterns. The therapist doesn't block patterns with advice giving, as much as reviewing options. Developing the will to change patterns is enhanced if these patterns can be uncovered and clearly connected in an experiential way to the past. This often facilitates the individual's "decision" to give up the goals that drive the patterns. Finally, Benjamin advocates traditional techniques from other approaches that can be utilized to build new patterns and ways of functioning, once the "unconscious underbrush" has been cleared away. Warmth, active listening, and support are keys to successful therapy. The therapist must remain a loyal and optimistic ally in treatment.

Group Therapy

The literature on the histrionic personality is quite interesting with regard to treatability of this disorder in group settings. There are clear warnings in the older psychoanalytic literature about the impact of these patients on other group members. Slavson (1939) cautioned that their changeability and unpredictability would engender stress and anxiety in a group. Thus, he believed these patients should be treated only in individual therapy. On the other hand, contemporary clinicians like Gabbard (1990, 1994) contend that histrionic patients that are appropriate for individual dynamic psychotherapy are also appropriate for dynamic group psychotherapy. In fact, Gabbard finds these patients are highly valued by other group members for their ability to express affects directly, and because of their concern for other group members. Rutan, Stone, and Shay (2014) provide a detailed analysis of a mixed diagnosis psychodynamic therapy group with a histrionic member. They draw attention to the strong negative reactions these individuals can have on the group facilitator and fellow members, as well as the benefits of having the histrionic patient's honesty.

The group treatment format has a number of advantages over individual treatment. First, a group setting frustrates the wish and demand these patients have for the exclusive attention of the therapist who now must inevitably challenge the approval-seeking posture of these patients. Thus, the risk of an eroticized transference developing is relatively small in contrast with individual therapy.

Second, their global cognitive style and associated defenses of repression and denial can be more effectively treated in a group setting. Group members will confront the distorted manner in which histrionic patients new themselves and others by their style, omission of details, and focus on affects over thought.

Finally, histrionic patterns tend to form positive maternal transference and expect the group to make up for the maternal nurturance they missed as children (Gabbard, 1990). While this transference is particularly challenging for the clinician in individual therapy, it is considerably "diluted" in a group treatment format.

Relatively little has been published about the effectiveness of group treatment of histrionic patients. But one study is encouraging. Cass et al. (1972) reported a behavioral group treatment significantly modified inappropriate passivity, manipulativeness, and acting out, replaced by more effective assertive interpersonal behavior.

The question of indication and contraindication has been addressed by some writers (Ogrodniczuk, Uliaszek, Lebow, & Kealy, 2021). Halleck (1978) notes that histrionic patients who cannot participate in a group process without monopolizing or disrupting it, should be excluded. Similarly, Gabbard (1990) cautions that individuals might still be candidates for group therapy if they are concurrently in individual psychotherapy. Scheidlinger and Porter (1979) indicated that combined treatment: individual plus group therapy, may be the treatment of choice for such histrionic patients.

Marital and Family Therapy

There are no reports of family therapy, per se, with histrionic patients. However, there are a number of case reports on marital therapy with these patients. Typically, the marriage consists of an obsessive compulsive husband and a histrionic wife, wherein the obsessive compulsive spouse tends to assume increasing responsibility while the histrionic spouse becomes increasingly helpless (Berman, 1983). Treatment may be sought following some primitive outburst which can include some threat of self-destructive behavior, typically during separation or divorce. The loss of a stable dependent figure is a major stressor for the histrionic patient who may exhibit aggressive attention seeking behavior, increased affective display and seductiveness and/or possibly promiscuity, in an effort to make the other spouse jealous, etc. (Harbir, 1981).

The general goal of treatment is to facilitate changing this pattern in both spouses (Ogrodniczuk, Uliaszek, Lebow, & Kealy, 2021). This is better accomplished in a couples format rather than in individual session. Harbir (1981) offers a treatment protocol for couples wherein divorce and child custody are issues.

Nichols (1996) describes the interactional patterns and symptomatology of individuals with Histrionic Personality Disorders and Antisocial Personality Disorders in close interpersonal relationships as well as a suggested treatment plan protocol and strategies for dealing with such couples in a therapeutic context.

An integrative marital therapy approach involving dynamic, cognitive-behavioral, and systemic interventions is described by Sperry and Maniacci (1996) for couples in which one partner presents with Histrionic Personality Disorder and the other with Obsessive-Compulsive Personality Disorder. Three phases of the treatment process are discussed and illustrated: establishing a therapeutic alliance, restoring balance to the couple relationship, and modifying individual partner dynamics. The first two phases involve conjoint couple's sessions, while much of the third phase involves individual sessions (Sperry & Maniacci, 1996).

Links and Stockwell (2004) point to the apparent paradox of the histrionic/obsessive-compulsive couple. Despite the fact that they demonstrate healthier personality styles compared to other personality disorders, they are often more difficult to engage in treatment than those with more severe forms of psychopathology. This paradox is explained by these individuals' particular attachment styles. Couples with histrionic/obsessive-compulsive styles are able to form attachment relationships; however, when their attachment needs are left unsatisfied, they look for compromises or alternatives that can be damaging to the relationship. These include leaving the relationship for another individual or forming triangulated relationship with a third party to maintain stability. Because of these additional options, these individuals may present as more ambivalent about couples therapy or change. As such, the authors point to the importance of evaluating these possibilities when determining the appropriateness of couple's therapy. The specific style of the histrionic/obsessive-compulsive couple are further illustrated by Landucci and Foley (2014). Couples of this composition are polar opposites: spontaneous v. controlled; vague v. detailed and rational. These two individuals are said to form one full person when taken together, so it is not surprising that there is often an instant attraction between these opposites. However, these dramatic differences are also the source of conflict. Couples therapists should normalize the belief that the other partner is "crazy" by discussing these dynamics.

Medication

Generally, speaking, there are no psychotropic medications specifically indicated for treating individuals with histrionic personality disorder (Silk & Feurino, 2012). Histrionic personality-disordered individuals may exhibit anxiety disorders, depressive disorders or somatoforms symptoms. Nevertheless, medications are used that target specific troubling symptoms associated with the disorder, such as depression, anxiety, or sleep problems.

Generally, these medications are used as an adjunct to psychotherapy and skills training. Because troubling symptoms often respond to medications sooner than most psychological interventions, medications are usually prescribed at the onset of treatment (Sperry, 1995b; Nelson & Tsheringld, 2021). Unfortunately, there is little research evidence to provide guidelines for the use of such medications (Silk & Feurino, 2012). However, there appears to be an exception: One variant of the histrionic personalities, called the "hysteroid dysphoria," has responded to certain antidepressant agents, specifically Parnate and Nardil (Liebowitz & Klein, 1979).

Integrated and Combined Treatment Approach

The basic premise of the book is that symptomatic and lower functioning personality-disordered individuals are less likely to respond to single treatment approach or modality. Since personality disorders are biopsychosocial phenomenon (Pies, 1992), combined or integrative, tailored treatment is indicated, particularly for the more symptomatic and severe presentations. Stone (1992) advocates combined treatments, wherein two or more approaches or modalities are utilized concurrently or in tandem.

Previously, it was mentioned that combining individual psychotherapy with group therapy concurrent was indicated for histrionic patients who monopolized or were disruptive in group settings (Sheidlinger & Porter, 1980). It has also been noted that behavioral techniques may be integrated with psychodynamic or a cognitive approach. Finally, medications may be a useful adjunct to psychotherapy (Winkeller & Schlesinger, 2021).

Horowitz (1997) discusses guidelines for the psychotherapeutic treatment for the Histrionic Personality Disorder that integrates cognitive and psychodynamic principles and methods. This personality disorder is formulated in terms levels: states of mind, defensive control processes and schemas. A phase-oriented treatment plan is linked to these three formulation levels. Specific psychotherapeutic guidelines for each of these phases are described.

Dorfman (2000) provides a case study with a 49-year-old histrionic woman who sought treatment for severe depression, anxiety, and problems with her boyfriend. The time-limited nature of the treatment included elements from a combination of models with three specific treatment goals. First, the therapist dealt with acute emotional distress by developing a supportive and empathic therapeutic relationship to help the patient contain and modulate her emotions. Second, a combination of cognitive challenges, communication skills training, and insight-oriented interpretations of the patient's childhood addressed her distorted self-concept and maladaptive style. Finally, the treatment focused on developing the confidence necessary to resume appropriate functioning at work and achieve some degree of independence.

Chapter 9

Narcissistic Personality Disorder

Individuals with narcissistic personalities tend to be grandiose, entitled, and self-centered. They are often impulsive and anxious, have ideas of grandiosity and "specialness," become quickly dissatisfied with others, and maintain superficial, exploitative interpersonal relationships (Ronningstam, 2012; Skodol, Bender, & Oldham, 2019; American Psychiatric Association, 2022).

While treatment of such individuals involves a number of unique therapeutic challenges, it can be highly effective and successful.

This chapter describes a framework for the assessment and effective treatment of this disorder. It includes sections on diagnosis, psychological assessment, case conceptualization, and treatment interventions. It begins with background information on the disorder as well as the DSM-5-TR description, prototypic description, associated features, and the Alternative Model of Personality Disorders description of this disorder. The section on case conceptualization provides five common clinical formulations of this disorder: psychodynamic, biosocial, cognitive-behavioral, interpersonal, and an integrative conceptualization of this disorder. Several treatment approaches, modalities, and intervention strategies are also described. These includes individual psychotherapy, group therapy, marital and family therapy, medication, and integrative and combined treatment.

Description of the Narcissistic Personality Disorders

The Narcissistic Personality Disorder can be recognized by the following descriptors and characteristics: styles vs. disorders, triggering event, behavioral styles, interpersonal styles, cognitive styles, affective styles, attachment style, and optimal criterion.

Style vs. Disorder. The narcissistic personality is quite common in western culture particularly among certain occupations and professions such as law, medicine, entertainment and sports, and politics. The narcissistic personality can be thought of as spanning a continuum from healthy to the pathological, with the narcissistic personality style on the healthy end and the personality disorder on the pathological end. Table 9.1 compares and contrasts differences between the narcissistic style and disorder.

The following two case examples illustrates the differences between the narcissistic personality style—Mr. J.—and the Narcissistic Personality Disorder—Mr. C.

> **Case Study: Narcissistic Personality Disorder**
>
> Mr. C. is a 41-year-old male who presented for therapy after his wife of six years threatened to leave him and because his employer was pressuring him to resign his position as a sales executive for a condominium project. Apparently, Mrs. C. had told her husband that he loved himself "a hundred times more than you love me." Mr. C. dismissed this by saying he needed to buy $600 suits because his job demanded that he look his best at all times and that he was "tall, dark, handsome and sexy, all any woman could want in a man." Mr. C. denied that he used scare tactics, exaggerated claims, or other pressure selling techniques with customers. "Sure, I'm a bit aggressive, but you don't get into the 'Millionaire's Club' by being a wimp." He added that his employer would "go belly up without me," and that he was too important to be dismissed for such petty reasons.

> **Case Study Example: Narcissistic Personality Style**
>
> Mr. J. is chairman of his state's democratic party and caucus. Throughout most of his career, he had been incredibly successful and effective. He is extroverted, witty, and charming interpersonally, and astute, visionary and effective in mobilizing support for his party's political agenda. However, in graduate school a political science professor had criticized a first draft of his master's thesis evaluating his arguments as weak and conclusions only partially substantiated by the research cited. Prior to this, he had held the professor in high esteem, but questioned the professor's competence after this criticism. Nevertheless, he swallowed his pride and reworked the thesis according to the professor's suggestion and graduated. A short time after graduation Mr. J. lost his first job as a speech writer for a state senator because the opinions and conclusions cited in his drafts were not sufficiently well documented. Fortunately, Mr. J. took these lessons to heart and found others to research his own speeches when he ran for office. Mr. J. recognized that this was not one of this strengths and could delegate it while focusing on his real strengths which were envisioning policy and political agendas and galvanizing support for them.

Although DSM-5-TR only describes one type or presentation of the Narcissistic Personality Disorder in Section II, research describes three types: overt, covert, and the malignant (Caligor, Levy, & Yeomans, 2015). All three types are highly self-absorbed and have little genuine regard for the needs or feelings of others. Fortunately, the Alternative Model of Personality Disorders in Section III addresses all three.

Overt Type. This type presents as grandiose and thick-skinned and is the embodiment of DSM-5 criteria. These individuals are characterized by overt grandiosity, attention seeking, entitlement, arrogance, and little observable anxiety. They can be socially charming,

Table 9.1 Comparison of Narcissistic Personality Style and Disorder

Personality Style	Personality Disorder
Although emotionally vulnerable to negative assessments and reaction of others, they can handle these gracefully	Reacts to criticism with feelings of rage, stress, or humiliation (even if not expressed)
Shrewd in dealing with others, utilizing the strengths and advantages of others to achieve their own goals	Interpersonally exploitive, taking advantage of others to achieve his or her own ends
Can energetically sell themselves, their ideas and their projects	Grandiose sense of self-importance
Tend to be able competitors who love getting to the top and enjoy staying there	Believe their problems are unique and understood only by other special people
Can visualize themselves as the best or most accomplished in their field	Preoccupied by fantasies of unlimited success power, brilliance, beauty, or ideal love
They believe in themselves, their abilities and their uniqueness but do not demand special treatment or privilege	Have a sense of entitlement and unreasonable expectations of especially favorable treatment
Accept accomplishments, praise and admiration gracefully and with self-possession	Require constant attention and admiration
Possess a keen awareness of their thoughts and feelings and have some awareness of those of others	Lack of empathy; inability to recognize and experience how others feel
Expect others to treat them well at All times	Preoccupied with feelings of envy

despite being oblivious to the needs of others, and are interpersonally exploitative. The problem is that they have a fragile sense of self that is predicated on maintaining a self-view that they are exceptional. Because genuine engagement can result in the painful realization that others have attributes which they lack, these individuals engage in superficial relationships and seek out external feedback that support this grandiose self-definition (Levy, 2012).

Covert Type. This type presents as vulnerable, "fragile" and thin-skinned. These individuals are characterized as inhibited, manifestly distressed, hypersensitive to the evaluations of others while chronically envious and evaluating themselves in relation to others. Interpersonally they tend to be shy, outwardly self-effacing, and hypersensitive to slights, but are covertly or secretly grandiose and jealous. Unlike the overt type, these tend to withdraw from social situations (Levy, 2012).

Malignant Type. This type is also referred to as "malignant narcissism" (Kernberg, 1984). These individuals are characterized by the typical symptoms of narcissistic personality disorder, as well as prominent antisocial behavior, paranoid features, and sadism toward others. They may engage in chronic lying, intimidation, and financial or interpersonal secondary gains which maintain their malignant pattern (Caligor, Levy, & Yeomans, 2015).

Triggering Event. The typical situation, circumstance or event that most likely triggers or activates the characteristic maladaptive response of the Narcissistic Personality Disorder (Othmer & Othmer, 2002), as noted in behavioral, interpersonal, cognitive, and feeling styles, is: "evaluation of self."

Behavioral Style. Behaviorally, narcissistic individuals are seen as conceited, boastful, and snobbish. They appear self-assured and self- centered, and they tend to dominate conversation, seek admiration, and act in a pompous and exhibitionistic fashion. They are also impatient, arrogant, and thin-skinned or hypersensitive.

Interpersonal Style. Interpersonally, they are exploitive and use others to indulge themselves and their desires. Their behavior is socially facile, pleasant, and endearing. However, they are unable to respond with true empathy to others. When stressed, they can be disdainful, exploitive, and generally irresponsible in their behavior.

Cognitive Style. Their thinking style is one of cognitive expansiveness and exaggeration. They tend to focus on images and themes rather than on facts and issues. In fact, they take liberties with the facts, distort them, and even engage in prevarication and self-deception to preserve their own illusions about themselves and the projects in which they are involved. Their cognitive style is also marked by inflexibility. In addition they have an exaggerated sense of self-importance and establish unrealistic goals of power, wealth, and ability. They justify all of this with their sense of entitlement and exaggerated sense of their own self-importance.

Affective Style. Their emotional or affective style is characterized by an aura of self-confidence and nonchalance which is present in most situations except when their narcissistic confidence is shaken. Then they are likely to respond with rage at criticism. Their feelings toward others shift and vacillate between overidealization and devaluation. Finally, their inability to show empathy is reflected in their superficial relationships with minimal emotional ties or commitments.

Attachment Style. Individuals with a view of others that is negative and a self-view that vacillates between positive and negative exhibit a composite fearful–dismissing style of attachment. They tend to view themselves as special and entitled but are also mindful of their need for others who can potentially hurt them. Accordingly, they use others to meet their needs while being wary and dismissive of them. The Fearful–Dismissing Attachment Style is common in individuals with this disorder.

Optimal Diagnostic Criterion. Of all the diagnostic criteria for the Antisocial Personality Disorder, one has been found to be the most useful in diagnosing this disorder. The belief is that by beginning with this criterion, the clinician can test for the presence or absence of the criterion and more quickly diagnose the personality disorder (Allnutt & Links, 1996). The optimal criterion for this disorder is: has a grandiose sense of self-importance.

DSM-5 Description

Individuals with this personality disorder are characterized by an unremitting pattern of self-centeredness and grandiosity. More specifically, they have an exaggerated sense of their own abilities and achievements. They may have a constant need for attention, affirmation and praise. Typically, they believe they are unique or special and should only associate with others of the same status. They are likely to have persistent fantasies about attaining success and power. These individuals can exploit others for personal gain. A sense of entitlement and the expectation of special treatment is common. They may come across as snobbish or arrogant. They appear to be incapable of showing empathy for others. In addition, they can be envious or think that others are envious of them (American Psychiatric Association, 2022).

Prototypic Description

A prototype is a brief description that captures the essence of how a particular disorder commonly presents. Prototypic descriptions are useful and convenient, and clinicians commonly rely on them rather than lists of behavioral criteria or core beliefs (Westen, 2012). Here is a common prototypic description of the Narcissistic Personality Disorder: These individuals are the center of their worlds. They believe and act as if they are special in every way. They can be showoffs and name droppers. Without a doubt, they are legends in their own minds. There is no limit to their sense of self-importance and entitlement. They are haughty, high-handed, and superior and expect others to show deference and admiration. They seldom recognize the needs, concerns, or feelings of others. Not surprisingly, they experience disappointments and anger when others fail to live up to their highly unrealistic expectations (Francis, 2013).

Associated Features

Prevalence. NPD has been identified in 0.8 percent of the general population and 10.1 percent in clinical practice (Torgersen, 2021).

Differential Diagnosis. Other personality disorders, such as histrionic antisocial, and borderline, can be confused with NPD. The key discriminating feature with these disorders is grandiosity. Also, self-destructiveness, separation insecurity, impulsivity, and emotional hyperreactivity distinguish it from BPD (American Psychiatric Association, 2022).

Development and Course. While narcissistic traits are common in adolescents, NPD is more likely to develop in adulthood often in the context of very challenging life crises like bankruptcies, divorce, or job loss. Such individuals may have difficulty adjusting to health or occupational limitations inherent with old age. Nevertheless, tolerable disappointments and setbacks can be corrective and contribute to improvements in those with this disorder (American Psychiatric Association, 2022).

Culture, Sex, and Gender. Narcissistic traits may be acceptable in cultures that emphasize individualism and personal autonomy than in collectivist cultures. Similarly in individualist cultures such traits less frequently lead to social impairment and warrant less clinical attention. While males tend to exhibit more reactivity to stress and compromised empathy, females tend to exhibit more self-focus and withdrawal. Nevertheless, males are more likely to receive this diagnosis (American Psychiatric Association, 2022).

Alternative Model of Narcissistic Personality Disorder

The Alternative Model of Personality Disorders (AMPD) offers a clinically useful description of the Narcissistic Personality Disorder in terms of typical features and trait facets.

Table 9.2 Characteristics of Narcissistic Personality Disorder

Triggering Event(s)	Evaluation of self
Behavioral Style:	Sense of entitlement
	Arrogant, thin-skinned
	Self-assured and pompous
Interpersonal Style:	Requires excessive admiration
	Lacks empathy
	Envies or feels envied
	Arrogant and haughty
	Exploits others
Cognitive Style:	Cognitive expansiveness and exaggeration
	Takes liberties with facts
	Impatient, persistent, and inflexible
Feeling Style:	Self-confident
	Narcissistic rage
Temperament:	Active and responsive
	Special talents and early language development
Attachment Style	Fearful and dismissing
Parental Injunction:	"Grow up and be wonderful, for me"
Self View:	"I'm special and unique, and I'm entitled to extraordinary rights and privileges whether I've earned them or not"
World View:	"Life is a banquet table to be sampled at will. People owe me admiration and privilege. Therefore, I'll expect and demand this specialness"
Maladaptive Schemas	Entitlement; Defectiveness; Emotional Deprivation; Insufficient Self-Control; Unrelenting Standards
Optimal Diagnostic Criteria	Has grandiose sense of self-importance

Typical features are variable and vulnerable self-esteem, with attempts at regulation through attention and approval seeking, and either overt or covert grandiosity. As noted earlier in this chapter this refers to the manner in which they exhibit a sense of entitlement, either directly or covertly, or indirectly or covertly. This distinction is clinically useful since overt grandiosity has too often been considered the only presentation of NPD. Trait facet criteria include Grandiosity and Attention seeking; and both are required. The alternative model also includes a "specifier" for *Malignant Narcissism* when the additional criteria of Manipulativeness, Deceitfulness, and Callousness are present (American Psychiatric Association, 2022). Table 9.2 summarizes the characteristics of this disorder.

Conceptualizations of the Narcissistic Personality Disorder

Psychodynamic Case Conceptualizations

Freud (1914/1976) described the original psychoanalytic formulation of narcissistic personality. For Freud, parental overevaluation or erratic, unreliable caretaking in early life were factors disrupting the development of object love in the child providing. As a result of this fixation or arrest at the narcissistic phase of development, Freud posited that narcissists would be unable to form lasting relationships. In other words, the etiology of the Narcissistic Personality Disorder is that it is the outcome of insufficient gratification of the normal narcissistic needs of infancy and childhood. The contrary hypothesis is that the disorder stems from narcissistic overgratification during childhood and because of this fixation interferes with the normal maturation and integration of the superego leading to difficulties in regulation of self-esteem (Fernando, 1998). Another common belief is that the disorder arises from faulty parenting or disturbed object relations. Imbesi (2000) suggests this hypothesis is the common etiology of most personality disorders and instead proposes that the caretaker's failure to provide optimal frustrating experiences necessary to foster the development of a more realistic self-image in the child is the etiology of the narcissistic personality.

In the past two decades the formulations of the narcissistic personality by Kohut and Kernberg have become the dominant models. Kohut (1971, 1977) believed the narcissistic is developmentally arrested at the stage which requires specific responses from individuals in their environment to maintain cohesive selves. i.e., the structures of the grandiose self and the idealized parental image are not integrated. He described the formulation of self-object transferences—both mirroring and idealizing—that recreate the situation with parents that was not fully successful during childhood. When such responses are not forthcoming (an empathic deficits) the narcissistic is prone to fragmentation of the self (narcissistic injury).

Unlike Kohut, who worked with high functioning professionals in psychoanalysis, Kernberg (1975, 1984) based his conceptualization of narcissistic pathology on his work with inpatients as well as outpatients. He views the narcissist's grandiosity and exploitation as evidence of oral rage which he believes results from the emotional deprivation caused by on indifferent and covertly spiteful mother figure. Concurrently, some unique attribute talent or role provides the child with a sense of being special which provides an emotional escape valve in a world of perceived threat or indifference. Thus, grandiosity and entitlement shelter a "real self" that is "split off," i.e., outside consciousness. Parenthetically for Kernberg, the real self contains strong but unconscious feelings of envy, deprivation, fear and rage. Finally, Kernberg (1975) views defensive structure of the narcissist as remarkably similar to the borderline differentiating the two on the basis of their integrated but pathological grandiose self.

Biosocial Case Conceptualizations

According to Millon and Everly (1985) the Narcissistic Personality Disorder primarily arises from environment factors, since the role of biogenic factors is unclear. The principal environmental factors are parental indulgence and overvaluation, learned exploitive behavior and only-child status. Essentially then, children are pampered and given special treatment by the parents such that they learn to believe the world revolves around them. They become egotistical in their perspectives and narcissistic in their expressions of love and emotion. Not surprisingly, they come to expect special treatment from others outside the home. When special treatment is not forthcoming the children experiments with demanding and exploitive tactics and subsequently develops considerable skill in manipulating others so as to receive the special consideration, they believe they deserve. At the same time, they come to believe that most others are inferior, weak and exploitable. Furthermore, Millon (Millon & Everly, 1985; Millon & Davis, 2000) indicate that parental overindulgence is particularly likely with only with children. Finally, the narcissistic pattern is self-perpetuated through their illusion of their superiority, a lack of self-control manifested by their disdain for situations and persons that do not support their exalted beliefs, deficient social responsibility and the self-reinforcement of the narcissistic pattern itself.

Cognitive Behavioral Case Conceptualizations

According to Beck (2015) the key feature of this disorder is self-aggrandizement. Individual with this disorder can be characterized by specific core, conditional, and instrumental beliefs. Their *core beliefs* include deserving special treatment and dispensations because of their specialness. They also include believing that they are not bound by the rules and social conventions that govern others. Their *conditional beliefs* are that others should be punished if they do not recognize their special status, and that to maintain their special status, others must be subservient to them. Their *instrumental belief* is to continually strive to demonstrate their superiority. Underlying these various beliefs are their beliefs about self and the world. These individuals tend to view themselves as special, superior, entitled to special favors and treatment, and vulnerable to loss of status. They view others as inferior but also potential admirers who recognize their superiority and grandiosity. Not surprisingly, such beliefs are reflected in their main strategy or pattern of seeking prestige, power, position, and wealth as a way of reinforcing their image of superiority. If necessary, they will use manipulation and guile to achieve these goals (Beck, 2015; Behary & Davis, 2015).

Specific schemas characterize this disorder. The central schema is the superior/special schema which develops from direct and indirect messages from parents, siblings, and significant others as well as by experiences that mold beliefs about personal uniqueness and self-importance. The schema of being superior can be shaped by flattery, indulgence and favoritism. Similarly, the schema of being special can be shaped by experiences of rejection, limitations, exclusion or deficits. The common denominator for such beliefs about self is that the individual perceives himself or herself as different from others in significant ways (Behary & Davis, 2015).

Taking a more behavioral tact, Turkat (1990) differentiates this disorder into three types: the self-centered impulsive type, the ruthless impression management type, and the acceptance-oriented impression-management type. Of these, he considers the last type to have the best therapeutic prognosis. Nevertheless, he formulates each type as behavioral manifestations of an impulse control deficit which is learned in early childhood. Specifically, these individuals learned to seek reinforcers without having to work for them. This resulted in their development as self-indulgent, egocentric, and impulsive individuals. Individuals with the second and third types focus on creating a favorable impression on others. However, they are unable to maintain close relationships because while they have excellent skills at reading superficial cues, they have empathic deficits (Turkat, 1990).

Interpersonal Case Conceptualizations

For Benjamin (1996), persons with Narcissistic Personality Disorder typically was raised in an environment of selfless no contingent love and adoration. Unfortunately, this adoration was not accompanied by genuine self-disclosure. As a result, those developing a narcissistic personality learn to be insensitive to others' needs and views. The adoring parent is likely to have been consistently differential and nurturant to the narcissistic-in-training. As a result, is that the adult narcissist hold the arrogant expectation that others will continue to provide these emotional supplies. Along with this nurturance and adoration is the ever-present threat of a fall from grace. As such the narcissistic individual who is simply "normal" and ordinary creates unbearable disappointment for the parent(s). Thus, the burden of being special or perfect can be overwhelming for the narcissistic individual. Since this individual's self-concept derives from an internalization of unrealistic adoration and nurturance, the substitution of criticism or disappointment for love can be particularly devastating. Thus, the narcissistically disordered individual can "dish it out" but is not well equipped "to take it." In short, there is extreme vulnerability to criticism or being ignored, together with a strong wish for love, support and admiration from others. Noncontingent love and presumptive control of others is expected and even demanded. If support is withdrawn or lack of perfection is evident, the self-concept degrades into severe self-criticism. Totally devoid of empathy, these individuals tend to treat others with contempt and rage of entitlement fail.

Integrative Case Conceptualizations

The following integrative formulation provides a biopsychosocial explanation for how this personality is likely to have developed and how it is maintained. Biologically narcissistic personalities tend to have hyperresponsive temperaments (Millon, 1981). As young children they were viewed by others as being special in terms of looks, talents, or "promise." Often as young children they had early and exceptional speech development. In addition, they were likely keenly aware of interpersonal cues.

Psychologically, the narcissists' view of themselves, others, the world and life's purpose can be articulated in terms of the following themes: "I'm special and unique, and I am entitled to extraordinary rights and privileges whether I have earned them or not." Their world view is a variant of the theme: "Life is a banquet table to be sampled at will. People owe me admiration and privilege." Their goal is, "Therefore, I'll expect and demand this specialness." Common defense mechanisms utilized by the narcissistic personality involve rationalization and projective identification.

Socially, predictable parental patterns and environmental factors can be noted for the narcissistic personality. Parental indulgence and overevaluation characterize the narcissistic personality. The parental injunction was likely: "Grow up and be wonderful—for me." Often, they were only children, and, in addition, may have sustained early losses in childhood. From an early age they learned exploitive and manipulative behavior from their parents. This narcissistic pattern is confirmed, reinforced, and perpetuated by certain individual and systems factors. The illusion of specialness, disdain for others' views, and a sense of entitlement lead to an underdeveloped sense of social interest and responsibility. This, in turn, leads to increased self-absorption and confirmation of narcissistic beliefs (Sperry & Mosak, 1996, Sperry, 2016).

Assessment of Narcissistic Personality Disorder

Several sources of information are useful in establishing a diagnosis and treatment plan for personality disorders. Observation, collateral information, and psychological testing are important adjuncts to the patient's self-report in the clinical interview. This section briefly describes some characteristic observations that the clinician makes and the nature of the rapport likely to develop in initial encounters with specific personality-disordered individuals. Characteristic response patterns on various objective (i.e., MMPI-2 and MCMI-IV) and projective tests (i.e., Rorschach and TAT) are also described.

Interview Behavior and Rapport. Interviewing Narcissistic Personality Disordered individuals is singularly different than interviewing other personality-disordered individuals. Throughout the interview, these individuals give clinicians the impression that the interview has only one purpose: to endorse their self-promoted importance (Othmer & Othmer,

2002). These individuals typically present themselves as self-assured, pretentious and unwilling to adapt to the basic cultural differences customary to the patient role. They behave as though they are indifferent to the clinician's perspective (Soloff, 1985). As long as the clinician plays the expected role, they are idealized as a marvelous clinician. However, confronting their grandiosity early in the treatment process will inevitably lead to rage and possibly premature termination. They prefer open ended questions which permit them extended descriptions of their many talents, accomplishments and future plans. Rapport is established after a considerable period of mirroring and soothing. Typical clinician countertransference in the initial interviews are boredom, frustration, and anger. To the extent the clinician can patiently wait through this period of mirroring, the work of confronting and interpreting their grandiosity can begin.

Psychological Testing Data. This section describes typical themes and patterns noted for the narcissistic personality on the Minnesota Multiphasic Personality Inventory (MMPI-2), the Millon Clinical Multiaxial Inventory (MCMI-IV), the Rorschach Psychodiagnostic Test, and the Thematic Apperception Test (TAT). This data has been useful in diagnosing the Narcissistic Personality Disorder as well as the narcissistic personality style or trait.

On the MMPI-2 a 4-9 (Psychopathic Deviant-Hypomania) profile or an elevation on scale 4 is most likely. Since they develop only superficial relationships, a low score on 0 (Social Introversion) might also be noted (Graham, 2011). And, since they often fit stereotypic sexual roles, scale 5 (Masculinity-Femininity) may be low particularly in narcissistic males. If they also tend to be suspicious or irritable, an elevation on scale 6 (Paranoia) may be noted (Meyer, 1995).

On the MCMI-IV elevation on scale 5 (Narcissistic) is expected. Scales 4A (Histrionic), 6A (Antisocial), and 6B (Sadistic) could also be elevated. During periods of stress, elevations on P (Paranoid) and PP (Delusional Disorder) may be noted. Since these individuals are adverse to admitting psychic distress or personal weakness, elevations on scales A (Generalized anxiety disorder) and D (Dysthymia disorder) and S (Schizotypal) are not likely (Choca & Denburg, 1997).

On the Rorschach, these individuals are likely to produce records with a high number of C (Pure Color) and CF (Color Form) responses. The seldom respond directly to Shading (Y, YF, or FY) but often make texture (T, TF, or FT) responses (Myers, 1993). Responses that reflect the ornate, the exotic, or the expensive and characteristics of narcissism (Shafer, 1954). The new Rorschach Performance Assessment System (R-PAS) is an improved method for scoring and interpreting the Rorschach Inkblot Test. Besides being evidence based and internationally normed, it increases clinical utility and is easier to use than Exner's Comprehensive System (Mihura & Meyer, 2018).

On the TAT, these individuals tend to avoid the essential features of the cards and thus their stories may be void of meaningful content. Cards that demand a response to potentially anxiety-producing fantasy, such as 13 MF, may yield a superficially avoidant story or are with blatant shocking or lewd content (Bellak, 1997).

Treatment Approaches and Interventions

Treatment Considerations

Included in the differential diagnosis of the Narcissistic Personality Disorder are the following personality disorders: Histrionic Personality Disorder, Antisocial Personality Disorder, and Paranoid Personality Disorder. The most common concurrent symptom disorders are Anxiety Disorders, Persistent Depressive Disorder, Somatic Symptom Disorders, and Delusional Disorders.

The efficacy of psychotherapeutic and psychopharmacological treatment approaches for narcissistic personality disorder has not been systematically or empirically investigated (Caligor, Levy, & Yeomans, 2015). Clinical practice guidelines for the disorder have yet to be formulated, and psychopharmacologic intervention is often symptom driven. Regardless of severity, the grandiosity and defensiveness that characterize narcissistic personality disorder make engagement in any form of psychotherapy difficult (Ronningstam, 2011).

Treatment recommendations for the narcissistic personality are currently based on clinical experience and theoretical formulations (Caligor, Levy, & Yeomans, 2015). In the absence of empirically supported treatments for this disorder, it is common practice to utilize efficacious treatments for similar disorders, typically with treatment modifications based on theoretical and clinical rationales regarding differences in the disorders (Levy, 2012). These include empirically supported treatments for borderline personality disorder that have adaptations for narcissistic personality such as mentalization-based therapy (Allen & Fonagy, 2006), transference-focused psychotherapy (Stern et al., 2012), and schema-focused psychotherapy (Young et al., 2003). All three treatments target psychological capacities thought to underlie and organize descriptive features of narcissistic personality disorder. Dialectical behavioral therapy (Linehan, 2015) is another option for those with significant self-destructive behaviors.

Individual Psychotherapy

Alone, or in conjunction with group or marital and family therapy, individual psychotherapy is viewed by many as the basic treatment of choice for individuals with Narcissistic Personality Disorder. Indeed, some have argued that this disorder and psychotherapy itself are both products of the modern world's intense focus on the self (Paris, 2014). Because of their empathic deficit and proclivity to devalue others, psychotherapy with these individuals can be very trying, giving little, treating others shabbily, and demanding much tends to frustrate the natural inclination of therapists to respond empathically. And although the literature is divided over whether to utilize either confrontation or mirroring techniques, both approaches must be part of the therapist's armamentarium. Generally speaking, higher functioning narcissistic personalities eventually do well in psychotherapy as their sense of entitlement gives way to emulation. On the other hand, lower functioning narcissistic personalities have fewer of the necessary personality assets and relational skills for changing, and unless the therapeutic process address these deficits, these individuals may predictably leave treatment precipitously to avoid the humiliation of admitting how ill-equipped they are to achieve realistic treatment goals. Psychodynamic, Cognitive Behavioral and Interpersonal approaches are briefly described.

Psychodynamic Psychotherapy Approaches

Psychodynamic therapies are often utilized with this disorder (Yeomans, Clarkin, & Levy, 2021).

This section will briefly outline the various psychodynamic approaches: psychoanalysis, psychoanalytic psychotherapy, supportive psychotherapy, and brief psychoanalytic psychotherapy.

Psychoanalysis: Although Freud (1914/1976) was not optimistic about the treatability of the narcissistic personality, Kernberg (1984) and Kohut (1972) believe that higher functioning Narcissistic Personality Disordered individuals are particularly suited for psychoanalysis. Kernberg views the core of the disorder as involving anger, envy and distorted self-sufficiency, and so emphasizes an active interpretation and confrontation of the individual's defenses. Kohut, on the other hand, views the core of the disorder as stunted development of the grandiose self. As such, he emphasizes that by establishment of self-object transference both mirroring and idealizing the functions for the individual in ways that fill in missing self-structure. When a correct empathic interpretation is made, the individual reintegrates by way of the reestablishment of the self-object transference—cohesion—and the disappearance of figmentation. In short then, Kernberg's goal of psychoanalysis is to effect a significant personality change so that envy and rage no longer overwhelm the individual and lead to a protective need to withdraw to a self-sufficient position. For Kohut, the goal is to heal the individual's incomplete self-structure and increase self-esteem through transmuting internalization, i.e., taking in of missing functions from the self-object analyst. The process of psychoanalysis for both Kohut and Kernberg are expected to take several years since significant personality change is the goal. Kernberg (2010) maintains that psychoanalysis is preferable for higher functioning narcissistic patients, as cognitive-behavioral or supportive modalities may successfully reduce symptoms but do not address the unconscious dynamics behind them. However, he states that psychoanalytically oriented psychotherapy is contraindicated for overwhelming negative prognostic indicators.

Psychoanalytic Psychotherapy: In what he calls expressive psychotherapy, Kernberg (1984) describes a modified psychoanalytic treatment as an alternative to psychoanalysis and supportive psychotherapy. In expressive psychotherapy the therapeutic effort focuses on the negative transference in which early manifestations of anger toward the therapist are explored and interpreted. Also included are the defenses of splitting, projection, and projective identification. Masterson (1981) and Rinsley (1982) further emphasize the value of this approach in the development of a therapeutic alliance. Masterson also emphasizes the importance of exploring the individual's exquisite sensitivity to the therapist's empathic failures and the importance of therapeutically exploring this vulnerability. Although Kohut did not describe a psychotherapeutic treatment of the Narcissistic Personality Disorder, Goldberg (1973) and Chessick (1985) have shown that self-object transference do become established in psychotherapy and can be interpreted in light of Kohut's approach. Goldberg (1989) describes the use of the mirroring idealizing, and twinship transference in a self-psychology approach of the narcissistic patient.

Psychoanalytically oriented psychotherapy of narcissistically disordered individuals typically involves one to three sessions a week for two or more years. Kantor (1992) offers a number of proactive suggestions for use in the course of psychotherapy. Among them is the use of predictive interpretation. He points out how painful therapy will be as the individual feels forced to abandon their entitlement and grandiosity. Such forewarning of the individual is less likely to leave therapy precipitously.

The idea of dependence on another person for help is anathema to the narcissistic individual. Kernberg (2010) notes that this dependence is often seen as humiliating, and the narcissist's defense mechanisms are activated in order to protect against this feeling. Individuals may attempt to wrest control of the treatment from the therapist by engaging in "self-analysis." They treat therapists as "vending machines" of interpretations, accepting those with which they agree and rejecting others. Narcissistic patients may alternatively compete with and idealize their therapists, both of which are intended to create distance and assume control. Treatment is filled with feelings of envy and hostility on the part of the patient. These may manifest in attempts to seduce the therapist or self-injurious behaviors intended to destroy the legitimacy of the therapist's role. As such, psychoanalytically oriented psychotherapy with narcissistic individuals must account for these particular defenses.

Supportive Psychotherapy. According to Kernberg (1984), supportive psychotherapy emphasizes an avoidance of working with the negative transference, and instead focuses on supporting the individual in developing expanding ego functions, skills and capacities. According to Kernberg, rapid symptomatic improvement is more likely in supportive psychotherapy than in more expressive approaches. The reader is referred to Kernberg's (1984) chapter on "Supportive Psychotherapy" for an extended discussion of treatment goals and techniques. Kantor (1992) recommends palliation as the goal of supportive psychotherapy wherein the disordered narcissistic personality is maintained while reducing or eliminating its destructive sequelae. He recommends a number of palliative strategies such as teaching the individual to become a better narcissist. For instance, Kantor shows the individual how excessive self-adoration actually interferes with the ability to receive more realistic, wanted and needed adoration from others.

Brief Psychoanalytically Oriented Psychotherapy. Not surprisingly, the least explored treatment modality of the psychodynamic therapies of the disorder narcissistic personality are the shorter-term and brief approaches. Until recently, a self-deficit disorder like the narcissistic personality was considered unamenable to any but long-term treatment. However, as economic realities collide with ideology, this view may be changing somewhat. Kernberg (1984) describes a short-term crisis intervention for the Narcissistic Personality Disorder until the individual is ready and motivated for long-term treatment. Lazarus (1982) and Binder (1979) reports utilizing an brief approach for increasing the individual's self-esteem and self-cohesion, again as preparation for longer-term treatment. Klein (1989) describes a shorter-term treatment which is not a preparation for longer-term therapy. Admittedly, the goals are not ego repair, but are more limited. The goals are learning: increased awareness and anticipation of personal vulnerability to injury, shame and disappointment; containment: increased ability to modulate affects, especially narcissistic rage; and adaptation, i.e., seriously taking into account those aspects of realistic previously ignored and their destructive consequences. Interpretation of narcissistic vulnerability and clarification of the need for containment of defensive devaluation and withdrawal are the cornerstones of this approach. Klein, a colleague of Masterson, describes two selection criteria: an acute interruption of narcissistic "supply lives" (i.e., interpersonal rejection or disappointment) resulting in narcissistic injury amenable to a substitute "supply line" (i.e., the therapist's mirroring). Second, when the narcissistic injury milieus conscious a persistent vulnerability (often experienced as depression or somatic preoccupation) and these individuals are motivated to learn more adaptive ways of managing their environment. Klein specifically excludes individuals who present or are referred with chronic, nonspecific, vague or ego-syntonic symptoms form his brief approach. He describes a course of time-limited treatment (i.e., six months) with a young male which effected symptom relief and circumscribed improvement in functioning. Oldham (1988) describes a 24-session treatment strategy that he describes as a dynamically informed directive approach with limited, focused treatment goals. Marmar and Freeman (1988) also describe a brief dynamic approach, as does Trujillo (2013).

Cognitive Behavioral Therapy Approaches

Cognitive Therapy. Beck, Freeman, and associates (2004) provide an in-depth discussion of the Cognitive Therapy approach to Narcissistic Personality Disordered individuals. Early in the course of therapy with these individuals, three treatment objectives must be met: developing a collaborative working relationship, socializing the individuals to the cognitive theory and model of treatment, and agreeing on treatment goals. Narcissistic individuals often arrive to treatment somewhere between pre-contemplation and contemplation in a stance that is opposed to change. Even while experiencing distress, these individuals are ambivalent about accepting help or examining their own thoughts and behaviors because this may activate their core negative belief of inferiority. Forming a collaborative relationship is challenging in that narcissistic individuals are deeply invested in being special and superior, and usually have a limited capacity for working collaboratively. These self-protective strategies can easily provoke strong reactions in the therapist, such as annoyance, anxiety, defensiveness, or lapses in judgment. Establishing and maintaining firm treatment guidelines and limits, in a neutral, matter-of-fact tone is necessary. Pointing out that sticking to an agreed upon agenda allows the therapist to more effectively address the narcissistic individual's important concerns. Similarly, the therapist can approach other counterproductive behaviors in therapy by appealing to the individual's self-interest. With these particular individuals, it is important to offer praise and support for their strengths in order to meet their expectations for the relationship and keep them engaged in treatment. Of course, this must be done strategically to reinforce desired behaviors without contributing to problem ones.

Because disclosing shortcomings and weaknesses are alien to the narcissist's style, behavioral interventions are usually easier to implement earlier in treatment since they require less self-disclosure than most cognitive techniques (Fowler, Orme, & Hart, 2021). The rhythm of treatment with narcissistic individuals alternates focus among increasing responsibility for behavior, decreasing cognitive distortions and dysfunctional affects—such as rage reactions—and developing healthier attitudes and beliefs. The challenge of treatment with these individuals is to tailor treatment for the three components of grandiosity, hypersensitivity to criticism, and empathic deficits. Cognitive techniques are useful in revising their distorted self-view, particularly with dichotomous, black-white thinking. Furthermore, magical restructuring methods wherein a realistic and pleasurable fantasy replaces a grandiose one are useful. Systematic desensitization and role reversal can be used to address hypersensitivity. Working with empathy deficits is a major focus of treatment and involves several techniques. After bringing these deficits to the attention of the individual, emotional schemas related to the feelings and reactions of others are activated, usually through role plays including role reversal. Then alternative ways of relating to others can be discussed, and new statements of belief, such as "other's feelings count too," are formulated. The use of significant others in therapy—such as in couples sessions—has been found useful in developing and practicing empathy and in reinforcing changes, as well as helping the significant other cope more affectively with the narcissistic individual.

According to Behary & Davis (2014), five key treatment goals are: recognize maladaptive coping modes and weaken their predominance; build affect regulation skills, emphasizing tolerance of frustration and imperfection; increase respect and empathy for others; increase attunement to natural strengths rather than contingent self-worth; and increase role involvement and appropriate reciprocity. The ultimate purpose of these goals is not to create homogenous individuals who are unfalteringly loving and tolerant; rather, it is to allow narcissistic individuals the capacity to be more flexible and adaptive manner.

In summary, cognitive therapy with the Narcissistic Personality Disordered individual can be most challenging, nevertheless, they can make significant changes. Beck indicates that the best predictor of success are the degree of narcissism and the therapist's ability to withstand the individual's demands for approval and special treatment. To the extent that a collaborative working relationship is established, limits are set and maintained regarding the control of therapy and special treatment, and schemas of regarding grandiosity, hypersensitivity and empathy are changed and associated behaviors and affects modulated, positive treatment outcomes are likely.

Schema Therapy. Schema Therapy is an elaboration of cognitive therapy that has been developed by Young (1994; 1999) specifically for personality disorders, and other difficult individual and couples problems. Schema Therapy involves identifying maladaptive schemas and planning specific strategies and interventions. Four main strategies are cognitive, experiential, behavioral and the therapeutic relationship itself. Cognitive restructuring, i.e., modification of maladaptive schemas, is an important cognitive strategy, but is combined with imagery exercises, empathic confrontation, homework assignments and "limited re-parenting," i.e., a form of corrective emotional experience (Young, 1999).

Maladaptive schemas typically associated with Narcissistic Personality Disorder include: *entitlement,* i.e., the belief that one is superior to others and not bound by the rules and norms that govern normal social interaction; *emotional deprivation,* i.e., the belief that one's desire for emotional support will not be met by others; *defectiveness*: i.e., the belief that one is defective, bad, unwanted, or inferior in important respects; *unrelenting standards*, i.e., the belief that striving to meet unrealistically high standards of performance is essential to be accepted and to avoid criticism; and *insufficient self-control*, i.e., the belief that one is incapable of self-control and frustration tolerance (Bernstein, 2002). Young et al. (2003) provide a detailed treatment protocol for treating the Narcissistic Personality Disorder.

Interpersonal Psychotherapy

For Benjamin (2003) psychotherapeutic interventions with Narcissistic Personality Disordered individuals can be planned and evaluated in terms of whether they enhance collaboration, facilitate learning about maladaptive patterns and their roots, block these patterns, enhance the will to change, and effectively encourage new patterns. As with other Interpersonal Psychotherapy applications, the success of interventions aimed at treating narcissistic personality disorder should be evaluated in terms of their impact on the patient and not the therapist's intention. This means the occurrence of rage, angry withdrawal from the therapist, or regal autonomy signal that an error has been made. Any subtle suggestion of blame may elicit problem patterns.

Facilitating collaboration with narcissistic individuals in rooted in accurate, consistent empathy. Consistent empathy provides the affirmation and soothing needed to learn self-regulation. Through the experience of being accurately mirrored, able to internalize this empathic affirmation of self. Another important aspect of collaboration involves the individual's learning to tolerate his or her faults. This is facilitated through modelling as the therapist acknowledged mistakes or error, such as an occasional minor lapse in understanding the individual. In therapy, narcissistic individuals must learn to recognize and block the patterns of entitlement, grandiosity and envy of other's success. Gentle confrontations embedded in strong support are utilized for this purpose. Benjamin considers this a fragile practice, one that may easily result in a hurt narcissistic individual abandoning treatment. To accomplish this successfully, the therapist must master the delicate art of pushing the edge of awareness without destroying the therapeutic relationship. Couples therapy can be useful in the recognition and blocking of maladaptive patterns.

Once these individuals understand their maladaptive patterns and choose to relinquish the quest for unattainable or maladaptive goals, new learning is relatively easy. According to Benjamin, the basic focus of interpersonal learning is empathy. Empathy can effectively be taught in couple's therapy. Role playing and other empathy training approaches can be particularly useful. Benjamin contends that when utilizing role playing, it is important that a collaborative and benign use of the individual's exact words and inflections be employed, as inexact mirroring can elicit rage and withdrawal.

Group Therapy

There is growing literature in the treatment of this and other personality disorders in group therapy formats (Ogrodniczuk, Uliaszek, Lebow, & Kealy, 2021). Many of the recent reports are based on object relations and/or self-psychology approaches (Leszcz, 1989). Outcome research demonstrates that group therapy is as effective as any other therapy in treating the Narcissistic Personality Disorder. (Alonzo, 1992). A number of factors contribute to the effectiveness of groups with this personality disorder. First, peer rather than therapist feedback is likely to be more acceptable to the individual. Second, transference are likely to be less intense than in individual therapy. Working through intense affects is more possible because of the individual's positive attachments within the group and because of peer group scrutiny of the individual's disavowed affects. Third, group membership provides the narcissist individual with three unique needs: mirroring of needs, objects for idealization, and opportunities for peer relationships (Grotjahn, 1984). Finally, the group provides individuals with opportunities to increase their capacity to empathize with others, as well as enhance self-esteem and self-cohesion.

Most of the recent reports suggest that groups consisting exclusively of narcissistic individuals can have successful therapeutic outcomes. Alonzo (1992) notes that while narcissistic pathology undermines the usual forces that lead to group cohesion, a properly run group can function as a container for splitting and oscillation of self-love and hate. She also notes that a high drop out rate is common in groups for Narcissistic Personality Disordered individuals with up to 50 percent of the individuals dropping out in ongoing—rather than time-limited—groups. Alonzo recommends intermittent individual therapy focused on helping individuals remain in the group. Horowitz (1987) describes the indication and contraindications for group treatment of narcissistic individuals. He notes four indications: demandingness, egocentrism, social isolation and withdrawal, and socially deviant behavior. Even though these traits may be taxing to both therapist and group members. Horowitz believes individuals with such traits are quite amenable to group treatment. Stone and Whiteman (1980) note that attention to the unique needs of the individual might warrant a deemphasis on interpretations geared to the entire groups with a focus on an individual member's needs or capacities that are different from that of the group. Finally, Rutan, Stone, & Shay (2014) maintain that group therapy does not provide narcissistic individuals with the safety of individual psychotherapy. The presence of others triggers fears of non-responsiveness and, as such, presents a serious danger to the self. Groups provide an opportunity for narcissistic individuals to face their difficulties *in vivo*, gaining valuable reparative experiences in self–other interactions. While all group members may suffer narcissistic injury for time to time, it is important to distinguish between the narcissistic needs of all individuals and the pathology of this disorder.

Marital and Family Therapy

The early family therapy literature emphasized the treatment of adolescents in families with severe narcissistic pathology (Shapiro, 1982; Berkowitz et al., 1974). Typically, such families identify the adolescent as the patient and project onto him or her their own devalued view of themselves. Not surprisingly, when the adolescent attempts to separate and individualize, the parent's rage and projections intensify. In a family therapy format, the therapist functions to contain displaced, projected and acted out impulses and affects. Furthermore, the therapist must acknowledge, work through and redirect these responses and so provide the family an opportunity to restore previously severed communication and mutual support during this critical phase of adolescent development.

More recent applications of family therapy to Narcissistic Personality Disorder treats entire family systems for one or both parents (Ogrodniczuk, Uliaszek, Lebow & Kealy, 2021).

Jones (1987) advocates family systems approach to the narcissistic family. He suggests several strategies, particularly, determining the dilemma the family faces regarding change by analyzing the metaphorical themes that paradoxically bind the family to resist change. Subsequently, the therapist must join—rather than challenge or confront—the family's resistance. Such an empathic relationship is useful in understanding how resistance can be lowered. Usually, family sessions are scheduled weekly for ninety minutes with all family members. Such family treatment has been described as up to or more than a year's duration.

Considerably more has been published about marital therapy with the narcissistic spouse or couple. Berkowitz (1985) has described a couple's therapy protocol based on Kohut's view of narcissistic vulnerability, self-object needs and projective identification. The couple is seen conjointly in weekly sessions—usually 75 to 90 minutes—with the goal of "owning" projections and internalizing needed self-object functions. Lachkar (1986; 1992) describes a common spousal bond: the narcissistic dominated by mirroring needs and the others by fears of abandonment. She describes a psychoanalytic treatment approach—combining both object relations theory and self-psychology—in which the therapist functions as a self-object so that the exhibitionistic/bonding expectations can become channeled into more realistic goals. Therapy is envisioned as involving three developmental phases: fusion, separation, and interaction. It should be noted that Lachkar views conjoint marital therapy as a precursor to individual psychotherapy or psychoanalysis of one or both spouses.

Furthermore, she adds that in conjoint work, the therapeutic alliance must be joined with the spouse who is predominately narcissistic because of their tendency to flee, isolation and withdraw from therapy.

Solomon (1989) describes marital therapy wherein one or both spouses meet criteria for the Narcissistic Personality Disorder. Elucidating a self-psychology perspective of narcissism in marriage, she described a conjoint treatment protocol wherein marital therapy session functions as a "holding environment." Furthermore, she believes that distorted conscious and unconscious communication is central to marital conflict and its resolution. Finally, she describes the therapist's empathic self as the basic tool of treatment. Masterson and Orcutt (1989) describe a conjoint approach to working with the narcissistic couple.

Relationship Enhancement Therapy. This approach has recently been adapted to couple's therapy with narcissistic spouses (Snyder, 1994). Relationship enhancement therapy is a unique blending of object relationship theory, social learning theory, interpersonal theory, and system theory which provides a psychoeducational format for incorporating skill training in an individual psychotherapy of conjoint couple therapy.

Relationship Enhancement couples therapy focuses on the learning and application of four care interpersonal skills; empathy; effective expression; discussion-mode switching between empathic and expressor roles, and problem solving/conflict resolution. The therapist explains, demonstrates and coaches each skill in the conjoint session, and the spouse then practices these skills during and between sessions with progressively difficult issues. Not surprisingly, the empathic skills and the subjective aspect of the expressor skill are notably deficient for the narcissistically vulnerable couple. Furthermore, the therapist provides a "holding" environment" in which narcissistic vulnerability is minimally acted out and instead is experienced and addressed productively. As a result, both spouses learn to express feelings with less risk of shaming the other and more able to empathize with the feelings of the other spouse that previously evoked defensive reactions. Snyder (1994) provides a detailed case example of this promising approach.

There have been a number of recent developments in couple's therapy wherein one or both partners present with narcissistic personality issues or the full blown personality disorder. Kalojera et al. (1999) provide a detailed rationale and treatment strategy for approaching such couples from a self-psychology perspective that incorporate systemic dynamics. These authors present a useful flow chart of the process of relational work with such couples and a detailed case example illustrating the application of this approach.

Lachkar (1999) offers additional insight into the psychoanalytic treatment of couples in which one partner has a narcissistic personality structure while the other partner presents with a borderline personality pattern or meets criteria for the Borderline Personality Disorder. Solomon (1999) also addresses the treatment of the narcissistic-borderline couple from a somewhat different psychoanalytic perspective. This line of research has been continued by Landucci and Foley (2014). They note that the therapist's job in working with the narcissistic-borderline couple is to assist the couple in understanding how their dysfunctional interactions replay developmental problems and do not necessarily signal problems in the relationship itself. Therapist empathy and the ability to contain the narcissistic partner's rage enable the other partner to feel safe in the session and thereby rekindles the developmental process for both. Another common relational pattern is the dependent/narcissistic couple. Nurse (1998) provides a detailed rationale and treatment protocol for working with such couples based on Millon's theory of personality disorders (Millon & Davis, 1996).

Medication

Currently, there are no psychotropic medications specifically indicated for treating individuals with dependent personality disorder (Silk & Feurino, 2012). Nevertheless, medications are used that target specific troubling symptoms associated with the disorder, such as depression, anxiety, or sleep problems. Generally, these medications are used as an adjunct to psychotherapy and skills training (Nelson & Tsheringld, 2021). Because troubling symptoms often respond to medications sooner than most psychological interventions, medications are usually prescribed at the onset of treatment (Sperry, 1995b). Unfortunately, there is little research evidence to provide guidelines for the use of such medications with this disorder (Silk & Feurino, 2012).

Combined and Integrative Treatment Approaches

As noted in the opening chapter of this book, there is seldom a single treatment of choice, be it specifically method—i.e., mirroring—or general approach—i.e., psychoanalysis—that can ensure positive treatment outcomes with personality-disordered individuals. Rather, depending on the individual's overall level of functioning, temperamental patterns, defensive style, and skill deficits, a focused, specific and sequentially coordinated tailored treatment protocol is usually necessary to accomplish treatment goals and objectives in a timely matter and fashion (Winkeller & Schlesinger, 2021). Pincus, Wright, and Cain (2014) describe narcissistic grandiosity and narcissistic vulnerability in the context of psychotherapy, with links to the previous discussion of overt and covert narcissism. Symptoms of social anxiety, depression, and suicidality often drive narcissistic individuals into treatment seeking relief and addressing these with a combined/integrative treatment strategy is particularly useful. Roche, Pincus, Lukowitsky, Ménard, and Conroy (2013) also provide an integrative approach to the assessment of this disorder.

Several treatment approaches and interventions applicable to the Narcissistic Personality Disorder have now been described by orientation (i.e., psychodynamic, cognitive) (behavior/psychoeducational, interpersonal) or format (i.e., individual, group, marital/family, or medication). This final section offers another treatment perspective: an integrative and combined approach. Again, as described in the opening chapter, the highest functioning individuals who meet either DSM-5-TR or dynamic criteria for a personality disorder, are more likely to have few rather than many troubling temperamental patterns, skill deficits, and defensive styles, than the lower functioning individual. And, repeating the basic premise of the book: the higher the functioning and fewer skill deficits the personality-disordered individual the more likely a single approach will be effective, while the lower the functioning and the more skill deficits and under- or overmodulated temperament patterns the personality-disordered individual, the more an integrative, tailored and combined sequential approach is necessary.

Chapter 10

Obsessive-Compulsive Personality Disorder

Individuals with obsessive compulsive personalities often present themselves as inhibited, stubborn, perfectionistic, judgmental, overconscientious, rigid, and chronically anxious. They tend to avoid intimacy and experience little pleasure from life. They may be successful, but at the same time can be indecisive and demanding (Samuels & Costa, 2012; Skodol, Bender, & Oldham, 2019; American Psychiatric Association, 2022). All of these factors can impede personal change. However, despite a number of unique therapeutic challenges, it can be highly effective and successful. Furthermore, although there are some similarities, this disorder differs from the Obsessive-Compulsive Personality Disorder which is characterized by ritualistic compulsions and obsessions (Samuels & Costa, 2012).

This chapter describes a framework for the assessment and effective treatment of this disorder. It includes sections on diagnosis, psychological assessment, case conceptualization, and treatment interventions. It begins with background information on the disorder as well as the DSM-5-TR description, prototypic description, associated features, and the Alternative Model of Personality Disorders description of this disorder. The section on case conceptualization provides five common clinical formulations of this disorder: psychodynamic, biosocial, cognitive-behavioral, interpersonal, and an integrative conceptualization of this disorder. Several treatment approaches, modalities, and intervention strategies are also described. These include individual psychotherapy, group therapy, marital and family therapy, medication, and integrative and combined treatment.

Description of the Obsessive-Compulsive Personality Disorder

The Obsessive-Compulsive Personality Disorder can be recognized by the following descriptors and characteristics: styles vs. disorders, triggering event, behavioral styles, interpersonal styles, cognitive styles, affective styles, attachment style, and optimal criterion.

Style vs. Disorder. The obsessive compulsive personality can be thought of as spanning a continuum from healthy to pathological, with the obsessive personality style on the healthy, and the Obsessive-Compulsive Personality Disorder on the pathological end. Table 10.1 compares and contrasts differences between the obsessive compulsive style and disorder.

Table 10.1 A Comparison of the Obsessive-Compulsive Personality Style and Disorder

Personality Style	Personality Disorder
Desires to complete tasks and projects without flaws or errors	Perfectionism that interferes with task completion
Take pride in doing all job or tasks well, including the smallest details of it	Preoccupation with details, rules, lists, order, organization, or schedules to the extent that the major point of the activity is lost
Tend to want things to be done "just right" and in a specific manner, but has some tolerance for things being done	Unreasonable insistence that others submit exactly to their way of doing things, or unreasonable reluctance to allow others to do things because of the conviction that they will not do them correctly
Dedicate to work and working hard capable of intense, single-minded effort	Excessive devotion to work and productivity to the exclusion of leisure activities and friendships (not accounted for by obvious economic necessity)
Carefully considers alternatives and their consequences in making decisions	Indecisive: decision making either avoided, postponed or prolonged (but not due to excessive need for advice or reassurance from others)
Tend to have strong moral principles and strongly desires to do the right thing	Overconscientious, scrupulous and inflexible about matters of morality, ethics or values
No-nonsense individuals who do their work without much emotional expenditure	Restructured expression of affection
Generally, careful thrifty and cautious, but able to share from their abundance	Lack of generosity in giving time, money or gifts when no personal gain is likely to result
Tend to save and collect objects and is reluctant to discard objects that have, formerly had or someday may have value for them	Unable to discard worn-out or worthless objects even when they have no sentimental value

The following case examples further illustrate the differences between the personality disorder (Mr. Z.) and the personality style (Mr. C.).

Case Study: Obsessive-Compulsive Personality Disorder

Mr. Z. is a 39-year-old male business executive who wanted to begin a course of psychotherapy because his "whole world was closing in." He gave a history of long-standing feelings of dissatisfaction with his marriage which had worsened in the past two years. He described his wife's increasing demands for time and affection from him, which he believed was a weakness she had. His professional life also had become conflicted when his partner of ten years wanted to expand their accounting firm to another city. Mr. Z believed this proposal was fraught with dangers and had come to the point of selling out his share of the business to his partner. He knew he had to make some decisions about his marriage and his business but found himself unable to do so. He hoped therapy would help with these decisions. He presented as neatly dressed in a conservative three-piece blue suit. His posture was rigid and he spoke in a formal and controlled tone with constricted affect. His thinking was characterized by preoccupation with details and was somewhat circumstantial.

> **Case Study: Obsessive Compulsive Personality Style**
>
> Mr. C. is a 41-year-old assistant vice president of personnel for a public utility. He rose through the ranks because of his loyalty and accomplishments above and beyond the call of duty. Because of his thoroughness and attention to detail he has saved his corporation nearly $3 million in the past two years on insurance and health benefits for the employees of the utility. Most evenings Mr. C. takes a briefcase of work home with him. Although he didn't really mind this intrusion into his family life, his wife of eighteen years did. Accordingly, they've reached an agreement that Mr. C. will spend at least two hours with his wife and three kinds before turning to his briefcase.

Triggering Event. The typical situation, circumstance or event that most likely triggers or activates the characteristic maladaptive response of the Dependent Personality Disorder (Othmer & Othmer, 2002), as noted in behavioral, interpersonal, cognitive, and feeling styles, is: "authority; unstructured situations, and/or demands of intimate and close relations."

Behavioral Style. Behaviorally, this disorder is characterized by perfectionism. Individuals with this disorder are likely to be workaholics. In addition to dependability, they tend to be stubborn and possessive. They tend to be indecisive and procrastinating.

Interpersonal Style. Interpersonally, these individuals are exquisitely conscious of social rank and status and modify their behavior accordingly. That is, they tend to be deferential and obsequious to superiors, and haughty and autocratic to subordinates and peers. They can be doggedly insistent that others do things their way without an appreciation or awareness of how others react to this insistence. At their best they are polite and loyal to the organizations and ideals they espouse.

Cognitive Style. Their thinking style can be characterized as constricted and rule-based. They have difficulty establishing priorities and perspective. They are "detail" people and often lose sight of the larger project. In other words, they "can't see the forest for the trees." Their indecisiveness and doubts make decision making difficult. Their mental inflexibility is matched by their nonsuggestible and unimaginative style, suggesting they have a restricted fantasy life. Like passive aggressive individuals, obsessive compulsive individuals have conflicts between assertiveness and defiance, and pleasing and obedience, but for different reasons.

Affective Style. Their affective or emotional style is characterized as grim and cheerless. They have difficulty with the expression of intimate feelings such as warmth and tenderness. They tend to avoid the "softer" feelings, although they may express anger, frustration, and irritability quite freely. This grim, feeling-avoidant demeanor shows itself in stilted, stiff relationship behaviors.

Attachment Style. The preoccupied attachment dimension is characterized by a sense of personal unworthiness and a positive evaluation of others. These individuals tend to be very externally oriented in their self-definitions. This Preoccupied Attachment Style is common in individuals with Obsessive-Compulsive Personality Disorder.

Optimal Diagnostic Criterion. Of all the diagnostic criteria for the Dependent Personality Disorder, one has been found to be the most useful in diagnosing this disorder. The belief is that by beginning with this criterion, the clinician can test for the presence or absence of this criterion and more quickly diagnose the personality disorder (Allnutt & Links, 1996). The optimal criterion for this disorder is: shows perfectionism that interferes with task completion.

DSM-5-TR Description

Individuals with this personality disorder are characterized by an unremitting pattern of perfectionism, orderliness, and control instead of flexibility, openness, and efficiency. They are overly preoccupied with details, rules, and schedules. Their perfectionism interferes with completing tasks, owing to their overly strict standards. They are overly devoted to work and productivity to the exclusion of leisure activities and friendships. When it comes to matters of values, morality, or ethics, these individuals are inflexible, scrupulous, and overconscientious. Often, they are unable to discard worn-out or worthless objects that have no sentimental value. They will not delegate tasks or work with others unless it can be on their terms. Not surprisingly, these individuals are also rigid and stubborn. Finally, they are misers with money, and it is hoarded in the event of future catastrophes (American Psychiatric Association, 2022).

The "Alternative DSM-5 Model for Personality Disorders" provides another description of this disorder (American Psychiatric Association, 2022). It is described as making it difficult for an individual to establish and maintain close personal relationships, associated with perfectionism, restricted emotional expression, and inflexibility. Characteristic difficulties are noted in identity, self-direction, empathy, and intimacy, as well as restricted affect, intimacy avoidance, perseveration, and rigid perfectionism.

Prototypic Description

A prototype is a brief description that captures the essence of how a particular disorder commonly presents. Prototypic descriptions are useful and convenient, and clinicians commonly rely on them rather than lists of behavioral criteria and core and instrumental beliefs (Westen, 2012). Here is a common prototypic description of the Obsessive-Compulsive Personality Disorder: These individuals are perfectionists and unyielding control freaks. They cannot rest until they get every detail exactly right. Because they insist that others can never be careful or competent enough, they never delegate or trust important matters to others. Their lives are controlled by schedules, rules, and rigid routines. Because of their scrupulous attention to details and their projects, they cannot relax, be spontaneous, or enjoy close and intimate relationships. They are unusually tight with money, feelings, and affection. They make it clear they must always have their way or else (Francis, 2013).

Associated Features

Prevalence. This disorder has been identified in 2.5 percent of the general population and 10.1 percent in clinical practice (Torgersen, 2021).

Differential Diagnosis. Obsessive Compulsive Disorder (OCD) can easily be confused with OCPD. True obsessions and compulsions are distinguishing feature for OCD. When criteria for both OCD and OCPD are met, both diagnoses are to be reported (American Psychiatric Association, 2022).

Development and Course. OCPD appears to develop as a result of both genetics and childhood experiences. In some case studies, adults can recall experiencing OCPD from a very early age. Typically, these individuals felt that they needed to follow rules, be a perfect or perfectly obedient to be accepted by their parents and caregivers. This need for rule following, perfectionism, being right, and doing their best followed over into adulthood. Left untreated, OCPD can worsen with age (Diedrich & Voderholzer, 2015).

Culture, Sex, and Gender. Awareness of specific cultural values and norms is critical in the diagnosis of this disorder. Certain cultures highly regard work and productivity. Some of its members may emphasize over conscientiousness, striving for perfection, and moral superiority and be reinforced by such a culture. But such behaviors on their own are not necessarily indicative of OCPD. This disorder is equally prevalent in males and females (American Psychiatric Association, 2022).

Alternative Model of Obsessive-Compulsive Personality Disorder

The Alternative Model of Personality Disorders (AMPD) offers a clinically useful description of the Obsessive-Compulsive Personality Disorder in terms of typical features and trait facets. Typical features are difficulties in establishing and sustaining close relationships, associated with rigid perfectionism, inflexibility, and restricted emotional expression. Trait facet criteria include Rigid perfectionism, Perseveration, Intimacy avoidance, and Restricted affectivity. Three or more are required and must include Rigid Perfectionism (American Psychiatric Association, 2022).

Conceptualizations of Obsessive-Compulsive Personality Disorder

Psychodynamic Case Conceptualizations

Early psychoanalytic writers formulated the obsessive compulsive personality as a regression from the oedipal phase to the anal phase of development. Because of punitive superego, these obsessive compulsive individuals employed intellectualization, isolation of affect, undoing, development and reaction formation as defense. Presumably, these individuals experienced difficulty expressing aggression as a result of power struggle with maternal figures over toilet training.

However, contemporary writers formulate this pattern much broader than anal fixation. As children these individuals were not sufficiently valued or loved by their caretakers and subsequently developed overwhelming doubt. Salzman (1980) believes the obsessive pattern is basically a device for preventing any thought or feeling that could produce shame, loss of pride or status, or a feeling of deficiency or weakness, irrespective of whether the feelings are hostile, sexual or otherwise. He views obsessive compulsivity as a neurotic strategic which protects these individuals from exposure of any thoughts or feelings that could endanger their physical or psychological existence. This overriding need to control their inner and outer world requires these individuals to lead overly structured and manageable lives. They tend to maintain doubts, are willing to make commitments, and strive for perfection. Thus, it is necessary for them to know everything to predict the future and prepare for every exigency. To maintain the fiction of perfection, they must never make an error or admit any deficiency. Furthermore, their tendency to procrastinate is related to their tendency to doubt as a means of guaranteeing their omniscience when life forces a decision or choice. As such, they are deeply ambivalent, which allows them to maintain security, but at the price of productivity and positive feelings and attitudes. These individuals find both anger and dependency consciously unacceptable and so defend against these feelings with defenses like reaction formation and isolation of affect as well as differential and obsequious behaviors. Intimacy poses major concerns for these individuals who fear being overwhelmed by powerful wishes to be taken care of while also experiencing the frustration of those wishes along with the fear of being out of control. In addition, these individuals harbor the secret conviction that if they could become perfect, they would finally receive the parental approved and esteem they missed in early life. Finally, psychodynamic writers have noted the unique cognitive style of obsessive compulsive individuals (Shapiro, 1965; Horowitz, 1988; Horowitz et al., 1984) characterized by drivenness, careful attention to detail and lack of spontaneity, and ruminative thinking.

Biosocial Case Conceptualization

To date there is no research evidence that biological predisposing factors underlie this disorder (Millon & Davis, 1996). Nonetheless, clinical observations suggest that many obsessive compulsive individuals display an anhedonic temperament (Millon, 1981) and tend to be first born in their families of origin (Toman, 1961). Certain environmental factors may be etiologic: parental overcontrol, learned compulsive behavior and responsibility training. Rather than being overprotective, parents of obsessive compulsive individuals overcontrol with firmness and punitiveness. This attempt to prevent their children from causing trouble for themselves or others and is punitive when the child misbehaves or fails to meet expectations. These children learn compulsive behavior directly and indirectly within the family matrix. They learn to avoid punishment by accepting and meeting the demands and expectations of perfectionistic and punitive parents. Furthermore, they learn compulsivity by imitating the compulsive behaviors modelled by one or both parents. As a result, they do not develop the ability to generate options and explore alternatives and thus fail to function autonomously. Obsessive compulsive individuals are regularly exposed to conditions that teach them to overvalue a sense of responsibility to others. They are taught to feel guilt when these responsibilities are not met, and shame when they act impulsively or even playfully. Instead, they learn to be polite, pleasing, and loyal to superiors. These influences typically yield individuals who are hard driving, perfectionistic, and seemingly polite and pleasing individuals who lead rather restrictive, tentative, colorless lives.

This obsessive compulsive pattern is self-perpetuated through an interaction of cognitive and behavioral rigidity, strict adherence of roles, regulations and social convention, and a tendency to be highly self-critical. While their cognitive rigidity serves to reduce anxiety associated with flexibility and ambivalence, they tend to lead overstructured, one-sided lives. Self-criticism serves to keep them in line, while striving for perfection reduces opportunities for risk taking and adventure.

Behavioral Case Conceptualizations

Beck (2015) identified the core beliefs or schemas held by obsessive compulsive individuals: perfectionism and control. The perfectionism schema involves beliefs such as: "To be worthwhile I must avoid making mistakes because to make a mistake is to fail which would be intolerable," and "If the perfect course of action is unclear, it is better to do nothing." The control schema involves beliefs such as: "I must be perfectly in control of myself and my environment, because loss of control is intolerable and dangerous". "Without my rules and rituals, I'll collapse into an inert pile," "Magical rituals or obsessive ruminations prevent the occurrence of catastrophes." Typically, they view themselves as responsible and accountable for most everything in their lives. At the same time, they believe they are inadequate, helpless, or defective. They view others as incompetent, careless, and less concerned about matters than they are. Related beliefs include needing rules and regulations in order to survive. Because of their beliefs about control and perfect, should they fail at a task, they are likely to conclude that they must be failures and worthless. Not surprisingly, such beliefs are reflected in their main strategy or pattern of exercising maximum control over themselves and others through the use of directiveness, coercion, and disapproval (Beck, 2015; Simon, 2015).

Guidano and Liotti (1983) provide a similar but different cognitive formulation which involves three maladaptive schemas. They are: perfectionism, the need for certainty, and the belief that there is an absolute correct solution for human problems. Guidano and Liotti note that these individuals received mixed, contradictory messages from at least one parent. They also describe typical automatic thoughts of obsessive compulsive individuals. "I need to get this assignment done perfectly"; "I have to do this project myself or it won't be done right"; "That person misbehaved and should be punished"; and "I should keep these old reports because I might need them some day." In addition to these schemas and automatic thoughts, individuals with this personality pattern often utilize the cognitive distortions of dichotomous thinking and magnification or catastrophizing.

Turkat (1990) and Turkat and Maisto (1985) suggest a behavioral formulation of this pattern. These individuals are noted to have been reared in families that emphasized productivity and rule-following at the expense of emotional expressivity and interpersonal relationships. Accordingly, these individuals did not acquire adequate levels of empathy skills or skills in interacting with others on an emotional basis.

Interpersonal Case Conceptualizations

According to Benjamin (1996) persons diagnosed with Obsessive-Compulsive Personality Disorder were likely raised in an atmosphere of unreasonable and relentless coercion to perform correctly and follow rules regardless of personal cost. As a consequence, the obsessive compulsive individual has an unbalanced devotion to perfection of self and others. These parents typically held extremely high expectations for self-control and perfection, and not only punished their children for not being perfect but give them little or no reward for success. Subsequently, a focus on mistakes and self-criticism on the adult consequences. Furthermore, there tended to be little warmth in these households. Laughter, hugging, holding and other signs of affection were seldom, if ever, modelled. Expression of feelings were considered dangerous. The adult consequences of their lack of warmth and demand for perfection is social correctness albeit inaccessibility of feelings. Finally, there is a fear of making mistakes and a penchant for rule following. A quest for order underlies blame and inconsiderate control of others with control alternating with blind obedience to authority of principle. This stance is supported by excessive self-discipline, restraint by excessive feelings, and self-criticism, as well as neglect of the self.

Integrative Case Conceptualizations

The following integrative formulation provides a biopsychosocial explanation for how this personality is likely to have developed and how it is maintained. Biologically, these individuals were likely to have exhibited an anhedonic temperament as children. Not surprisingly, firstborn children have a greater propensity for developing a compulsive style than other siblings.

Psychologically, these individuals view themselves, others, the world, and life's purpose in terms of the following themes. They tend to view themselves with some variant of the theme: "I'm responsible if something goes wrong, so I have to be reliable, competent, and righteous." Their world view is some variant of the theme: "Life is unpredictable and expects too much." As such, they are likely to conclude, "Therefore, be in control, right, and proper at all times."

Socially, predictable patterns of parenting and environmental conditioning are noted for this personality. The parenting style they experienced could be characterized as both consistent and overcontrolled. As children they were trained to be overly responsible for their actions and to feel guilty and worthless if they were not obedient, achievement-oriented, or "good." The parental injunction to which they were most likely exposed was "You must do and be better to be worthwhile."

This obsessive compulsive pattern is confirmed, reinforced, and perpetuated by a number of factors: exceedingly high expectations plus harshly rigid behavior and beliefs, along with a tendency to be self-critical, lead to rigid rule-based behavior and avoidance of social, professional, and moral unacceptability. This in turn further reconfirms the harshly rigid behaviors and beliefs of this personality pattern (Sperry, 2015).

Table 10.2 summarizes the characteristics of this disorder.

Assessment of Obsessive-Compulsive Personality Disorder

Several sources of information are useful in establishing a diagnosis and treatment plan for personality disorders. Observation, collateral information, and psychological testing are important adjuncts to the patient's self-report in the clinical interview. This section briefly describes some characteristic observations that the clinician makes and the nature of the rapport likely to develop in initial encounters with specific personality disordered individuals. Characteristic response patterns on various objective (i.e., MMPI-2 and MCMI-IV) and projective tests (i.e., Rorschach and TAT) are also described.

Interview Behavior and Rapport. The obsessive compulsive's dynamics of circumstantiality, perfectionism, and ambivalence make interviewing these individuals difficult and challenging. Their preoccupation with and focus on details and need for control leads to a seemingly endless struggle about words, issues, and who is in charge without being able to develop an atmosphere of understanding and cooperation. Open ended questions leads them to confusion. Instead they want more focused questions, but interpret them too narrowly when this

Table 10.2 Characteristics of Obsessive-Compulsive Personality Disorder

Triggering Event(s)	Demands of authority figures; unstructured situations, and/or demands of intimate and close relations
Behavioral Appearance:	Perfectionistic and righteous
	Workaholic
	Dependable, reliable, and overly conscientious
	Indecisive and procrastinates
Interpersonal Behavior:	Devotion to tasks or work limits relationships
	Unwillingness to delegate or collaborate
	Rigid and stubborn
	Judgmental
	Autocratic to subordinates but deferential to superiors
	Polite and loyal
Cognitive Style:	Constricted—rule-based
	Inflexibility
	Unimaginative
Feeling Style:	Grim and cheerless
	Feeling avoidance
Temperament:	Irritable, difficult, or anxious
Attachment Style:	Preoccupied
Parental Injunction:	"You must do/be better to be worthwhile"
Self-View:	"I'm responsible if something goes wrong"
World View:	"Life is unpredictable and expects too much. Therefore, be in control, be right and proper and don't make mistakes"
Maladaptive Schemas	Unrelenting Standards; Punitiveness; Emotional Inhibition
Optimal Diagnostic Criteria	Shows perfectionism that interferes with task completion

kind of question is asked. They may bring a notebook of their medical history, diet and exercise pattern, or even dreams, expecting to review these details with you. And while they may admit that affects and feelings are associated with the details, they are unwilling to admit the value of expressing those affects, much less talking about them. Their ambivalence is difficult to overcome since they cannot accept others' assurances that their problems are solvable or that they can tolerate less control in their lives.

The clinician's expression of empathy is problematic for them, since they insist they are objective and have no feelings. Thus, they are perturbed at the expression of empathy and reject it as irrelevant. They may insist that their problems, not their suffering, are important. Yet, their problems are unsolvable! The only therapeutic leverage for the clinician is to attempt to get and keep this individual in touch with their anger and other feelings. But this is difficult as they will attempt to defend or deny affects, and put forth even more obstructive obsessive thinking to neutralize such therapeutic leverage. Needless to say, forming a therapeutic alliance is difficult and the interview often consists of aborted attempts, frustrations and struggles (Othmer & Othmer, 2002).

Psychological Testing Data. The Minnesota Multiphase Personality Inventory (MMPI-2), the Millon Clinical Multiaxial Inventory (MCMI-IV), the Rorschach Psychodiagnostic Test, and the Thematic Apperception Test (TAT) can be useful in diagnosing the Compulsive Personality Disorder as well as the personality style (Groth-Marnat, 2009).

On the MMPI-2 there is likely to be a moderately high K (Correction) scale. Since individuals with obsessive compulsive features are not inclined to self-disclosure, they seldom leave elevated profiles. However, scales 1 (Hypochondriasis) and 3 (Hysteria) tend to be elevated. If physical complaints are the focus of the distress scale 1 may be particularly elevated. An elevation on scale 9 (Hypomania) usually reflects the degree to which these individuals are autocratic and dominant in interpersonal relationships. Since scale 7 (Psychasthenia) reflects obsessionalism, elevation of this scale usually indicates a complaining and querulous attitude in them (Meyer, 1995; Graham, 2011).

On the MCMI-IV, a high score on scale 7 (Compulsive) is likely (Millon et al., 2016). Elevations on scale a (anxiety), are not likely since these individuals tend to express anxiety somatically, thus scale H is likely to be elevated (Somatic symptom disorder) (Choca & Denburg, 1997).

On the Rorschach test there is likely to be an emphasis on Dd (Unusual Detail) and D (Common Detail) responses on the Also, a high F+% (Form Plus) and fewer W (Whole) response and color-based responses. Obsessive compulsive individuals tend to describe some responses in overly specific detail and make criticisms of the ink blots (Meyer, 1995). The new Rorschach Performance Assessment System (R-PAS) is an improved method for scoring and interpreting the Rorschach Inkblot Test. Besides being evidence-based and internationally normed, it increases clinical utility and is easier to use than Exner's Comprehensive System (Mihura & Meyer, 2018).

The TAT stories of these individuals tend to be lengthy with a variety of themes. Sometimes the primary theme is lost amid the detailing of their response. This is particularly likely on card 2 and 13 MF (Bellak, 1993).

Treatment Approaches and Interventions

Treatment Considerations

Included in the differential diagnosis of this disorder is the Dependent Personality Disorder, and the so called Passive Aggressive Personality Disorder. Common symptom diagnoses that are associated with the Dependent Personality Disorder include the Anxiety Disorders, particularly Simple Phobia, Social Anxiety Disorder, and Panic Disorder. Other common DSM-5-TR disorders include Conversion Disorders and Somatic Symptom Disorders.

The Obsessive Compulsive Disorder (OCD) has a long tradition of treatment dating back to Freud's case of the "Rat Man" and Adler's "Case of Mrs. A." Note that OCD is a symptom disorder while the Obsessive-Compulsive Personality Disorder is a personality disorder. Since the "Rat Man" exhibited both a symptom disorder and a personality disorder, many who have read Freud's account of this case and its treatment have incorrectly assumed that both disorders are the same and are treated the same. They are not the same disorder, but in about one-third of cases, both disorders have been shown to be present (Jenike, Baer, & Minichiello, 1998; Phillips & Stein, 2015). When both disorders are present together, treatment has been shown to be much more challenging than if only OCD is present.

The goals of treatment include increased cognitive constriction and increased feeling expression, so that a more reasonable balance can be obtained between thoughts and feelings. Treatment strategies for the Obsessive-Compulsive Personality Disorder usually involve long-term, insight-oriented therapy. Unlike the Obsessive Compulsive Disorder, where antidepressants plus behavior therapy can result in amelioration of obsessions and compulsions in a relatively short period of time, the Obsessive-Compulsive Personality Disorder does not lend itself to short-term treatment outcomes. However, psychodynamic and cognitive behavioral intervention appear to be effective. Medication is usually not needed with this disorder if the restitution of the accompanying symptom disorder is attainted (Sperry, 2015).

Individual Psychotherapy

Psychodynamic Psychotherapy Approach

The therapy of the obsessive compulsive patients involves exposing the patient's extreme feelings of insecurity and uncertainty. As they come to identify their neurotic structure as a defense against recognizing these weaknesses, they can begin to develop a more adaptive security system. At the outset of treatment, these patients are unable to abandon their obsessive compulsive defense fearing unspeakable consequences. However, as their esteem grow and awareness of their strengths increase, they are able to take the risks of abandoning these patterns and are thus freer to function more productively. The goal of therapy is to switch from impossible expectations for self and others to more realistic achievable ones (Yeomans, Clarkin, & Levy, 2021).

In short, these individuals come to learn that by relinquishing their rigid, inflexible patterns of control and protection, they can actually feel more productive as well. Doing psychodynamically oriented psychotherapy with obsessive compulsive patients requires a number of modifications. The modification involves the clinician's level of activity. The clinician must be active from the beginning through the end of treatment. Clinician passivity, according to Salzman, can lead only to interminable analysis an atmosphere of confusion. Specifically, free association and a tendency to endless detail and circumstantiality must be controlled and limited. Because of these patients' need for perfection, they tend to qualify and quantify their descriptions, which rather than clarifying confuses and obfuscates. The free association process tends to defeat its own purpose. Thus, the clinician must be active to prevent this tangentiality and distraction by attempting to interrupt the irrelevances and avoidances. Of course, the major avoidance is affects. While these patients may talk about feelings and emotions, and even about transference and countertransference, they assiduously avoid the expression of affect. The clinician must, therefore, focus on real feelings and their expression, and limit intellectual discussion of affects.

Another modification from traditional analytic methods involves a focus on recent events. While obsessive compulsive individuals can discuss anger and hostile behavior associated with past events, they find it very difficult to disclose tender impurities and feelings with recent and here-and-now experiences. Such tender impulses and feelings are viewed as threatening and dangerous, and Salzman contend this is the essence of obsessive compulsive defenses. It is the failure to express these feelings, rather than their hostile behavior, that initiated retaliatory behavior from others which in turn stirs up their wrath and hostile responders.

Finally, the usual instruction to forego major decisions during the course of therapy must be modified. Because of their fear of making mistakes, such instruction can serve to reinforce their pathological pattern. Rather, risk taking and decision making must be promoted. The techniques for dealing with their indeciveness is clarification and interpretation of their need for absolutes and certainties. If dream material is utilized the emphasis must be in the here-and-now, and dream content treated as data dealt with in the same manner as their other production.

The outcome goal of treatment is that these individuals achieve some degree of balance and compromise, and instead of needing to be superhuman, be able to function as fallible human persons. Because of their anticipatory anxiety, termination issues abound with these patients. It must be clearly understood by both patients and clinicians that anxiety episodes will occur throughout life, and that continuation in therapy is no guarantee against life's distress.

A related goal is superego modification so much that these patients can accept that their wish to transcend such feelings as anger, lust, and dependency are doomed to failure and must be integrated rather than disowned. Gabbard (1994) notes that such changes occur through detailed interpretation of conflicts around aggression, sexuality, and dependence.

There is a consensus that long-term psychodynamic treatment is needed with these patients. This is because of their constricted emotionality and their vulnerability to deflation of self-esteem under their rigid exterior. Treatment typically lasts two to three years of one or two session per week. The prevailing wisdom is that dynamic psychotherapy with the ancillary support of medication and behavioral interventions are effective (Salzman, 1989).

Svartberg & McCullough (2010) provide a useful discussion of Cluster C personality disorders from a psychodynamic perspective, including commentary on treatment for Obsessive-Compulsive Personality Disorder.

Time-limited Supportive-Expressive Therapy. Supportive-expressive therapy was provided to individuals with both obsessive-compulsive and avoidant personality-disordered individuals. Those with Obsessive-Compulsive Personality Disorder lost their personality disorder diagnosis in a significantly shorter period of time than those with Avoidant Personality Disorder. While both groups responded to this time-limited therapy on measures of personality disorder, depression, anxiety, general functioning and interpersonal problems, those with Obsessive-Compulsive Personality Disorder no longer met personality disorder criteria within the first 17 sessions (Barber et al., 1997).

Cognitive Behavioral Therapy Approaches

The cognitive behavioral approaches for Obsessive-Compulsive Personality Disorder are quite promising (Fowler, Orme, & Hart, 2021). Young's schema-focused approach and Beck's cognitive therapy approach were the first of these approaches. Kyrios (1999) describes several cognitive behavioral treatment targets in treating Obsessive-Compulsive Personality Disorder. These include targeting dysfunctional cognitions, restricted behavioral repertoires, negative affective dispositions, and issues related to attachment and identity. Until research-based guidelines are forthcoming, a careful assessment of client and situational attributes and clinician judgment must continue to guide treatment decisions.

Cognitive Therapy Approach. Beck, Freeman, and associates (2004) provide an extended discussion of the Cognitive Therapy approach with Obsessive-Compulsive Personality Disordered individuals. The general outcome goal in working therapeutically with these individuals is helping them modify and restructure their maladaptive schemas which underlie behaviors and effects. Establishing a collaborative working relationship is the first task of therapy. This can be quite difficult for these individuals because of their rigidity, feeling avoidance and tendency to minimize the importance of interpersonal relationships. Therefore, rapport is based on the individual's respect for the therapist's competence and the belief that the therapist will be respecting and helpful. Efforts to develop a closer emotional relationship early in treatment may result in premature termination. However, Strauss et al. (2006) conducted a non-randomized trial of cognitive therapy for Obsessive-Compulsive Personality Disorder and Avoidant Personality Disorder and found that stronger early therapeutic alliances predicted more improvement in symptoms. Even ruptures in the relationship later in therapy may be used as learning experiences if they are managed property. As a result, there are both risks and rewards to early investments in the alliance with these clients. It is also essential to introduce the obsessive-compulsive individual to the cognitive theory of emotion early in the course of therapy, as well as establishing therapeutic goals. Usually these involve presenting problems. After collaboratively establishing these, they are ranked in the order they are to be addressed. A given problem is monitored between sessions with the Dysfunctional Thought Record which includes the situation as well as the feelings and thoughts to when the problem occurred. The record is reviewed at the next session which is the basis for discussing automatic thoughts and the assumptions or schemas underlying the thoughts. In this collaborative relationship, the individual can identify and understand the negative consequences of the schema and ways of refuting them. This process of cognitive disputation and restructuring is particularly useful and well received by obsessive compulsive individuals because of its structured and problem-centered, here-and-now focus.

Several specific strategies and techniques have been found to be particularly useful with these individuals as adjunctive to cognitive therapy. Setting an agenda, prioritizing problems, utilizing problem-solving and thought stopping techniques are effective with issues of rumination, procrastination, and indecisiveness. Salzman (1989) reports that flooding, desensitization, response prevention and satiation training have been used in treating this disorder. Relaxation training is useful with anxiety and psycho-somatic symptoms, while behavioral experiments can be used instead of direct disputation of maladaptive beliefs. Because of their difficulty in attending to their emotions and those of others, empathy training and role reversal have been used effectively. In sum, Obsessive-Compulsive Personality Disorder is a challenging but very treatable disorder. With collaboration, cognitive restructuring and systematic application of cognitive and behavioral strategies and techniques, the obsessive compulsive individual's automatic thoughts and schemas that underlie their maladaptive behavior and affects can be effectively modified and changed.

Turkat (1990) concludes that behavioral modification alone is not sufficient for effective treatment outcomes with most of these patients. Turkat's treatment regimen involved social skills training to increase pleasure and emotion-related experience and to decrease their over commitment to work. He note that while these patients would agree with the clinical formulation and treatment plan, most would not agree to undergo the training. Turkat and Maisto (1985) report similar experience, leading them to conclude that behavior modification alone was not effective for Obsessive-Compulsive Personality Disorder.

Simon (2015) identifies four main goals in the cognitive treatment of OCPD: educate the patient about the role of perfectionism in the development and maintenance of symptoms; testing the rigidity of long-held rules and routines by evaluating whether or not they are working; evaluating the automatic thoughts, underlying assumptions, and core beliefs that maintain perfectionism; and, finally, linking all of the above goals to work and interpersonal relationships to develop more targeting treatment goals.

Schema Therapy. Schema Therapy is an elaboration of cognitive therapy that has been developed by Young (Young, Klosko, & Weishaar, 2003) specifically for personality disorders, and other difficult individual and couples problems. Schema Therapy involves identifying maladaptive schemas and planning specific strategies and interventions. Four main strategies are cognitive, experiential, behavioral and the therapeutic relationship itself. Cognitive restructuring, modification of maladaptive schemas, is an important cognitive strategy, but is combined with imagery exercises, empathic confrontation, homework assignments and "limited reparenting," i.e., a form of corrective emotional experience (Young et al., 2003).

Maladaptive schemas typically associated with this disorder include: *unrelenting standards, i.e.,* the belief that striving to meet unrealistically high standards of performance is essential to be accepted and to avoid criticism; *punitiveness,* i.e., the belief that others should be harshly punished for making errors; and *emotional inhibition,* i.e., the excessive inhibition of spontaneous action, feeling, or communication—usually to avoid disapproval by others, feelings of shame, or losing control of one's impulses (Bernstein, 2002).

Interpersonal Approach

For Benjamin (2003), psychotherapeutic interventions with Obsessive-Compulsive Personality Disordered individuals can be planned and evaluated in terms of whether they enhance collaboration, facilitate learning about maladaptive patterns and their roots, block these patterns, enhance the will to change, and effectively encourage new patterns.

Because of the centrality of control in their lives, obsessive compulsive individuals find collaboration difficult. These individuals are often inconsistent in their attitudes about control of the therapy, sometimes wanting to take control, and other times wanting the clinician to take it. Benjamin suggests breaking through a potential power struggle by describing their typical patterns of control, submission and self-control and their opposites: affirmation, disclosure, and self-affirmation and how and why the obsessive compulsive patterns developed. She notes that these individuals quickly grasp—intellectually—the idea of friendly differentiation as the opposite of hostile control and will develop an interest in collaboration. After this shared goal of openness and warmth has been established, they can begin working in experiencing feeling and changing their relational behaviors. Not surprisingly, the work of learning to let go is not easy.

As these individuals begin seeking connections between early life experiences and present difficulties, they must be helped to develop compassion and empathy for themselves as children. Benjamin notes that couples therapy is a particularly potent format for learning about and changing maladaptive patterns in obsessive compulsive individuals. Dealing with control and power struggles between partners is aided by reframing and paradoxical injunctions. A paradoxical use of their preference for rule following would involve the clinician "ordering" the obsessive compulsive individual to collimate with the partner to develop "rules" for dealing with the problematic relational issues.

Therapeutic efforts to block maladaptive patterns should be targeted to power struggles, feeling avoidance and perfectionism. With regard to perfectionism, undercutting the need to reach perfection through control usually results in anger reduction. As the obsessive compulsive individual no longer needs to make others perfect, there is no need to be angry at them. Similarly, with the anxiety that comes from fear of not reaching perfection. Since the individual does not need to be perfect to survive, the individual no longer needs to be anxious about not being perfect. As these individuals come to understand the origins of their quest for perfection, and compare their early life situations with the present, they are better able to relinquish their past neurotic strivings. Developing empathy for the self as a child and for the parent at that distant time can strengthen their will to give up their maladaptive patterns.

Cognitive therapy is particularly useful in modifying their constricted cognitive style and self-criticism. Likewise, insight can increase the probability these individuals will become more comfortable with fallibility and ordinariness. Benjamin concludes that both insight and transference are important parts of the process of change for obsessive-compulsive individuals. A caring, benevolent relationship with the therapist as a trustworthy caregiver who accurately responds to the individual's needs enhances the insight. However, she cautions that treating this disorder, as with the other personality disorders, is a long-term process with no easy shortcuts.

Group Therapy

Because a major deficit of the obsessive compulsive personality is the inability to share tenderly and spontaneously with others, group treatment has particular advantages with such patients (Ogrodniczuk, Uliaszek, Lebow, & Kealy, 2021).Nonetheless, there are certain complications, because of these patients' tendency to competitiveness and control of situations. Yalom (1995) uses the description "monopolist" to refer to this obsessive compulsive pattern in group therapy. They can easily dominate a group with their rambling and excessive speech patterns. They may find the affective atmosphere in psychotherapy group particularly overwhelming at first, resulting in either further isolation or detached intellectualization. The group leader may need to intervene and to avoid unnecessary power struggles. If this is achieved, these patients may be able to vicariously model the emotional expressiveness of other group members.

Actually, group therapy offers a number of advantages over individual therapy as the obsessive compulsive personality pattern tends to make the dyadic therapy process tedious, difficult and unrewarding, particularly during the inevitable "constipated" period of treatment when clinicians commonly err with premature interpretations or behavioral prescriptions (Salzman, 1980; Wells, Glickhauf-Hughes, & Buzzel, 1990).

A group format can diffuse intensity of the patient's impact, particularly in a heterogeneous group (Frances, Clarkin, & Perry, 1984). Group treatment can also reduce transference and countertransference traps because patients are more likely to accept feedback from peers without the same power struggle that often accompanies feedback from the clinician (Gabbard, 1994). Furthermore, group therapy propels these patients into having problems rather than just talking about them (Alonso & Rutan, 1984). Rutan, Stone, & Shay (2014) also echo this notion from a psychodynamic perspective. Their review suggests that group therapy is particularly helpful for those with strict or otherwise problematic superegos. These individuals may use the group members to offset the intensity of transference found in individual therapy, allowing them to work on issues without this disruption.

Wells, Glickhauf-Hughes, and Buzzell (1990) note the following contraindications for group therapy for these patients. They are severe depression or strong suicidal potential, impulsive dyscontrol, strong paranoid propensities, acute crisis, difficulty in establishing trust, fear of relinquishing obsessive compulsive defenses, the need to establish superiority, and the use of "pseudo insight" to avoid dealing with both hostile and tender feelings.

These authors have described a unique group approach combining interpersonal and psychodynamic principles based on the premise that this personality disorder arises from the unsuccessful resolution of the developmental tasks of autonomy vs. shame and doubt. The process of treatment involves six goals: 1) modifying cognitive style; 2) augmenting decision making and action taking; 3) modifying harsh superego; 4) increasing comfort with emotional expression; 5) resolving control issues and modifying interpersonal style.

Marital and Family Therapy

Some of the dynamics and treatment discussed regarding group therapy are relevant in a family treatment context (Ogrodniczuk, Uliaszek, Lebow, & Kealy, 2021). For instance, Harbir (1981) notes that obsessive compulsive personality-disordered individuals typically enter family treatment because close family members are angry with their rigidity, procrastination, constricted affect, perfectionism, and somber or joyless outlook. The spouse of an obsessive compulsive individual may threaten divorce if the individual does not change. Often, such a threat of separation or divorce is the only motivation for treatment. The anxiety of the complaining spouse may be the only leverage for treatment, and the clinician may need to work with that spouse to deal more effectively with the other spouse's obsessive compulsive personality pattern. Harbir adds that it is not uncommon for an obsessive compulsive individual to marry an individual with a histrionic personality.

Salzman (1989) cautions that obsessive compulsive patients who are particularly anxious may not be able to participate in family therapy until their anxiety has been sufficiently ameliorated in individual psychotherapy or combined psychotherapeutic and psychopharmacological treatment. Even when excessive anxiety is not a particular concern, these patients are often tyrants in family sessions. They may immobilize other family members to such an extent that treatment is jeopardized. The use of structural and strategic intervention directed at redistributing power may be particularly advantageous in such situations (Minuchin, 1974).

Regarding treatment outcomes, no controlled research studies have been published. However, Minuchin (1974) and Haley and Hoffman (1967) have reported favorable outcomes with family therapy interventions with obsessive compulsive personalities and particularly those with permanent eating disorders. Harbir (1981) and Perry, Frances, and Clarkin (1989) present a case example of marital therapy wherein one partner exhibits an obsessive compulsive personality and the other a histrionic personality. This case is quite instructive with regard to treatment strategy and technique.

An integrative approach involving dynamic, cognitive-behavioral, and systemic interventions is described for couples in which one partner presents with Obsessive-Compulsive Personality Disorder and the other with Histrionic Personality Disorder. Three stages of the treatment process are discussed and illustrated: establishing a therapeutic alliance, restoring balance to the couple's relationship, and modifying individual partner dynamics. The first two phases involve conjoint couple's sessions, while much of the third phase involves individual sessions (Sperry & Maniacci, 1996). This particular relationship configuration is also addressed by Landucci and Foley (2014). They state that the spontaneity and liveliness of the histrionic partner provides the obsessive-compulsive individual with a welcome break from his or her mundane routines.

For additional commentary on family therapy with OCPD, refer to Benjamin (2003). She notes that many disorders are the result of patients' desire to gain the approval of a critical parent. This dream of reconciliation is rarely realized as a clinical goal, however. The likelihood of the patient's own internalizations or the family members themselves undermining the process is high. Rather, Benjamin suggests that family therapy may accomplish change only when the obsessive-compulsive patient gives up this fantasy.

Medication

Currently, there are no psychotropic medications specifically indicated for treating this personality disorder (Silk & Feurino, 2012). Nevertheless, medications are used that target specific troubling symptoms associated with the disorder, such as depression, anxiety, or sleep problems. Generally, these medications are used as an adjunct to psychotherapy and skills training (Nelson & Tsheringld, 2021).

Because troubling symptoms often respond to medications sooner than most psychological interventions, medications are usually prescribed at the onset of treatment (Sperry, 1995b). Because antidepressants have been effective in the treatment of Obsessive Compulsive Disorder, it was expected that these medications might also reduce the symptoms of this personality disorder. However, there is no evidence to support this expectation. Furthermore, there is little research evidence to even provide guidelines for the use of any medications with this disorder (Silk & Feurino, 2012).

Integrated and Combined Treatment Approach

Salzman (1989) elegantly makes the case for a combined/integrated approach to the treatment of the obsessive compulsive disorder, particularly for the more severe cases. He argues that the various treatment modalities and approaches are supplementary rather than mutually exclusive.

Combining treatment should follow a protocol (Winkeller & Schlesinger, 2021). Since high levels of anxiety or depression may limit participation in psychotherapy, an appropriate medication trial may be useful at the onset of treatment. If rituals or obsessions are prominent, specific behavior interventions—such as response prevention, exposure, habituation, and thought stopping (Salkovskis & Kirk, 1989)—are indicated. The basic dynamics of perfectionism, indecisiveness, and isolation of affect are best reached by psychotherapeutic approaches. Decisions about whether individual, group, or a marital and module format, or a combination of modalities are based on severity of the disorder, the particular treatment target, and specific contraindications. For instance, where isolation of affect and perfectionism manifest primarily as rambling speech pattern, integrative group therapy approach, such as described by Wells et al. (1990) may greatly delimit resistance and subsequent countertransference so common in dynamic treatment formats. Where indecisiveness is a prominent issue, modelling and other behavioral methods, as well as role playing might be incorporated in individual treatment formats. In general, the more severe the disorder, the more treatment needs to be tailored an multimodal.

Salzman (1989) concludes that a true understanding and appreciation of the obsessive compulsive personality "requires an integration of psychodynamic, pharmacologic, and behavior therapies, because the resolution of the disabling disorder demands cognitive clarity plus behavioral and physiologic alterations. Each modality alone deals with only a piece of the puzzle. A therapist who can combine all these approaches will be the most effective" (Salzman, 1989, p. 2782).

Developmental Therapy. Developmental approaches to therapy focus on fostering optimal functioning. For individuals with Obsessive-Compulsive Personality Style who seek to development beyond the adequate level of functioning, the current endpoint of therapy, a developmental-focused therapy utilizes a variety of interventions to facilitate this process and goal. Various developmental approaches have been proposed (Cortright, 1997; Blocher, 2000; Sperry, 2002). A protocol for conducting developmental therapy for individuals with Obsessive-Compulsive Personality is described and illustrated by Sperry (2002).

Manduchi and Schoendorff (2012) provide a case study of a 36-year-old mother of three undergoing Functional Analytic Psychotherapy (FAP) for a diagnosis of OCPD with borderline features. This type of treatment involves using the therapist's in-the-moment private experiences regarding the client to promote changes in behavior. It is an integrative approach that may include exploration of past significant relationships as well as the practice of new interpersonal skills in the session. This is accomplished through the analysis of three types of Clinically Relevant Behaviors (CRBs). CRB1s are behaviors which are directly observable in session and linked to client reports of outside-of-session problems; CRB2s are in-session behaviors that represent improvements over CRB1s; finally, CRB3s are the client's functional explanations for his or her behavior, including antecedents and consequences.

Chapter 11

Paranoid Personality Disorder

Individuals with paranoid personalities are aloof, emotionally cold individuals who display unjustified suspiciousness, hypersensitivity, jealousy, and a fear of intimacy. In addition, they can be grandiose, rigid, contentious, and litigious. Because of their hypersensitivity to criticism and tendency to project blame on others, they tend to lead isolated lives and are often disliked by others (Hopwood & Thomas, 2012; Skodol, Bender, & Oldham, 2019; American Psychiatric Association, 2022). Paranoid Personality Disorder can be thought of as a paranoid spectrum disorder ranging from this personality disorder through the delusional disorder to paranoid schizophrenia. The distinguishing feature of this personality disorder from others on the spectrum is the lack of clearcut delusions, hallucination, or other psychotic features.

This chapter describes a framework for the assessment and effective treatment of this disorder. It includes sections on its description, assessment, case conceptualization, and treatment interventions. It begins with background information on the disorder as well as the DSM-5-TR description, prototypic description, associated features, and the Alternative Model of Personality Disorders description of this disorder. The section on case conceptualization provides five common clinical formulations of this disorder: psychodynamic, biosocial, cognitive-behavioral, interpersonal, and an integrative conceptualization of this disorder. Several treatment approaches, modalities, and intervention strategies are also described. These includes individual psychotherapy, group therapy, marital and family therapy, medication, and integrative and combined treatment.

Description of the Paranoid Personality Disorder

The Paranoid Personality Disorder can be recognized by the following descriptors and characteristics: styles vs. disorders, triggering event, behavioral styles, interpersonal styles, cognitive styles, affective styles, attachment style, and optimal criterion.

Style vs. Disorder. The paranoid personality can be thought of as spanning a continuum rom healthy to the pathological, with the paranoid personality style on the healthy end, and the Paranoid Personality Disorder on the pathological end. Table 11.1 compares and contrasts differences between the paranoid personality style and disorder.

The following two cases further illustrate differences between the Paranoid Personality Disorder (Mr. W.) and the paranoid personality style (Janice L.).

Case Study: Paranoid Personality Disorder

Mr. W. is a 53-year-old male referred for psychiatric evaluation by his attorney to rule out a treatable psychiatric disorder. Mr. W. had entered into five lawsuits in the past two and one-half years. His attorney believed that each suit was of questionable validity. Mr. W. was described as an unemotional, highly controlled male who was now suing a local men's clothing store "for conspiring to deprive me of my consumer rights." He contends that the store manager had consistently issued bad credit reports on him. The consulting psychiatrist elicited other examples of similar concerns. Mr. W. had long distrusted his neighbors across the street and regularly monitors their activity since one of his garbage cans disappeared two years ago. He took an early retirement from his accounting job one year ago because he could not get along with his supervisor, whom he believed was faulting him about his accounts and paperwork. He contends he was faultless. On examination, Mr. W.'s mental status is unremarkable except for constriction of affect and for a certain hesitation and guardedness in his response to questions.

Case Study: Paranoid Personality Style

Janice L is a 46-year-old tax attorney for a major corporation. Although she had been reluctant to leave her private law practice, the corporation had courted her for several years. They really needed a skilled and successful female to round out their legal team. They made her an offer she couldn't refuse, and after ensuring that she could maintain sufficient independence in the job, she accepted. Although she had a loose reporting relationship to the chief counsel and two corporate vice-presidents, from the beginning Janice maintained cordial but somewhat distant relationships with them. She attended only those meetings and social gatherings that were absolutely required. She kept small talk to a minimum and went about her work with a single-minded and vigor that others came to respect although they couldn't quite understand her style of relation. When others began to question her standoffish manner, she replied she was hired "to be a competent litigator, not a social butterfly." In the courtroom she was an awesome sight: cool, calm and collected. She was totally in charge of examining and cross examining witnesses, and in her opening and closing statements. No stone was left unturned, and no verbal or non-verbal cue was missed. She instinctively went to "juggler" as her peers would say, and seldom lost a judgement. They was never a question about her worth or loyalty to the corporation, and in time, her peers and superior came to accept her unique style.

Triggering Event. The typical situation, circumstance or event that most likely triggers or activates the characteristic maladaptive response of the Paranoid Personality Disorder (Othmer & Othmer, 2002), as noted in behavioral, interpersonal, cognitive, and feeling styles, is: "close interpersonal relationships and/or personal queries."

Table 11.1 Comparison of Paranoid Personality Style and Disorder

Personality Style	Personality Disorder
Self-assured and confident in their ability to make decisions and take care of themselves	Reluctant to confide in others because of unwarranted fear that the information will be used against them
Good listeners and observers, keenly aware of subtlety, tone and multiple levels of meaning	Reads hidden meanings or threatening into benign remarks or events, i.e., suspects that a neighbor put out trash early to annoy them
Take criticism rather seriously without becoming intimidated	Bears grudges or is unforgiving of insults or slights
Place a high premium on loyalty, fidelity, working hard to earn and maintain it and never taking it for granted	Questions, without justification, the fidelity of spouse or sexual partner, friends and associates
Careful in dealings with other people, preferring to size up individuals before entering into relationships with them	Expects, without sufficient basis, to be exploited or harmed by others
Are assertive and can defend themselves without losing control and becoming aggressive	Are easily slighted and quick to react with anger or to counterattack

Behavioral Style. Behaviorally, paranoid individuals are resistive of external influences. They tend to be chronically tense because they are constantly mobilized against perceived threats from their environment. Their behavior also is marked by guardedness, defensiveness, argumentativeness, and litigiousness.

Interpersonal Style. Interpersonally, these individuals tend to be distrustful, secretive, and isolative. They are deeply suspicious of others' motives. They are also intimacy-avoiders by nature and repudiate nurturant overtures by others.

Cognitive Style. Their cognitive style is characterized by mistrusting preconceptions. They carefully scrutinize every situation and scan the environment for "clues" or "evidence" to confirm their preconceptions rather than objectively focusing on data. Thus, while their perception may be accurate, their judgment often is not. The paranoid personalities' prejudices mold the perceived data to fit their preconceptions. Thus, they tend to disregard evidence that does not fit their preconceptions. When under stress their thinking can take on a conspiratorial or even delusional flavor. Their hypervigilance and need to seek evidence to confirm their beliefs lead them to have a rather authoritarian and mistrustful outlook on life.

Affective Style. Their emotional or affective style is characterized as cold, aloof, unemotional, and humorless. In addition, they lack deep sense of affection, warmth, and sentimentality. Because of their hypersensitivity to real or imagined slights, and their subsequent anger at what they believe to be deceptions and betrayals, they tend to have few, if any, friends. The two emotions they experience and express with some depth are anger and intense jealousies.

Attachment Style. Individuals with a fearful attachment style exhibit a sense of personal unworthiness combined with an expectation that other people will be rejecting and untrustworthy.

They trust neither their own internal cognitions or feelings nor other's intentions. While they believe themselves to be special and different from others, they guard against threats and unexpected circumstances since they cannot trust that others will protect them. This Fearful Attachment Style is common in individuals with Paranoid Personality Disorder.

Optimal Diagnostic Criterion. Of all the diagnostic criteria for the Dependent Personality Disorder, one has been found to be the most useful in diagnosing this disorder. The belief is that by beginning with this criterion, the clinician can test for the presence or absence of the criterion and more quickly diagnose the personality disorder (Allnutt & Links, 1996). The optimal criterion for this disorder is: suspects, without sufficient basis, that others are exploiting, harming or deceiving him or her.

DSM-5-TR Characterization

Individuals with this personality disorder are characterized by an unremitting pattern of distrust and suspicion and interpret others' motives as harmful. Without sufficient basis, they suspect that others are exploiting, harming, or deceiving them. They are obsessed with unfounded doubts about the loyalty of friends and associates. Because of their unfounded fears, they are reluctant to confide in others. They are likely to interpret otherwise benign remarks and situations as threatening and dangerous. Not surprisingly, they are unforgiving of slights, insults, and injuries. These individuals are quick to react angrily or to counterattack when they believe that their character or reputation is being attacked. They are likely to continually suspect, without justification, that their spouse or sexual partner is unfaithful (American Psychiatric Association, 2022).

Prototypic Description

A prototype is a brief description that captures the essence of how a particular disorder commonly presents. Prototypic descriptions are useful and convenient, and clinicians commonly rely on them rather than lists of behavioral criteria and core and instrumental beliefs (Westen, 2012). Here is a common prototypic description of the Paranoid Personality Disorder: These individuals grew up believing that the world is dangerous and that others—particularly those closest to them—are never to be trusted. They are constantly checking to make sure that no one takes advantage of them, makes fun of them, or plots against them. Convinced that it will be used against them, they will not share their thoughts or feelings. They hold on to grudges, never forget a slight, nor pass up a chance for revenge.

Associated Features

Prevalence. PPD has been identified in 1.7 percent of the general population and 9.6 percent in clinical practice (Torgersen, 2021).

Differential Diagnosis. Because features of suspiciousness and insensitivity characterize other mental disorders, PPD should be diagnosed only when the defining features appeared before early adulthood, are typical of long-term functioning, and do not occur exclusively during an episode of another disorder. Accordingly, it is essential to rule out psychotic disorders or persistent substance use as part of the differential diagnosis (American Psychiatric Association, 2022).

Development and Course. PPD appears to develop as a result of both genetics and childhood experiences. It may first appear in childhood with solitariness, social anxiety, poor peer relations, underachievement, and interpersonal hypersensitivity. Adolescent onset is usually associated with externalizing symptoms, peer bullying, and a history of child maltreatment.

Interpersonal aggression appears in adulthood. While traits of this disorder may appear in childhood they often do not persist in adulthood. Such traits must be distinguished from characteristics that emerge in response to specific stressors or transient mental states like bipolar disorder or substance intoxication (American Psychiatric Association, 2022).

Culture, Sex, and Gender. PPD should not confused with problems associated with acculturation following migration or the expression of customs, or religious, political or cultural values. Cultural groups that face social adversity may show low trust especially to outgroup members which may lead to behaviors that can be misjudged as paranoid. Such behaviors generate anger and frustration in others, including clinicians, resulting in a vicious cycle of mistrust. This should not be confused with PPD. This disorder appears to be slightly more common in females (American Psychiatric Association, 2022).

Alternative Model of Paranoid Personality Disorder

The Alternative Model of Personality Disorders (AMPD) offers a clinically useful description of the Paranoid Personality Disorder in terms of typical features and trait facets. Typical features are Pervasive distrust and suspiciousness of others such that their motives are interpreted as malevolent (American Psychiatric Association, 2022). Trait facet criteria include Withdrawal; Intimacy avoidance; Anhedonia, and Restricted affectivity (Skodol, 2021).

Conceptualizations of the Paranoid Personality Disorder

Psychodynamic Case Conceptualizations

Psychoanalytic formulations of the paranoid personality focus on the phenomenon of projection. Essentially, paranoid individuals inaccurately perceive in others that which is true of them, and, as by projecting unacceptable feelings and impulses onto these experiences reduction of anxiety and distress (Shapiro, 1965).

The self-representation of the paranoid personality involves the coexistence of a special, entitled grandiose self with a weak, worthless, inferior polar opposite (Gabbard, 1990). Developmentally, individuals with Paranoid Personality Disorder are likely to have grown up in an atmosphere charged with criticism, blame and hostility, and to have identified with a critical parent. Identification with such critical parents suppresses these individuals' feelings of inadequacy and insures the continuing importance of the mode of criticalness in the development and functioning of the personality. Through their identifications paranoid individuals learn hypervigilance, suspiciousness and blaming. Hypervigilance and suspiciousness prevent self-criticism, while blaming—considered an identification with the aggressor—serves to erase possible experience of humiliation (Kellerman & Burry, 1989).

Paranoid individuals focus on seeing imperfection in the world around them. This externalization permits a denial of any personal imperfection. Essentially, paranoid individuals feel inferior, weak and ineffective, thus, grandiosity and specialness allow to be understood as a compensatory defense against feelings of inferiority (Gabbard, 1990).

The primary defense mechanisms of this disorder are then projection and projective identification. In addition to externalizing threats with projection, projective identification additionally serves to control others in the environment by binding them to paranoid individuals in pathological ways. This need to control others reflects low self-esteem which is at the heart of the Paranoid Personality Disorder. Basically, it sensitizes these individuals to concerns about all passive surrender to all impulses and to all persons (Shapiro, 1965). Finally, rationalization, reaction formation, and displacement are secondary defense mechanisms.

In short, the need to criticize the world and external objects allows paranoid individuals to maintain an anxiety-free existence in the face of personal imperfections and a grave sense of inadequacy. Profound inferiority feelings are projected onto the "inferior" world which is then related to in a consistently critical manner. The self can be then viewed as "good" and "badness" split off and projected outward.

Cognitive Behavioral Case Conceptualizations

According to Beck (2015), individuals with paranoid personality are distrustful of others in most circumstances. They are identifiable by their characteristic core, conditional, and instrumental beliefs. Their *core beliefs* include: "Other people can't be trusted," "Others ulterior motives (or bad intentions)s toward me," and "Others are deceptive, and are out to hurt or undermine me." Their *conditional belief* is that if they are not careful others will abuse, manipulate, or take advantage of them, and that if others act friendly it is only because they have an ulterior motive. Their *instrumental belief* is to be on guard, look for hidden meaning, trust no one, and not get taken in. Underlying these various beliefs are their beliefs about self and the world.

These individuals typically view themselves as righteous and mistreated by others. They tend to view others as devious, treacherous, manipulative, and discriminatory. They may believe that others form secret coalitions against them. Based on belief that others are against them, these individuals are driven to be hypervigilant and on guard. Their strategy is to be wary, vigilant, and counterattack. When they confront their "adversaries" they often provoke the hostility that they believed already existed (Renton & Mankiewicz, 2015).

From a more behavioral perspective, Turkat (1990) contends there is no single formulation for this disorder. However, hypersensitivity to criticism is characteristic. Such individuals receiving early training to be frightened at what others think of them. These individuals also learn that they are different than others, and that they must not make mistakes. As a result of these two beliefs, paranoid individuals become overly concerned about the evaluations of others, constrained to conform to parental expectations, and hypersensitive to other's evaluation. This, of course, often interferes with acceptance by their peers. Eventually, they are humiliated and ostracized by their peers, in part, because they lack the interpersonal skills necessary to overcome this ostracism. Consequently, they excessively engage in ruminating about their isolation and mistreatment by others. From this, they conclude that the reason for this rejection and persecution is because they are special and others are jealous of them. Accordingly, they act in ways to avoid negative evaluations from others, but these attempts lead them to act differently which invites social criticism. In their isolation they brood about their predicament which engenders persecutory and grandiose thoughts, which further maintain their social isolation. Accordingly, these individuals are caught in a vicious cycle that perpetuates the disorder (Turkat, 1990).

Interpersonal Case Conceptualizations

According to Benjamin (1996), persons diagnosed Paranoid Personality Disorder were likely to have experienced sadistic, controlling and degrading parenting. Typically abused children themselves, parents of paranoid disordered individuals believed that children are basically evil or bad, require containment, and deserve retribution. Family loyalty was a basic value, and sharing family secrets with others was not tolerated. The adult consequences of such harsh upbringing is that paranoid disordered individuals expect attack and abuse even from those close to them. As children they were harshly punished for dependency, and even attached when they were sick, hurt, or cried. As a result, they learned not to cry, not to ask for help even if injured or sick, and not to trust anyone. Subsequently, as adults they tend to avoid intimacy unless they can control their partner. Often these individuals were subjected to covert as well as overt invidious comparisons within the family, and later among peers. They learned that mistakes and hurts were seldom forgotten and that grudges were long lasting. Not surprisingly, paranoid individuals are exquisitely sensitive and angry about exclusion, slights, and even whispering. They tend to be keenly aware of any inequalities in punishments or privileges, and they are likely to sustain grudges for long periods. Furthermore, as children they were rewarded for competence in helping the family while "staying out of the way." While they were given permission and support to do well, they were degraded and humiliated for venturing out of an assigned area. They came to believe that being a good and lovable person was outside their reach. Subsequently, as adults they can function competently and independently but are interpersonally withdrawn. Their expectations of not being acknowledged inspires fear, resentment and alienation. Finally, they constantly fear that others will attack, blame or hurt them, while they continue to wish that others will affirm and understand them. Not expecting to be affirmed, they angrily withdraw and tightly control themselves and if they perceived attack will reflexively counterattack.

Biosocial Case Conceptualizations

In a marked departure from other formulations of Paranoid Personality Disorder, Millon (Millon & Davis, 1996) and Millon and Everly (1985) conceive of the Paranoid Personality Disorder as a severe form of character pathology. More specifically, Millon and Everly describe it as syndromal continuation of three less severe disorders: narcissistic, antisocial or compulsive. Based on their clinical research, individuals with Paranoid Personalities develop in one of these three syndromal patterns based on their unique biogenic and environmental histories. The narcissistic variation of the paranoid disorder is largely shaped by parental overvaluation and indulgence. As a result, these individuals fail to adequately learn interpersonal responsibility, cooperation and interpersonal skills. They are often perceived by others as selfish and egotistical. Furthermore, lack of parental controls can give rise to grandiose fantasies of success, power, beauty or brilliance. As a result they tend to be rejected and humiliated by their peers. These interpersonal rebuffs and followed by increased fantasy and isolation from which a propensity for paranoia emerges.

The antisocial variant of the Paranoid Personality exhibit high levels of activation and impulsive high energy temperaments. The principal environmental determinant seems to be harsh parental treatment. Consequently, they develop a deep abiding mistrust of others and manifest a strong self-directedness and arrogance. Because of their tendency to reject both parental and social controls, they also develop an aggressive, impulsive, hedonistic lifestyle. Anticipating the attacks of others, paranoid-antisocial individuals react irrationally and vindictively. Since they are unable to cope directly with perceived threats, they often erupt in overt hostility.

Individuals with the paranoid-compulsive pattern have developmental histories quite similar to the Obsessive-Compulsive Personality Disorder. However, they exhibit more irrationally rigid and inflexible behavior (Millon & Everly, 1985). These three version of the paranoid disorder appear to be self-perpetuated by their own rigidity and suspiciousness. By ascribing slanderous and malevolent motives to others, paranoid individuals remain in a defensive and vindictive posture most of the time. Furthermore, keeping distance from others fosters the maintenance of their illusion of superiority which allows a self-fulfilling pattern: as they expect others to be hostile and malevolent, others often become so.

Integrative Case Conceptualizations

The following integrative formulation provides a biopsychosocial explanation for how this personality is likely to have developed and how it is maintained. Biologically, a low threshold for limbic system stimulation and deficiencies in inhibitory centers seem to influence the behavior of the paranoid personality. The underlying temperament can best be understood in terms of the subtypes of the paranoid disorder. Each of three subtypes are briefly described in terms of their underlying temperament, and correlative parental and environmental factors. In the narcissistic type, a hyperresponsive temperament and precociousness, parental overvaluation and indulgence, as well as the individual's sense of grandiosity and self-importance probably result in deficits in social interest and limited interpersonal skills. The antisocial type of the paranoid personality is likely to possess a hyperresponsive temperament. This, plus harsh parental treatment, probably contributes to the impulsive, hedonistic, and aggressive style of this type. In the compulsive type, the underlying temperament may have been anhedonic. This, as well as parental rigidity and overcontrol, largely accounts for the development of this type. Finally, a less common variant is the paranoid-passive aggressive type. As infants, the individuals usually demonstrated the "difficult child" temperament, and later temperament characterized by affective irritability. This plus parental inconsistency probably accounts in large part for the development of this type (Millon, 1981).

Psychologically, paranoid individuals view themselves, others, the world, and life's purpose in terms of the following themes. They tend to view themselves by some variant of the theme: "I'm special and different. I'm alone and no one likes me because I'm better than others." Life and the world are viewed by some variant of the theme: "Life is unfair, unpredictable and demanding. It can and will sneak up and harm you when you are least expecting it." As such, they are likely to conclude "Therefore, be wary, counterattack, trust no one, and excuse yourself from failure by blaming others." The most common defensive mechanism associated with the paranoid disorder is projection.

Socially, predictable patterns of parenting and environmental factors can be noted for this disorder. For all the subtypes the parental injunction appears to be "You're different.

Don't make mistakes." Paranoid personality-disordered individuals tend to have perfectionistic parents who expose these children to specialness training. This, plus the parental style that has been articulated for the subtypes of the disorder and parental criticism leads to an attitude of social isolation and hypervigilant behavior. To make sense of the apparent contradiction between being special and being ridiculed, the children creatively conclude that the reason they are special and that no one likes them is because they are better than other people. This explanation serves the purpose of reducing their anxiety and allowing them to develop some sense of self and belonging.

This paranoid pattern is confirmed, reinforced, and perpetuated by the following individual and systems factors: A sense of specialness, rigidity, attributing malevolence to others, blaming others, and misinterpreting motives of others leads to social alienation and isolation, which further confirms the individual's persecutory stance (Sperry & Mosak, 1996; Sperry, 2015). Table 11.2 summarizes the characteristics of this disorder.

Assessment of Paranoid Personality Disorder

Several sources of information are useful in establishing a diagnosis and treatment plan for personality disorders. Observation, collateral information, and psychological testing are important adjuncts to the patient's self-report in the clinical interview. This section briefly

Table 11.2 Characteristic of Paranoid Personality Disorder

Triggering Event(s)	Close interpersonal relationships and/or personal queries
Behavioral Appearance:	Guarded and defensive
	Resists external influence
	Hypervigilant and chronically tense
Interpersonal Behavior:	Distrustful and suspicion of others
	Reluctance to confide
	Bears grudges and blames
	Counterattacks for perceived slights
	Hypersensitive to slights and criticism
Cognitive Style:	Tends to disregard evidence to the contrary
	Quick to rationalize and hold to preconceptions
Feeling Style:	Restricted affect but easily provoked
	Aloof and humorless
	Jealous and envious
Temperament:	*Narcissistic type*: active, hyper-responsive
	Compulsive type: irritable
	Passive-Aggressive type: affective irritability
Attachment Style	Fearful
Parental Injunction:	"You're different. Keep alert. Don't make mistakes"
Self-View:	"I'm so special and different. I'm alone and no one likes me because I'm better than others."
World View:	"Life is unfair, unpredictable, and demanding. It will sneak up and harm you. Therefore, be wary, counterattack, trust no one, and excuse yourself from failure by blaming others"
Maladaptive Schemas	Abuse/Mistrust; Defectiveness
Optimal Diagnostic Criteria	Suspects, without sufficient basis, that others are exploiting, harming or deceiving him or her

describes some characteristic observations that the clinician makes and the nature of the rapport likely to develop in initial encounters with specific personality-disordered individuals. Characteristic response patterns on various objective (i.e., MMPI-2 and MCMI-IV) and projective tests (i.e., Rorschach and TAT) are also described.

Interview Behavior and Rapport. Interviewing Paranoid Personality Disordered individuals is a delicate challenge. Rapport with them is hampered by their pervasive belief that others will harm and exploit them. Therefore, they screen all questions for conspiratorial content and hidden meaning and assume that any kindness shown by the clinician is a cleaver maneuver to take advantage of their weakness. Similarly, they cannot allow themselves to relax in the interview, fearful that easing up would make them too vulnerable. And so, they justify their suspiciousness and hypervigilance. They can easily confront others but will not tolerate being confronted. Smooth transitions from topic to topic are essential. Any abruptness may be experienced as a unjustified attempt to trap them which could lead to anger, counter attack, or termination of the interview (Othmer & Othmer, 2000; Ackley, Mack, Beyer, & Erdberg, 2011).

Psychological Testing Data. The Minnesota Multiphase Personality Inventory (MMPI-2), the Millon Clinical Multiaxial Inventory (MCMI-IV), the Rorschach Psychodiagnostic Test, and the Thematic Apperception Test (TAT) can be useful in diagnosing the Compulsive Personality Disorder as well as the Obsessive Compulsive Personality style (Groth-Marnat, 2009).

On the MMPI-2, an elevation on the 6 scale (Paranoia) is common. However, since these individuals tend to be hyperalert about being perceived as paranoid, this scale may be greatly elevated (Graham, 2011). These individuals are easily irritated at the MMPI's forced choice format as well as the self-disclosure required of many of the items (Meyer, 1995). Scales 3 (Hysteria) and 1 (Hypochondriasis) and K (Correction) tend to be high in these individuals reflecting their use of denial and projection, their inclination to focus on somatic concerns, and their need to present a facade of adequacy (Graham, 2011).

On the MCMI-IV elevation on scale 6B (Sadistic) and P (Paranoid) are expected (Millon, Millon, Grossman, Boice, & Sinsabaugh, 2016). Since this personality pattern often overlaps with the antisocial, the narcissistic and the passive aggressive, elevations are likely on scales 6A (Antisocial), 5 (Narcissistic) and 8A (Negativistic-passive aggressive) (Choca & Denburg, 1997).

On the Rorschach, these individuals produce records that are generally constricted, but characterized by more P (Popular) and A (Animal) responses, than C (Pure color) and M (Human Movement) responses. These individuals typically resent ambiguous stimuli and so respond to the test with condescending criticism and flipping of cards, and a focus on D (Detail) responses. Occasionally they reject cards or refuse to continue with the examination (Meyer, 1995). The new Rorschach Performance Assessment System (R-PAS) is an improved method for scoring and interpreting the Rorschach Inkblot Test. Besides being evidence-based and internationally normed, it increases clinical utility and is easier to use than Exner's Comprehensive System (Mihura & Meyer, 2018).

On the TAT, suspiciousness may characterize their stories. This is particularly likely to occur on cards 9, G, F, 11, and 16 (Bellak, 1997).

Treatment Approaches and Interventions

Treatment Considerations

Included in the differential diagnosis of this disorder are the following personality disorders: Antisocial Personality Disorder, Narcissistic Personality Disorder, and Obsessive-Compulsive Personality Disorder. The most common symptom disorders associated with the Paranoid Personality Disorder are Generalized Anxiety Disorder, Panic Disorder, and Delusional Disorder. If a Bipolar Disorder is present, an irritable manic presentation is likely. Decompensation into Schizophrenic reaction is also likely. When this occurs, the paranoid and catatonic subtypes are most likely to be present (Sperry, 2015).

Until recently, the prognosis for treatment of the Paranoid Personality Disorder was considered guarded. Today more optimism prevails in achieving specific treatment goals such as increasing the benignness of perception and interpretation of reality and increasing trusting behavior. Several psychotherapeutic and psychoeducation interventions are useful in accomplishing these goals. Medication may be useful in decreasing anxiety associated with loss of control. To date, no controlled treatment outcomes studies have been completed for the Paranoid Personality Disorder (Crits-Christoph & Barber, 2002).

Individual Psychotherapy

Psychodynamically Oriented Psychotherapy

Patients with paranoid personalities tend to be individuals who lead reasonably adaptive and productive lives, and not surprisingly, are responsive to psychodynamic psychotherapy. Meissner (1978) contends, however, that their treatment is not easy but requires empathy, patience, and a great deal of sensitivity to their vulnerabilities. Meissner contends that the treatment process must be slowly paced with limited, long-term goals. Three treatment principles characterize such treatment (Meissner, 1978; 1986).

First a meaningful therapeutic alliance must be established and maintained (Yeomans, Clarkin, & Levy, 2021). The therapeutic alliance requires the patient to have a certain degree of trust in the clinician, which is considerably for paranoid patients. The clinician's empathic responsiveness and willingness to serve as a container for a range of negative affects is essential. The clinician must avoid responding defensively, nor challenge the patient's perception of events or of the clinician. Instead, the clinician asks for more details and empathizes with the patient's perceptions and affects. Most importantly, the clinician must resist the countertransference tendency to be rid of indescribable projection by deflecting them back to the patient with predictive interpretations (Epstein, 1984). In short, the patient must come to view the clinician as a benign, disinterested but friendly helper (Salzman, 1980).

Second, the essential treatment strategy is to convert paranoid manifestations into depression and work through the underlying mourning. Gradual undermining of paranoid defenses and attitudes leads to the emergence of a depressive core in which the patient's inner sense of weakness, defectiveness, vulnerability and powerlessness comes into focus. This is accomplished through the techniques of counterprojection and "creative doubt" (Meissner, 1986). Depressive elements are worked through in the transference, which allows them to begin the process of mourning their frustrated learning and disappointments with early objects.

Third, the clinician must respect the patient's fragile and threatened sense of autonomy and work toward building and reinforcing it in the therapeutic relationship. A commitment to openness, honesty, and confidentiality means that all decisions must be explored with the patient, and the ultimate choice must be the patient's. This even applies to decisions about medication, if, when and if they are indicated (Meissner, 1989).

Since these patients tend to be resistant, provocative and contentious, countertransference issues cannot be underestimated. Behind their defensiveness and arrogance are narcissistic vulnerability, core feelings of shame and humiliation, and passive longing for dependence. Thus, these patients attempt to counter their anxieties by "turning the tables" and making the clinician feel vulnerable, humiliated, and helpless. Clinicians may react with annoyance, impatience, confrontative and argumentative. Or they may experience frustration, discouragement and victimization. These reactions must be monitored, their impact on therapy analyzed, and efforts to rebalance the therapeutic alliance initiated (Meissner, 1989). Examples of these kinds of exchanges can be found in Williams (2010).

Metacognition-oriented therapy provides another treatment for personality disorders based on individual narrative and interpretation. Its goal is to progressively promote awareness of problems in subjective experience and schemas driving social behavior (Salvatore, Russo, Russo, Popolo, & Dimaggio, 2012). Therapists elicit patients' autobiographies, or narrative episodes, to identify the influences and theories behind their problems. This also includes work intended to develop the skills to understand the minds of others. The authors present a case study of an 8-month, ongoing course of metacognition-oriented treatment with a 31-year-old female law student diagnosed with paranoid personality disorder and delusional disorder.

A similar type of psychotherapy used for paranoid personality disorder is based on Dialogical Self Theory (DST), which examines the inner dialogue between different parts, or voices, of the self (Dimaggio, Catania, Salvatore, Carcione, & Nicolo, 2006).

Brief Psychodynamic Psychotherapy. Long-term psychodynamically oriented psychotherapy involves two or more sessions per week for three or more years. However, since Paranoid Personality Disordered individuals do not easily engage in the therapeutic process, they may have reluctance to such intensive long-term work. On the other hand, receptivity for treatment has increased during crisis period, usually the experience of acute anxiety or depression. Shorter-term therapy that is more crisis-oriented might be a preferable way of beginning treatment. These such crisis focused short-term therapy could be a prelude to longer-term treatment.

Malan (1976) and Balint et al. (1972) describe short-term psychotherapy with acute paranoid difficulties. While these treatments were effective with reactive paranoid presentations, it may not be for the enduring presentations, more typical of the Paranoid Personality Disorder. Currently, there are no published reports of completed successful treatments of Paranoid Personality Disorder in the context of brief dynamic psychotherapy.

Cognitive Analytic Therapy (CAT) (Ryle, 2004) is another time-limited model of psychodynamically oriented treatment that has been used for personality disorders. It consists of a narrative reformulation and the sequential diagrammatic reformulation (SDR). Patients receive 24 weekly sessions and four follow up sessions spread out over a six-month period. Following the first three assessment sessions, personality patients are read a letter from the therapist that reformulates the origins of their distress and identifies target problems and procedures. Kellet and Hardy (2014) conducted a mixed methods single-case study with a 36-year-old male diagnosed with paranoid personality disorder. The six target complaint measures were as follows: suspiciousness; hyper vigilance; dissociation; conspiracy; questioning; and anxiety. Cognitive Analytic Therapy ends with a "goodbye letter" jointly formulated by the patient and therapist to summarize achievements, prepare for future obstacles, and address any feelings of abandonment related to the termination of therapy. Results showed that five out of the six measures identified at the onset of treatment were extinguished during the treatment phase. The patient also attributed his changes to the CAT method.

Cognitive Behavioral Therapy Approaches

Cognitive Therapy Approach. Beck, Freeman, and Associates (2004) provide an extended discussion of the Cognitive Therapy approach with Paranoid Personality Disordered individuals. The initial phase of treatment can be exceedingly stressful for paranoid individuals in that participating in treatment requires self-disclosure, trusting another, and acknowledging weakness, all of which they experience as being quite dangerous. This stress can be reduced by focusing initially on less sensitive issues or by discussing issues directly, i.e., talking about how "some individuals" experience and react to such situations, or by beginning with a more problem- solving approach and behaviorally focused interventions on presenting problems. Such strategies, as well as giving the individual more than the usual amount of control over scheduling appointments or the content of sessions can facilitate development of a collaborative working relationship wherein, they will feel less distrustful, coerced, and vigilant. Trust can be engendered by explicitly acknowledging and accepting the individual's difficulty in trusting the therapist. As this becomes evident and gradually demonstrated through trustworthiness and actions, it provides the evidence on which trust can be based.

A guided discovery approach when working on treatment goals will reveal the manner in which their paranoid pattern contributes to their problems, facilitating collaborative work on their distrust of others, feelings, of vulnerability, and desire for retribution, rather than the therapist insisting that these issues be directly addressed. As treatment progresses to working on specific goals, emphasis should shift to increasing the individual's sense of self-efficacy before attempting to modify interpersonal behaviors, automatic thoughts or schemas. Developing an increased awareness of another's point of view and learning a more assertive approach to interpersonal conflict are other common treatment goals with these individuals. The use of traditional cognitive behavioral techniques such as assertive communication training and behavioral rehearsal are commonly employed to reverse the provocation of hostile reactions from others that previously confirmed the paranoid individuals view of self and others. In instances where hypervigilance and ideas of reference are particularly resistant, the information processing social skills intervention strategy described by Turkat and Maisto (1985) can be exceptionally useful.

The treatment goals are to decrease sensitivity to criticism and modify social behavior (Fowler, Orme, & Hart, 2021). Social skills training consists of instructional role playing, behavioral rehearsal, and videotaped feedback. The patient is taught to attend to more appropriate social stimuli; to interpret that information more accurately; to attack, criticize or single out the patient; and to receive other's feedback in a non-defensive way and utilize it constructively (Turkat, 1990). Turkat and Maisto (1985) present a detailed case report illustrating these treatment strategies.

Williams (1988) provides a detailed case report of time-limited cognitive therapy with a substance depressed college student who also met criteria for Paranoid Personality Disorder. The patient was distressed about poor interpersonal relations and drug use and was quite intelligent and motivated for therapy. Noteworthy about William's treatment protocol is that the only eleven session were available and needed to achieve three treatment goals: reduce depressive symptoms, less threatening perceptions of the world and other people, and increase skills in being more relaxed and comfortable with others. Cognitive restructuring and progressive muscle relaxation were the principal intervention strategies. Six month follow-up showed that all gains had been maintained. Williams concludes that brief cognitive therapy may be particularly well suited for the Paranoid Personality Disorder. Renton & Mankiewicz (2015) identify three key treatment goals for the treatment of any Cluster A disorder. There are: elicit trust in therapy by exploring ambivalence and respecting the individual's independence and boundaries; explore the influence of unhelpful beliefs about others in key social contexts while developing alternative, functional beliefs; and experiment with new social behaviors not based on suspicion and mistrust. They provide a case study of a 27-year-old female accountant diagnosed with paranoid personality disorder.

In short, the Cognitive Therapy approach to working with paranoid individuals focuses considerable effort on carefully developing a work collaborative relationship and increasing the individual's sense of self-efficacy early in treatment. It utilizes cognitive techniques and behavioral experiments to directly challenge the individual's remaining paranoid beliefs late in therapy.

Schema Therapy. Schema Therapy is an elaboration of cognitive therapy that has been developed by Young (1994; 1999; Young, Klosko, & Weishaar, 2003) specifically for personality disorders, and other difficult individual and couples problems. Schema Therapy involves identifying maladaptive schemas and planning specific strategies and interventions. Four main strategies are cognitive, experiential, behavioral and the therapeutic relationship itself. Cognitive restructuring, modification of maladaptive schemas, is an important cognitive strategy, but is combined with imagery exercises, empathic confrontation, homework assignments and "limited reparenting," i.e., a form of corrective emotional experience (Young, 1999; Young et al., 2003).

Maladaptive schemas typically associated with Paranoid Personality Disorder include: *mistrust/abuse*, i.e., the belief that others will abuse, humiliate, cheat, lie, manipulate, or take advantage; and *defectiveness*: i.e., the belief that one is defective, bad, unwanted, or inferior in important respects; and *approval-seeking* (Bernstein, 2002).

Interpersonal Approach

For Benjamin (2003) psychotherapeutic interventions with Paranoid Personality Disordered individuals can be planned and evaluated in terms of whether they enhance collaboration, facilitate learning about maladaptive patterns and their roots, block these patterns, enhance the will to change, and effectively encourage new patterns.

Benjamin notes that the major treatment problem with paranoid individuals is establishing a collaborative therapeutic relationship. To the extent that collaboration occurs, paranoia disappears. Accustomed to being abused and humiliated, paranoid individuals view therapists as critical and judgmental, look for "slip ups," and want them to leave. Patience and kindness without hints of coercion, criticism, or appeasement are essential for a considerable period during the early stages of therapy. Benjamin provides an excerpt from a session with a woman hospitalized with delusional disorder, suspicious type that illustrates the effectiveness of this kind of respectful, caring curiosity.

As treatment proceeds, they must learn that their expectations of attack and abusive control stem from past experiences. As such, they can begin appreciating that these expectations are not always appropriate in the present, and that hostility begets hostility. Furthermore, they must come to understand that their defenses of control, avoidance and anticipatory relation will elicit attack and alienation in others. Benjamin advocates the use of "verbal holding" as an antidote to their original abuse. Accurate empathy, genuine affirmation of accomplishments, and understanding constitute verbal holding. At the same time, therapists need to gently but firmly confront provocations. Since confrontation is likely to be threatening to them, therapists must carefully balance affirmation with confrontation. The goal here is for proactive criticism and these individuals to learn the meaning of feedback and that their feelings of vulnerability and fearfulness do not "prove" that others, including therapists, are attacking them.

Benjamin's discussion of blocking maladaptive patterns in paranoid individuals includes strategies for dealing with various crises such as aborting or redirecting rageful outburst at therapists, dealing with homicidal threats and abuse of their children. She believes that therapist's honesty, caring, calmness, attentiveness and clear commitment to resolving conflicts are extremely useful to paranoid individuals in crisis. Benjamin finds that the wish to relinquish patterns of alienation, hostile control, carrying grudges, and fearfulness do not develop until these individuals feel safe to do otherwise. As therapy proceeds, they are helped to lessen their enmeshment with early controlling, attacking figures. As they can see that they are acting like a hated parent, they may become interested in becoming different.

Once safer bases are established with significant others and or with their therapist, they can begin channeling their anger in a direction that encourages separation from earlier destructive patterns and beliefs. Finally, to the extent that therapeutic collaboration develops, considerably new learning about trust, giving and receiving positive and negative feedback from and to others, and thinking more benignly about people and life circumstances has already taken place. As these are mastered, any residual learning that remains by the last stage of therapy is relatively easy to implement. For paranoid individuals at the last stage of treatment, excursions into the social world further the idea that friendly approaches elicit friendly reaction can be slightly frightening but also exhilarating.

Group Therapy

Because of their hypersensitivity, suspiciousness, and tendency to misinterpret comments of others, paranoid personality-disordered individuals tend to avoid group therapy and other forms of group treatment (Ogrodniczuk, Uliaszek, Lebow, & Kealy, 2021).Similarly, the paranoid tendency to be accusatory, self-righteous, obstinate, hostile, and evasive has been a contraindication to heterogeneous intensive group therapy (Yalom, 1985; Francis, Clarkin, and Perry, 1984; Vinogradou & Yalom, 1989).

On the other hand, higher functioning paranoid patients who can maintain a degree of self-awareness and are able to tolerate a group confrontation of their paranoid distortion, may derive considerable benefit from participation in an established group that is sufficient cohesive and tolerant of divergent opinions (Meissner, 1989). Rutan, Stone, and Shay

(2014) provide an example of a patient sharing about, but not acting upon, his paranoid fantasies about the group facilitator's vacation being a covert attempt to get away from him. The patient connected this abandonment fantasy to being the only child in his family to be given up for adoption.

Marital and Family Therapy

There is relatively little published literature on therapy with the paranoid personality, per se. Nonetheless, either treatment modality can be used alone or concurrently with individual therapy. Meissner (1989) indicates that family therapy might be combined sometime during the course of long-term individual psychotherapy. Family therapy might be indicated for the paranoid adolescent whose family dynamics and interaction patterns interfere with or contribute to the patient's difficulties.

Harbir (1981) details some general principles for couple's therapy for the paranoid personality. He notes that paranoid features often lead to severe marital dysfunction. The paranoid partner's hypersensitivity, joyless intensity, hypervigilance, extreme mistrust and jealousy cause considerable suffering for their partner. Nevertheless, the non-paranoid partner also cause suffering because their action often exacerbate the paranoid condition. Typically, non-paranoid spouses react passively and secretively when accused or criticized. The more they withdraw and are evasive, the more their paranoid partner becomes suspicious and mistrustful. Therefore, the clinician who is treating a married paranoid patient in individual therapy should consider concurrent couples therapy or, at least, a conjoint session with the non-paranoid partner to modify the marital interaction pattern which seems to be maintaining the psychopathology.

The goal of marital therapy is to enhance the positive growth of the couple by reducing the personality pathology of either or both partners (Ogrodniczuk, Uliaszek, Lebow, & Kealy, 2021). Harbir (1981) reports that paranoid patients can progress in couple's therapy despite the inevitable issues of trust and confidentiality. The clinician needs to be constantly aware of the paranoid partner's close monitoring of the clinician's behavior. These patients invariably become angry if they perceive the clinician taking sides or become jealous of the clinician's relationship with their partner, if the clinician is of the opposite sex. Thus, the clinician, just as in individual psychotherapy, must be open and forthright about the specific therapeutic process and their rationale.

Once a therapeutic alliance has been established, the clinician can support the non-paranoid spouse to confront and challenge the constant mistrust of the paranoid partner. An angry response can be expected at first, but the paranoia will start decreasing. Obviously, such confrontation is only prescribed when the patient has adequate impulsive control and has not been violent. Harbir describes a detailed case example of conjoint couple's therapy involving a paranoid spouse. The treatment involves two stages and illustrates Harbir's therapy approach.

Benjamin (2003) also comments on the role of family in the treatment of this disorder. Damage caused by the controlling and attacking figures found in early life may be challenged by the rehabilitative presence of a spouse or child involved in sessions. The paranoid individual may come to see that their hostile behavior resembles that of their abuser, which can spark a desire to be different. She discusses the implications of child abuse by the paranoid individual at length, including the unintended effect of mandatory reporting laws that can lead to premature termination of treatment.

Medication

Currently, there are no psychotropic medications specifically indicated for treating this personality disorder (Silk & Feurino, 2012). Nevertheless, medications are used that target specific troubling symptoms associated with the disorder, such as depression, anxiety, or sleep problems. Generally, these medications are used as an adjunct to psychotherapy and skills training (Nelson & Tsheringld, 2021).

Because troubling symptoms often respond to medications sooner than most psychological interventions, medications are usually prescribed at the onset of treatment. Since antipsychotic medications are somewhat effective in paranoid schizophrenia, it was hoped that these medications would likewise be useful in the treatment of this personality disorder. Unfortunately, evidence does not support this hope. Furthermore, there is little research evidence to provide guidelines for the use of such medications (Silk & Feurino, 2012).

Combined and Integrative Treatment Approaches

There are sufficient data to suggest that the Paranoid Personality Disorder is no longer untreatable, as was previously believed, but can be successfully treated. Although treatment with psychodynamic and cognitive-behavioral approaches is considered long term, there has been at least one report of successful time-limited treatment (Williams, 1988). Currently, there is little published data on integrating and tailoring treatment with this disorder. Nevertheless, clinical experience shows that an integrative treatment approach probably can maximize therapeutic outcomes while decreasing the length of treatment (Winkeller & Schlesinger, 2021).

Conceptualizing personality disorder as having temperament and characterological dimensions, it appears that the dynamic approaches are particularly effective with the characterological dimensions, but less effective with the temperament/style dimension. It seems that cognitive restructuring and the behavioral information processing approach (Turkat & Maisto, 1985) are particularly effective with modifying the paranoid's cognitive style of hypervigilance. The cognitive-behavioral approach is also useful with difficulty relaxing and constricted affects. The interpersonal approach (Benjamin, 2003) seems particularly effective in reducing blame and hypersensitivity to criticism. Thus, integrating dynamic, cognitive-behavioral, and interpersonal approaches could have a synergistic effect at changing both temperamental and characterological dimensions of this disorder. It also appears that combining treatment modalities should increase treatment efficacy and cost effectiveness, especially for the more severe presentations of this disorder. The most obvious combined treatment involves the concurrent or sequential use of family, marital or group therapy with individual psychotherapy. Also, quite promising is the combination of medication, i.e., pimozide or serotonin reuptake inhibitors when they are indicated, with individual psychotherapy.

Chapter 12

Schizoid Personality Disorder

Individuals with schizoid personalities tend to be reclusive and have little desire or capacity for interpersonal relationships, primarily because they derive little pleasure from such relationships. Yet, they can perform well if left alone. For instance, they can effective night watchmen and security guards. Nevertheless, they have little emotional range, they daydream excessively, and appear to be humorless and aloof (Hopwood & Thomas, 2012; Skodol, Bender, & Oldham, 2019; American Psychiatric Association, 2022).

This chapter describes a framework for the assessment and effective treatment of this disorder. It includes sections on its description, assessment, case conceptualization, and treatment interventions. It begins with background information on the disorder as well as the DSM-5-TR description, prototypic description, associated features, and the Alternative Model of Personality Disorders description of this disorder. The section on case conceptualization provides five common clinical formulations of this disorder: psychodynamic, biosocial, cognitive-behavioral, interpersonal, and an integrative conceptualization of this disorder. Several treatment approaches, modalities, and intervention strategies are also described. These includes individual psychotherapy, group therapy, marital and family therapy, medication, and integrative and combined treatment.

Description of the Schizoid Personality Disorder

The Schizoid Personality Disorder can be recognized by the following descriptors and characteristics: styles vs. disorders, triggering event, behavioral styles, interpersonal styles, cognitive styles, affective styles, attachment style, and optimal criterion.

Style vs. Disorder. The schizoid personality can be thought of as spanning a continuum from healthy to pathological, with the dependent personality style at the healthy end and the Schizoid Personality Disorder at the pathological end. Table 10.1 compares and contrasts differences between the dependent style and the disorder.

The following case examples further illustrate the differences between the Schizoid Personality Disorder (Mr. Y.) and the schizoid personality style (Mr. P.).

Case Study: Schizoid Personality Disorder

Mr. Y. is a 20-year-old freshman who met with the director of the introductory psychology course program to arrange an individual assignment in lieu of participation in the small group research project course requirement. He told the course director that because of a daily two hour commute each way, he "wouldn't be available for the research project," and that he "wasn't really interested in psychology and was only taking the course because it was required." Upon further inquiry, Mr. Y. disclosed that he preferred to commute and live at home with his mother, even though he had the financial resources to live on campus. He admitted he had no close friend nor social contacts, and preferred being a "loner." He had graduated from high school with a "B" average, but did not date or participate in extracurricular activities, except the electronics club. He was a computer science major, and "hacking" was his only hobby. Mr. Y.'s affect was somewhat flattened and he appeared to have no sense of humor and failed to respond to attempts by the course director to make contact through humor. There was no indication of a thought nor perceptual disorder. The course director arranged for a individual project for the student.

Case Study: Schizoid Personality Style

Mr. P. is a 28-year and six-year veteran of the U.S. Department of the Interior. He has been a forest ranger since graduating from college. While in school he excelled in the classroom, but was considered a loner by others. Unlike most of his classmates he didn't pledge a fraternity feeling he really needed to live in a place that was quiet and distraction-free. Mr. P. enjoyed his work and has received commendations for it. A year ago, he was offered a promotion to field supervisor which he turned down since it would have required him to have regular voice or face-to-face contact with up to ten forest rangers that would report to him. Jeff had befriended a college friend whom he roomed with for three years whom he continues to have occasional contact with. He has never considered marriage or family so he has little interest in dating.

Triggering Event. The typical situation, circumstance or event that most likely triggers or activates the characteristic maladaptive response of the Schizoid Personality Disorder (Othmer & Othmer, 2002), as noted in behavioral, interpersonal, cognitive, and feeling styles, is: "close interpersonal relationships."

Behavioral Style. The behavioral pattern of schizoids can be described as lethargic, inattentive, and occasionally eccentric. They exhibit slow and monotonal speech and are generally non-spontaneous in both their behavior and speech.

Interpersonal Style. Interpersonally, they appear to be content to remain socially aloof and alone. These individuals prefer to engage in solitary pursuits, they are reserved and

Table 12.1 Comparison of Schizoid Personality Style and Disorder

Personality Style	Personality Disorder
Exhibit little need of companionship and are most comfortable alone	Neither desire nor enjoy close relationships including being part of a family; has one or no close friends or confidants other than first-degree relatives.
Tend to be self-contained, not requiring interaction with others in order to enjoy experiences or live their lives.	Nearly always choose solitary activities.
Even tempered, dispassionate, calm, unflappable and rarely sentimental.	Rarely, if ever, claim or appear to experience strong emotion, such as anger or joy.
Little driven by sexual needs, and while they can enjoy sex, do not suffer in its absence.	Little if any desire to have sexual experiences with another person.
Tend to be unswayed by either praise or criticism and can confidently come to terms with their own behavior.	Indifferent to the praise and criticism of others; displays constricted affects, e.g. is aloof, cold and rarely reciprocates gestures or facial expressions, such as smiles or nods.

reclusive, and rarely respond to others' feelings and actions. They tend to fade into the social backdrop and appear to others as "cold fish." They do not involve themselves in group or team activity. In short, they appear inept and awkward in social situations.

Cognitive Style. Their style of perceiving, thinking and information processing can be characterized as cognitively distracted. That is, their thinking and communication can easily become derailed through internal or external distraction. This is noted in clinical interviews when these patients have difficulty organizing their thoughts, are vague, or wander into irrelevance such as the shoes certain people prefer (Millon, 1981). They appear to have little ability for introspection, nor ability to articulate important aspects of interpersonal relationships. Their goals are vague and appear to be indecisive.

Affective Style. Their emotional or affective style is characterized as being humorless, cold, aloof, and unemotional. They appear to be indifferent to praise and criticism, and they lack spontaneity. Not surprisingly, their rapport and ability to empathize with others are poor. In short, they have a constricted range of affective response.

Attachment Style. Individuals with a dismissing attachment style are characterized by a sense of self that is worthy and positive as well as a low and negative evaluation of others which typically manifests as mistrust of others. Because they believe they are emotionally self-sufficient while other are emotionally unresponsive, they dismiss the need for friendship and contact with others. This Dismissing Attachment Style is common in individuals with Schizoid Personality Disorder (Lyddon & Sherry, 2001).

Optimal Diagnostic Criterion. Of all the diagnostic criteria for the Dependent Personality Disorder, one has been found to be the most useful in diagnosing this disorder. The belief is that by beginning with this criterion, the clinician can test for the presence or absence of the criterion and more quickly diagnose the personality disorder The optimal criterion for this disorder is: neither desires nor enjoys close relationships, including being part of a family (Allnutt & Links, 1996).

DSM-5-TR Characterization

Individuals with this personality disorder are characterized by an unremitting pattern of detachment from others and restricted emotional expression. They do not desire nor enjoy close relationships, including family relationships. Except for first-degree relatives, they are unlikely to have close friends or confidants. These individuals typically choose solitary activities, and have little, if any, interest in sexual relations. Not surprisingly, they seem indifferent to the feedback, including criticism, of others. They experience little, if any, pleasure in most activities. Instead, they exhibit emotional coldness, detachment, or flat affect (American Psychiatric Association, 2022).

Prototypic Presentation

A prototype is a brief description that captures the essence of how a particular disorder commonly presents. Prototypic descriptions are useful and convenient, and clinicians commonly rely on them rather than lists of behavioral criteria and core and instrumental beliefs (Westen, 2012). Here is a common prototypic description of the Schizoid Personality Disorder: These individuals just want to be left alone. Making and maintaining contact with others has little or no meaning and is without pleasure, comfort or emotion. Accordingly, they live alone, avoid dating, have no real friends, and have jobs that require little or contact with others. Others consider them awkward, distant, and overly formal in all social contacts. In short, they come across to others as "cold fish."

Associated Features

Prevalence. SZPD has been identified in 1.3 percent of the general population and 1.9 percent in clinical practice (Torgersen, 2021).

Differential Diagnosis. SZPD should be distinguished from schizophrenia, delusional disorder, and bipolar or depressive disorder with psychotic features since these disorders are characterized by a period of persistent psychotic symptoms of delusions and hallucinations. It is also critical to differentiate it from Autism Spectrum Disorder and persistent substance use (American Psychiatric Association, 2022).

Development and Course. SZPD appears to develop as a result of both genetics and childhood experiences. It appears in childhood and adolescence as solitariness, underachievement, and poor peer relationships that suggest that these individuals are different which can subject them to teasing and bullying (American Psychiatric Association, 2022).

Culture, Sex, and Gender. In contrast to those with an accurate diagnosis of SZPD, individuals from cultural groups who occasionally exhibit defensive behaviors may erroneously be labelled as "schizoid." For example, immigrants may be mistakenly perceived as cold, indifferent, or menacing in response to a hostile reception from the host country. Similarly, those moving from rural to metropolitan communities may react with "emotional freezing" that may last for several months with constricted affect, solitary activities, and communication deficits. There appears to be no gender difference with this disorder (American Psychiatric Association, 2022).

Alternative Model of Schizoid Personality Disorders

The Alternative Model of Personality Disorders (AMPD) offers a clinically useful description of the Schizoid Personality Disorder in terms of typical features and trait facets. Typical features are Pervasive distrust and suspiciousness of others such that their motives are interpreted as malevolent (American Psychiatric Association, 2022). Trait facet criteria include Withdrawal; Intimacy avoidance; Anhedonia, and Restricted affectivity (Skodol, 2021).

Conceptualizations of the Schizoid Personality Disorder

Psychodynamic Case Conceptualizations

The inner world of schizoid individuals appears to be different than their outward appearance. Akhtar (1987) describes them as overtly detached, asexual, self-sufficient, and uninteresting, while covertly emotionally needy, exquisitely sensitive and vulnerable, creative and acutely vigilant. These stark differences represent a splitting or fragmentation of different self-representations that remain integrated. The result is identity diffusion.

Balint (1968) and Nachmani (1984) believe that their difficulty relating to others stems from a deficit—inadequate mothering—rather than from an oedipal conflict. In short, these individuals base their decision to be isolative on the conviction that because they failed to receive maternal nurturance and support as infants, they cannot expect or attempt to receive any emotional supplies from subsequent significant figures. Fairburn (1954) views the isolation of schizoid individuals as a defense against a conflict between a wish to relate to others and a fear that their neediness will harm others. Thus, they vacillate between a fear of driving others away by their neediness, and the fear that others will smother or consume them. Consequently, all relationships are experienced as dangerous and must be avoided.

Kellerman and Burry (1989) view this isolation and social distancing as a way of managing anxiety. Schizoid individuals are remote, cool and aloof but not necessarily malicious toward others. Typically, schizoid individuals utilize the defenses of repression, suppression, isolation of fantasy affect, displacement and compensation to ensure distance from others and avoid anxiety.

Biosocial Case Conceptualization

Millon and Davis (1996) believes the schizoid personality is formed by an interaction of biogenic and environmental factors. Millon and Everly (1985) suggest that a proliferation of dopaminergic postsynaptic receptors in limbic and frontal cortical regions account for the unusual cognitive activity and inhibited emotional responses of schizoid individuals. Along with this excessive parasympathetic nervous system dampening could account for their apathy, flattened affect and under responsiveness. Finally, Millon and Everly note that an ectomorphic—thin and frail—body type which has been associated with shyness and introversion, is common among schizoid individuals.

Major environmental factors involve parental indifferences and fragmented communications patterns. Families of schizoid individuals are typically characterized by interpersonal reserve, formality, superficiality, and coldness. They tend to communicate in a fragmented, aborted and circumstantial fashion. Not surprisingly, individuals raised in such environments are likely to be vague, abortive and circumstantial in all their communications. These disjointed communication patterns tend to be confusing to others and foster misunderstanding, frustration, lack of tolerance and hostility on the part of others. Schizoid individuals are prone to be isolative and come to believe that others do not understand them. Furthermore, these individuals are usually incapable of correcting the problem.

They schizoid disorder is perpetuated by social distancing, by having their social isolation reinforced, and by their cognitive and social insensitivity. Their infrequent social activities limit their ability to grow, and their social isolation is frequently reinforced by others who ostracize isolative individuals. Furthermore, their social and cognitive insensitivity tends to oversimplify and make boring a world that is so rich and diverse to others.

Cognitive Behavioral Case Conceptualizations

According to Beck (2015) individuals with schizoid personality are, for all practical purposes, detached from others. There are characteristics core, conditional, and instrumental beliefs noted in individuals with this disorder. Their *core beliefs* are that they are misfits from life, that relationship take effort and are not worth the trouble, and that they are happier being alone. Their *conditional beliefs* are that if they get too close to others, they will be teased or imposed on by others, and there is no point in trying to connect with others. Their *instrumental beliefs* are don't get involved, say no to others' demand, and leave social situations quickly. Underlying these various beliefs are their beliefs about self and the world.

They typically view themselves as loners and oddballs who don't fit in. They tend to view others as demanding, hostile, and intrusive. Accordingly, their basic strategy is to keep their distance from others and avoid contact when others are around. While they may make contact with others as part of their job or meet basic needs, they typically avoid any form of intimacy (Renton & Mankiewicz, 2015)

From the behavioral perspective, Turkat (1990) does not offer a formulation for this disorder. However, it might be that parental indifference, emotional reserve, and little opportunity to develop interpersonal skills contribute to the development of this disorder.

Interpersonal Case Conceptualizations

According to Benjamin (1996) persons diagnosed with Schizoid Personality Disorders were likely to have been raised in a home that was orderly and formal. While these children's physical and educational needs were met, there was little warmth, play or social and emotional interaction within the family or elsewhere, for that matter. The schizoid individual would have modelled social isolation and colorless, unemotional functioning. Such identification with withdrawn parents, leads schizoid individuals to expect little and give little. Though they may be socialized for work, they are not predisposed to intimate contact, and prefer fantasy and solitary advocating instead. In short, they have neither fears of nor desires for others. Underdeveloped in social awareness and skills, they can meet social role expectations and employees or even as parents. They may be married but do not develop close, intimate relationships.

Integrative Case Conceptualization

The following integrative formulation provides a biopsychosocial explanation for how this personality is likely to have developed and how it is maintained. Biologically, the Schizoid

Personality was likely to have had a passive and anhedonic infantile pattern and temperament. Millon (1981) suggested that this pattern results, in part, from increased dopaminergic postsynaptic limbic and frontal lobe receptor activity. Constitutionally, the schizoid is likely to be characterized by an ectomorph body type (fragile and delicate) (Sheldon, Dupertius, & McDermott, 1954).

Psychologically, they view themselves, others, the world, and life's purpose in terms of the following themes. They view themselves by some variant of the theme: "I'm a misfit from life, so I don't need anybody. I am indifferent to everything." For schizoid personalities, the world and others are viewed by some variant of the theme: "Life is a difficult place and relating to people can be harmful." As a result, they are likely to conclude, "Therefore, trust nothing and keep a distance from others and you won't get hurt." Alexandra Adler (1956) further describes these life-style dynamics. The most common defense mechanism utilized by them is intellectualization.

Socially, predictable patterns of parenting and environmental factors can be noted in them. Parenting style is usually characterized by indifference and impoverishment. It is as if the parental injunction was: "You're a misfit" or "Who you, what do are you want?" Their family pattern is characterized by fragmented communications and rigid, unemotional responsiveness. Because of these conditions, schizoids are grossly under-socialized and develop few if any interpersonal relating and coping skills. This schizoid pattern is confirmed, reinforced, and perpetuated by the following individual and systems factors: Believing themselves to be misfits they shun social activity. This plus social insensitivity leads to reinforcement of social isolation and further confirmation of the schizoid style (Sperry & Mosak, 1996; Sperry, 2015). Table 12.2 summarizes the characteristic features of this disorder.

Table 12.2 Characteristics of Schizoid Personality Disorder

Triggering Event(s)	Close interpersonal relationships
Behavioral Style:	Slow and monotonous speech
	Lethargic and inattentive
	Non-spontaneous and indifferent
Interpersonal Style:	Minimal desire for relationships
	Choses solitude over social interaction
	Lacks confidants
	Fades into social background
	Isolative and content to remain aloof
Cognitive Style:	Cognitively distracted, easily derailed and tangential
	Absent minded
	Minimally introspective
Feeling Style:	Emotionally distant
	Rarely responsive to another's feelings
Temperament:	Passive and anhedonic infantile pattern
Attachment Style	Dismissing
Parental Injunction	"Who are you, what do you want?"
Self-View:	"I'm a misfit from live, so I don't need anybody." "I'm indifferent to everything."
World View:	"Life is a difficult place and can be harmful. Therefore, trust no one and keep distance from others and you won't get hurt"
Maladaptive Schemas	Social Isolation; Emotional Deprivation; Defectiveness; Subjugation; Undeveloped Self
Optimal Diagnostic Criteria	Neither desires nor enjoys close relationships, including being part of a family

Assessment of Schizoid Personality Disorder

Several sources of information are useful in establishing a diagnosis and treatment plan for personality disorders. Observation, collateral information, and psychological testing are important adjuncts to the patient's self-report in the clinical interview.

This section briefly describes some characteristic observations that the clinician makes and the nature of the rapport likely to develop in initial encounters with specific personality-disordered individuals. Characteristic response patterns on various objective (i.e., MMPI-2 and MCMI-IV) and projective tests (i.e., Rorschach and TAT) are also described.

Interview Behavior and Rapport. Interviewing the Schizoid Personality-Disordered individual can seem like an exercise in futility given their pervasive emotional withdrawal. They express little or no emotionality even when talking about anxious or depressed feelings. More intelligent individuals with this disorder may complain about anhedonia and may even use the label "depression" but seldom report associated sadness or guilt. Since emotional warmth is absent, it is difficult to judge whether problems or concerns are central to them. Typically, they have one word or short phrase answers to all questions. Neither open ended questions, structured questions, nor other interview strategies will change the flow of information or expression of affect. Unlike paranoid individuals, this restricted verbal and emotional expression is not due to self-protectiveness, but rather to emotional and mental emptiness. Rapport usually reflects a willingness to reveal symptoms, problems, and innermost feelings. Since these patients are so impoverished, rapport and engagement may seem impossible with these patients. Long periods of silence are not uncommon. If these patients return for sessions, it usually means they are "connecting" insofar as they know how. Thus, the clinician's persistence, patience, and tolerance for limited verbal interchange may have a therapeutic effect (Othmer & Othmer, 2002; Ackley, Mack, Beyer, & Erdberg, 2011).

Psychological Testing Data. The Minnesota Multiphase Personality Inventory (MMPI-2), the Millon Clinical Multiaxial Inventory (MCMI-IV), the Rorschach Psychodiagnostic Test, and the Thematic Apperception Test (TAT) can be useful in diagnosing the Schizoid Personality Disorder as well as the Schizoid Personality style or trait. On the MMPI-2, a normal profile is common for reasonably well integrated Schizoid individuals. In such instances O (Social Introversion) may be elevated (Lachar, 1974). As these individuals become distressed, a rise in F (Frequency), 2 (Depression) and 8 (Schizophrenia) are likely. Occasionally, a 1–8 (Hypochondriasis-Schizophrenia) "nomadic" profile is noted wherein interpersonal attraction is limited (Graham, 2011).

On the MCMI-IV an elevation on scale 1 (Schizoid) with low scores on 4A (Histrionic), 5 (Narcissistic) and N (Bipolar-Manic) are likely (Millon et al., 2016).

On the Rorschach, a high percentage of A (Animal) and few C (Color) responses are likely. The overall record tends to be constricted and certain blots may be rejected. Reaction time to many of the cards may be slow. There may be a higher Experience Potential than Experience Actual, and their M (Human Movement) production will be high relative to the overall quality of the protocol (Exner, 1986). The new Rorschach Performance Assessment System (R-PAS) is an improved method for scoring and interpreting the Rorschach Inkblot Test. Besides being evidence based and internationally normed, it increases clinical utility and is easier to use than Exner's Comprehensive System (Mihura & Meyer, 2018).

On the TAT, constricted response along with a blindness of theme is common. So also, is an impoverished portrayal of story characters (Bellack, 1997).

Treatment Approaches and Interventions

Treatment Considerations

Included in the differential diagnosis of this disorder are the following personality disorders: Avoidant Personality Disorder, Schizotypal Personality Disorder, and the Dependent Personality Disorder. The most common symptom disorders likely to be associated with this disorder are: Depersonalization Disorder, Bipolar Disorders, Obsessive Compulsive Disorder, Somatic Symptom Disorder, Schizophreniform, and Disorganized and Catatonic Schizophrenias.

Schizoid personalities rarely volunteer for treatment unless decompensation is present. However, they may accept treatment if someone, like a family member, demands it. Treatment goals are focused on symptom alleviation rather than on restructuring of personality. Common treatment strategies include crisis management and a consistent and supportive therapeutic interaction. Medications, particularly the antipsychotics, have not been shown to be useful with this disorder (Silk & Feurino, 2012).

Individual Psychotherapy

Some form of individual psychotherapy is indicated for the majority of the schizoid patients. Whether the clinician choose an active confrontative approach, or cognitive restructuring and social skills training approach, or one that is more supportive depends on a number of factors including a patient's psychological-mindedness, resilience, and treatment expectations, the clinician's therapeutic repertoire, and resources for treatment. This section briefly describes the psychodynamic, cognitive-behavioral, and interpersonal approaches to individual therapy.

Psychodynamic Psychotherapy Approaches

Because the dynamic understanding of both the schizoid and schizotypal personality are inherently similar, Gabbard (1990; 1994) proposes that their treatment is similar. Schizoid patients can be treated effectively with dynamically oriented psychotherapy, both expressive and supportive, depending on their level of functioning and treatment readiness (Gabbard, 1994). The basis for dynamic treatment is not interpretation of conflict but rather internalization of a therapeutic relationship (Stone, 1985).

Essentially, the clinician's task is to meet the patient's frozen internal object relations by providing a correct emotional experience (Yeomans, Clarkin, & Levy, 2021). The schizoid's style of relatedness results from inadequacies in early relationships with parental figures. As a result, these patients go through life distancing themselves from others. Therapy must therefore provide a new relationship for internalization (Gabbard, 1994). Thylstrup and Hesse (2009) suggest that the schizoid individual's outward emotional detachment from others actually conceals a deep inner longing for closeness. This ambivalence can be addressed within the context of therapy; however, because these patients are unable to adequately articulate their emotional needs, therapists tend to lose interest in them easily.

Therapists must pay particular attention to countertransference with these patients to avoid further alienation. Questions such as "do I feel like canceling appointments with my socially isolated patient, thinking it won't hurt him or her?" and "Do I find myself wondering if this patient has any problems at all, in spite of clear evidence that he does?" are useful guidelines. The authors present a case study of a 40-year-old unemployed male.

Kavaler-Adler (2004) presents the treatment of this disorder from an object-relations perspective. In this course of psychoanalysis, the schizoid individual is taken through a period of "developmental mourning" in order to grieve the loss of normal development in the separation-individuation process and understand how traumatic early childhood experiences influence current interpersonal problems. The schizoid patient may then work to confront and give up the regret associated with this. She presents a detailed case example of psychoanalysis with a female writer.

Supportive Therapy. Since their basic mode of functioning is non-relational, they find the task of therapy very challenging and difficult. Not surprisingly, they respond to the challenge with silence and emotional distancing. Clinicians need to adopt a permissive, accepting attitude, and must be exceedingly patient with these individuals. It is more helpful to understand silence as a nonverbal form of relating rather than as treatment resistance. By listening with a third ear, the clinician can learn much about these patients. Through projective identification they will evoke certain responses in that clinician that contain valuable diagnostic information regarding the patient's inner world (Gabbard, 1989). Dealing effectively with countertransference issues is critical in working with schizoid patients. Accepting silent non-relatedness is foreign to the clinician's psychological predisposition and training. Thus, when silence is prolonged, the clinician must guard against acting out and projecting their own self and object representations onto the patient. Accepting the silence and refraining from interpreting it, legitimizes the patient's private, noncommunicative core self. And it may be the only viable technique for building a therapeutic alliance (Gabbard, 1989).

The proper pace and depth of therapy is controversial. Bonime (1959) advocates an active, confrontative approach, while Gabbard (1990) and others maintain that a more restrained approach is more respectful and less threatening for these patients.

Supportive techniques can be utilized to encourage the lower functioning schizoid to become more active. For example, the patient is first urged to engage in activities where other are present, but where the patient's participation is minimal, for example at a sports event. If some level of comfort is achieved, further involvement may be encouraged. Involvement in a computer club, travel tour, or aerobics class risk them attending a sports event, but less than a social gathering or dance class. Kantor (1992) advocates the techniques of "productive substitution" and "modification total push" with these therapeutic tasks. In productive substitution the clinician suggests gratifying replacements for what is missing from the patient's life. Thus, relationships with peers in a therapy group substitutes for the unmarried patient. Using modified total push, the clinician urges the patient to become more socially active. Suggestions are presented tentatively, to test the patient's limits. Problems encountered are brought back into therapy and discussed. Treatment goals and outcomes may be quite limited: the patient may eventually work albeit in isolation, i.e. as a night watchman, may have one or two social friends, and possibly even a long-term relationship with someone who is willing to remain distant companions (Kantor, 1992).

Long-Term vs. Short-Term Dynamic Therapy: Decisions about the type and frequency of dynamic therapy should be based on the patient's level of functioning and motivation and readiness for treatment. Higher functioning schizoid patients who exhibit some depressive symptoms, or some capacity for empathy and emotional warmth tend to have better outcomes in dynamic psychotherapy (Stone, 1983).

Those patients who are highly motivated for exploratory psychotherapy can make dramatic gains in intense, long-term treatment of two to three sessions per week over several years. On the other hand, long-term supportive psychotherapy is indicated for the majority of schizotypal patients who present with major ego deficits and personal eccentricities. The goal of such treatment is improved adaptive functioning in day-to-day living. The frequency of sessions is one to two times per week for the majority of patients (Stone, 1989). Gamache and Diguer (2012) provide a case study of a 34-year-old male with schizoid personality treated for one year using psychodynamic psychotherapy.

Short-term dynamic therapy is indicated for crisis issues and situational difficulties related to job or personal life. It may also serve as follow-up for a previous course of long-term psychotherapy. Not surprisingly, there are no reports of short-term dynamic individual treatment as curative intervention.

Cognitive Behavioral Therapy Approaches

Cognitive Therapy Approach. Beck, Freeman, and Associates (2004) describe the Cognitive Therapy approach to working with Schizoid Personality-Disordered individuals. Since schizoid individuals tend to have limited motivation for social interaction, a principal treatment goal is to establish or increase positions of social interaction, as well as reduce social isolation. These individuals enter treatment largely because of symptom disorders, like an anxiety disorder, rather than to alter their manner of relating to others. Thus, the initial goal of treatment is a collaborative focus on presenting problems. As this occurs, the therapist can be commenting on the individual's relational patterns, discussing its advantages and disadvantages, and how this pattern effects the presenting problem.

The collaborative therapeutic relationship can itself serve as a prototype for other interpersonal relationships, as well as a basis for increasing the individual's range and frequency of interactions outside sessions (Fowler, Orme, & Hart, 2021). After rapport has been established, the therapist can point out the characteristic interaction pattern as well as give feedback on how this impacts other persons. As these individuals develop a greater awareness and understanding of interpersonal relating, they are guided in learning needed social skills and practicing them both within and outside the sessions. Given their lack of expressiveness, routinely soliciting feedback on their level of anxiety should reduce the likelihood of premature termination. Unlike work with other personality disorders where considerable therapeutic leverage and motivation for change are available, relatively little of either is likely with schizoid individuals besides reason. Accordingly, Freeman et al. (1990) advise therapists to clearly present the rationale for therapy, reasons for acting differently, the advantages and disadvantages of changing behavior, and the concrete gains possible. Presumably this strategy can induce these individuals to change.

Beck et al. (2004) indicates that the following techniques are effective with schizoid individuals. The Dysfunctional Thought record is not only useful in challenging dysfunctional automatic thoughts, but also in identifying a variety of affects and their subtle graduation in intensity, as well as indicating the reactions of others. Teaching social skills is best done directly through role playing, *in vivo* exposure and homework assignments. Helping these individuals become more attentive to and experience positive emotions can be facilitated by guided discovery. For example, as these individuals are helped to recognize their overgeneralized view of others: "I don't like people," they can learn to be specific about things they don't like, as well as things they do like about others after all.

As treatment needs termination, the matter of relapse prevention is discussed. Beck et al. (1990) reports that schizoid individuals are very likely to relapse into an isolative lifestyle after termination. Thus, they suggest maintaining contact with these individuals through booster sessions. Finally, although treatment with these individuals can be difficult, with persistence it is possible to improve their social skills, frequency of social interaction and decrease their "strangeness." However, the therapist should anticipate that schizoid individuals are likely to retain some distance and passivity in interpersonal relations after planned termination.

Renton & Mankiewicz (2015) echo the notion that these individuals rarely present for treatment of their own accord and, if doing so, it is likely to be short-lived and exclusively for the purpose of symptom relief or the resolution of specific problems related to changes in their environment. Therapy rarely extends to the examination and resolution of underlying cognitive factors, and ambivalence about change may be present throughout treatment. If these individuals can acknowledge the connection between their early experiences, maladaptive beliefs, and current problems, then they may be willing to reframe these beliefs.

Schema Therapy. Schema Therapy is an elaboration of cognitive therapy that has been developed by Young (1994; 1999; Young, Klosko, & Weishaar, 2003) specifically for personality disorders, and other difficult individual and couples problems. Schema Therapy involves identifying maladaptive schemas and planning specific strategies and interventions. Four main strategies are cognitive, experiential, behavioral and the therapeutic relationship itself. Cognitive restructuring, modification of maladaptive schemas, is an important cognitive strategy, but is combined with imagery exercises, empathic confrontation, homework assignments and "limited reparenting," i.e., a form of corrective emotional experience (Young, 1999; Young et al., 2003).

Maladaptive schemas typically associated with Schizoid Personality Disorder include: *social Isolation*, i.e., the belief that one is alienated, different from others, or not part of any group; *defectiveness*: i.e., the belief that one is defective, bad, unwanted, or inferior in important respects; *emotional deprivation*, i.e., the belief that one's desire for emotional support will not be met by others; *subjugation*, i.e., the belief that one's desires, needs, and feelings must be suppressed in order to meet the needs of others and avoid retaliation or criticism; and *undeveloped self*, i.e., the belief that one must be emotional close with others at the expense of full individuation or normal social development (Bernstein, 2002).

Interpersonal Approaches

There is very little in the literature about treatment of this disorder from an interpersonal perspective. For example, Benjamin (2003) provides no discussion of treatment goals or strategies for the Schizoid Personality Disorder. She notes that these individuals are socially withdrawn, do not desire social connections, and do not suffer from anger, fear, or depression. As such, they have little reason to present for treatment.

Group Therapy

Schizoid patients can profit from group therapy, particularly dynamic group therapy (Azima, 1983). Group therapy offers these patients a socialization experience, involving exposure to and feedback from others in a safe, controlled environment (Ogrodniczuk, Uliaszek, Lebow, & Kealy, 2021). It is an environment in which new parenting can occur. Here group members can function as a reconstructed family and provide a corrective emotional experience that can counterbalance the schizoid's negative and frightening internal objects (Appel, 1974). As their worst fears are not realized and they feel accepted, these patients gradually become more comfortable with others. Giles & Wienclaw (2008) note that the timing of group therapy is important to consider. They suggest that it is first better to develop a strong therapeutic alliance between the patient and the individual therapist before initiating group treatment, as these individuals generally avoid social contact.

From an object relations perspective, Leszcz (1989) contends that group's function as a holding environment which provide an opportunity for these patients to be initially involved in a "non-relate" way while slowly building trust. They do not have to leave their cocoon of self-sufficiency, but can observe how others related in the groups, how feelings make a difference, and how to deal with others related in the groups, how feelings make a difference, and how to deal with negative emotions. The wise group leader will permit this nonrelated position until this patient is better able to tolerate the ambiguities of the group.

From a systems perspective, Bogdanoff and Elbaum (1978) maintain that the schizoid's isolation is not simply due to a fragile ego but is also a function of the group's need to maintain that isolation. So, while the schizoid patient may provoke the group to make the schizoid talk, at other times the group effectively silences the schizoid by ragefulness or blaming that frightens the schizoid. Essentially, the schizoid is caught in an interpersonal trap—which they call a "role lock." On the other hand, successful group interaction can occur only when the role lock is broken. If the group is avoiding the schizoid, the therapeutic task is to focus the group's attention on the role lock. The aim is for group members to reveal their contribution of the lock and to relieve pressure on the locked member; and for the locked member or reveal how he or she sees the group process to isolate himself or herself.

From an interpersonal perspective, Yalom (1995) discusses other useful interventions for dealing with role lock. The schizoid is helped to differentiate responses to different group members, to take seriously feelings in the here-and-now, to become more aware of their specific avoidance strategies, and to become more aware of their bodily response. Yalom insists that these goals and strategies are preferable to cathartic methods which can drive the schizoid from the group. He cautions that this process is slow and that patients is essential for the clinician.

Finally, there seems to be a consensus of sorts, that heterogeneous groups are preferable to homogenous groups (Leszcz, 1989; Bogdanoff & Elbaum, 1978; Slavik, Sperry, & Carlson, 1992). Spotnitz (1957) suggests that the schizoid patient should be referred to a group that is homogeneity in terms of global functioning, but heterogeneous in terms of personality types.

Marital and Family Therapy

Schizoid patients, particularly males, do not marry and seldom become self-supporting. They may reside with and become dependent on their families. This can result in a vicious cycle in which limited motivation for social contacts and a job or career leads to interferences and bitterness on the part of the family, which is followed by lowered self-esteem, and an even greater reluctance to leave home (Stone, 1989).

Clinician's working with the schizoid patient still living at home often confronts family tension, impatience and discord arising from differences between parental expectations and the patient's capacities and motivation. Family therapy can be quite effective in addressing these expectational differences, discord, and impatience (Anderson, 1983). Shapiro (1982) describes how the family therapist can function to contain such displaced and projected affects and impulses, and acknowledge, bear, work through, and redirect them. Family treatment can also help family members reestablish more functional communication patterns between schizoid patients and their families (Ogrodniczuk, Uliaszek, Lebow, & Kealy, 2021).

McCormack (1989) describes a common marital constellation in which schizoid individuals marry borderline individuals. In discussing the treatment of the schizoid spouse, McCormack indicates that the core of the schizoid's difficulty is an overwhelming fear of attachments. Insecurity arises from escalating aggression because frustration of their dependency needs leads to marital dissatisfaction and discord. Schizoid spouses experience their love as lethal and then abort awareness of these feelings and dependency needs as a defense against them. Thus, they develop and maintain relationships in which they are never fully involved.

The treatment of the schizoid spouse emphasizes clarification and careful interpretation while deemphasizing confrontation. Exploration should involve their narcissistic vulnerability, legitimization of their needs, acknowledgement of the potential risks and gains attached to pursuing them, and the schizoid compromise. McCormack describes the "schizoid compromise" as a means of maintaining relationships which require limited emotional involvement, at the cost of limiting personality development. The clinician needs to acknowledge to these patients that this compromise has been adaptive but is a stage through they must pass before facing their fear of genuine, healthy relationships.

Schizoid spouses tend to treat others as they fear being treated, which is frustrating to those wanting an intimate relationship with them. In conjoint session the clinician helps both spouses to see that each suffers from difficulties that are both similar to and different from their own and that though these difficulties are fostered in the marriage relationship, that also exist independent of it.

Couple's therapy with the schizoid-borderline relationship may require referral of one spouse for individual therapy, the use of medication or hospitalization. Long-term couples treatment is usually necessary, if the goal is to foster separation and autonomy, increased marital satisfaction and harmony.

Medication

Currently, there are no psychotropic medications specifically indicated for treating individuals with dependent personality disorder (Silk & Feurino, 2012). Because there are some controlled trials that antipsychotics were useful in the treatment of Schizotypal Personality Disorder (Koenigsberg, Woo-Ming, & Siever, 2002), it was hoped that these medications might also be useful with the Schizoid Personality Disorder (Nelson & Tsheringld, 2021). Unfortunately, that hope has not been realized. Nevertheless, antipsychotics are still prescribed but are only likely to be useful if some psychotic decompensation has been noted

(Sperry, 1995b). Furthermore, there is little research evidence to provide guidelines for the use of medications for this personality disorder (Silk & Feurino, 2012).

Combined and Integrative Treatment Approaches

Schizoid patients tend to avoid mental health professional just as they avoid relationships in general. When they do present for help, often at the urging of their family, they have a tendency to prematurely terminate therapy after a short time (Stone, 1989). This means there is only a small window of opportunity to engage these patients in the therapeutic process. Combining treatment modalities and integrating treatment approaches can facilitate both commitment to treatment and positive treatment outcomes.

Gabbard (1994) advocates combining dynamic group therapy with dynamic individual psychotherapy as the treatment of choice for the majority of schizoid patients. However, he cautions that many of these patients will recoil at the recommendation for group therapy, even feeling betrayed by their clinician. Thus, Gabbard suggests that prior to making a group referral, fantasies about the group experience need to be explored and worked through. Stone (1989) also recommends combining individuals and group modalities. However, he proposes a developmental approach in which the patient first forms a stable dyadic relationship with the clinician and then proceeds to group therapy with the same clinician. In both instances the combined treatment is concurrent.

As noted earlier, McCormack (1989) makes the case for combining marital therapy with individual therapy, particularly when there is considerable splitting and projective identification. Combining family therapy and individual therapy has advantages, particularly if the schizoid patient is financially dependent on the family and/or resides with the family. Family can greatly influence the patient's continuation in individual and/or group treatment (Winkeller & Schlesinger, 2021).

Armstrong (2002) describes schizoid personality features in substance abusers. He echoes others when he suggests that these are individuals who want to relate, but whose social anxiety stands in the way of this. Substance abuse is one way in which these individuals actively isolate themselves from others while medicating their intense feelings. For these dually diagnosed individuals, the addition of treatments targeted at changing substance use behaviors, such as Motivational Interviewing, may be helpful.

Slavik, Sperry, and Carlson (1992) advocate both combining treatment modalities and integrating treatment approaches. They indicate the utility of concurrent individual and group treatment. And they describe how an Adlerian approach can be integrated with an object relations theory approach, social skills training, hypnosis and psychodrama depending on the patient's style, needs, and expectations. These authors believe that the Schizoid Personality Disorder is eminently treatable, and that these patients are largely untreatable because clinicians have not found sufficient ways to engage and encourage them in the change process.

Chapter 13

Schizotypal Personality Disorder

Individuals with schizotypal personalities share some features of the schizoid personality. In addition, they are characterized by eccentric behavior and peculiar thought content. Typically, they describe strange intrapsychic experiences, think in odd and unusual ways, and are difficult to engage. Yet, none of these features reach psychotic proportions. It has been suggested that the schizotypal personality is one of the schizophrenic spectrum disorders because schizophrenia occurs with increased frequency in family members of the schizotypal individual (Kwapil & Barrantes-Vidal, 2012; Skodol, Bender, & Oldham, 2019; American Psychiatric Association, 2022).

This chapter describes a framework for the assessment and effective treatment of this disorder. It includes sections on its description, assessment, case conceptualization, and treatment interventions. It begins with background information on the disorder as well as the DSM-5-TR description, prototypic description, associated features, and the Alternative Model of Personality Disorders description of this disorder. The section on case conceptualization provides five common clinical formulations of this disorder: psychodynamic, biosocial, cognitive-behavioral, interpersonal, and an integrative conceptualization of this disorder. Several treatment approaches, modalities, and intervention strategies are also described. These includes individual psychotherapy, group therapy, marital and family therapy, medication, and integrative and combined treatment.

Description of the Schizotypal Personality Disorder

The Schizotypal Personality Disorder can be recognized by the following descriptors and characteristics: styles vs. disorders; triggering event; behavioral styles; interpersonal styles; cognitive styles; affective styles; attachment style and optimal criterion.

Style vs. Disorder. The schizotypal personality can be thought of as spanning a continuum from healthy to pathological, wherein, the schizotypal personality style is closer to the healthy end and the schizotypal personality is on the pathological end. Table 13.1 compares and contrasts the schizotypal personality style and disorder.

The following two case examples further illustrate the differences between the Schizotypal Personality Disorder (Ms. S.) and the schizotypal personality style (Mr. P.)

Case Study: Schizotypal Personality Disorder

Ms. S. is a 41-year-old single female who was referred to a community mental health clinic by her mother because Ms. S. had no interests, friends, or outside activities and was considered by neighbors to be an "odd duck." Her father had recently retired, and because of a limited pension, the parents were having difficulty in making ends meet since Ms. S had been living with them for the past eight years after she had been laid off from an assembly line job she had held for about ten years. The patient readily admitted she preferred to be alone but denied that this was a problem for her. She believed that her mother was concerned about her because of what might happen to the patient after her parents' deaths. Ms. S. was an only child who had graduated from high school with average grades but had never been involved in extracurricular activities while in school. She had never dated, and mentioned she had a female friend whom she had not talked with in four years. Since moving back with her parents, she stayed in her room preoccupied with books about astrology and charting her astrological forecast. On examination, she was an alert, somewhat uncooperative female appearing older than her stated age, with moderately disheveled hair and clothing. Her speech was monotonal and deliberate. She achieved poor eye contact with the examiner. Her thinking was vague and tangential, and she expressed a belief that her fate lay in "the stars." She denied specific delusions or perceptual abnormalities. Ms. S's affect was constricted except for one episode of anger when she thought the therapist was being critical.

Case Study: Schizotypal Personality Style

Mr. P. is a 28-year-old and six-year veteran of the U.S. Department of the Interior. He has been a forest ranger since graduating from college. While in school he excelled in the classroom, but was considered a loner by others. Unlike most of his classmates he didn't pledge a fraternity feeling he really needed to live in a place that was quiet and distraction-free. Mr. P. enjoyed his work and has received commendations for it. A year ago, he was offered a promotion to field supervisor which he turned down since it would have required him to have regular voice or face-to-face contact with up to ten forest rangers that would report to him. Mr. P. had befriended a college friend whom he roomed with for three years whom he continues to have occasional contact with. He has never considered marriage or family so he has little interest in dating.

Triggering Event. The typical situation, circumstance or event that most likely triggers or activates the characteristic maladaptive response of the Schizotypal Personality Disorder (Othmer & Othmer, 2002), as noted in behavioral, interpersonal, cognitive, and feeling styles, is: "close interpersonal relationships."

Table 13.1 Comparison of Schizotypal Personality Style and Disorder

Personality Style	Personality Disorder
Tend to be tuned into and sustained by their own feelings and belief	Ideas of reference; suspicious or paranoid ideation; inappropriate or constricted affect
Keen observation of others and are particularly sensitive to how others react to them	Excessive society anxiety, e.g., extreme discomfort in social situations involving unfamiliar people
Tend to be drawn to abstract and speculative thinking	Odd beliefs or magical thinking, speculative thinking influencing behavior and inconsistent with subculture with norms, e.g., superstitiousness, belief in clairvoyance, telepathy or "sixth sense", others can feel my feelings.
Receptive and interested in the occult, extrasensory, and the supernatural	Unusual perceptual experiences, e.g., illusions, sensing the presence of a force or person not actually there (e.g., "I felt as if my dead mother were in the room with me")
Tend to be indifferent to social convention, and lead interesting and unusual lifestyle.	Odd or eccentric behavior or appearance, e.g., unkempt, unusual mannerisms, talks to self; odd speech (without loosening of association or incoherently) e.g., speech that is impoverished, digressive, vague or inappropriately abstract
Usually are self-directed and independent requiring few close relationships	No close friends or confidants (or only one) other than first-degree relatives

Behavioral Style. Behaviorally, schizotypals are noted for their eccentric, erratic, and bizarre mode of functioning. Their speech is markedly peculiar without being incoherent. Occupationally, they are inadequate, either quitting or being fired from jobs after short periods of time. Typically, they become drifters, moving from job to job and town to town. They tend to avoid enduring responsibilities and in the process lose touch with a sense of social propriety.

Interpersonal Style. Interpersonally, they are loners with few if any friends. Their solitary pursuits and social isolation may be the result of intense social anxiety which may be expressed with apprehensiveness. This apprehensiveness doesn't diminish with familiarity, and, is associated with paranoid features rather than negative self-appraisal. If married, their style of superficial and peripheral relating often leads to separation and divorce in a relatively short period of time. Their lives tend to be marginal, and they gravitate toward jobs that are below their capacity or demand little interaction with others.

Cognitive Style. The cognitive style of schizotypals is described as scattered and ruminative and is characterized by cognitive slippage. Presentations of superstitiousness, telepathy, and bizarre fantasies are characteristic. They may describe vague ideas of reference and recurrent illusions of depersonalizing, derealizing experiences without the experience of delusions of reference, or auditory or visual hallucinations.

Affective Style. Their affective style is described as cold, aloof, and unemotional with constricted affect. They can be humorless and difficult individuals to engage in conversation probably because of their general suspicious and mistrustful nature. In addition, they are hypersensitive to real or imagined slights.

Attachment Style. Individuals with an "other-view" that is negative and a "self-view" that vacillates between positive and negative exhibit a composite fearful–dismissive style of attachment. They tend to view themselves as special and entitled but are also mindful of their need for others who can potentially hurt them. Accordingly, they use others to meet their needs while being wary and dismissive of them. This fearful–dismissive attachment Style is common in individuals with Schizotypal Personality Disorder.

Optimal Diagnostic Criterion. Of all the stated DSM-IV-TR criteria for the Schizotypal Personality Disorder, one criterion has been found to be the most useful in diagnosing this disorder. The belief is that by beginning with this criterion, the clinician can test for the presence or absence of the criterion and quickly diagnose the personality disorder (Allnutt & Links, 1996). The "optimal criterion" for this disorder is: "odd thinking and speech: behavior or appearance that is odd, eccentric or peculiar."

DSM-5-TR Characterization

Individuals with this personality disorder are characterized by an unremitting pattern of social and interpersonal deficits with significant discomfort and limited capacity for relationships as well as by perceptual distortions and eccentric behavior. They experience ideas of reference as well as unusual beliefs and thinking that influences their behavior, and which is inconsistent with their subculture. They also experience unusual perception, such as bodily illusions, and odd speech thinking. These individuals are prone to suspiciousness and paranoid ideation. They exhibit inappropriate or constricted emotions, and behavior that is odd, peculiar, or eccentric. With few exceptions, they lack close friends or confidants except for first-degree relatives. When they are around others, they experience excessive social anxiety that is not diminished by familiarity and is associated with suspicion and fears (American Psychiatric Association, 2022).

The "Alternative DSM-5 Model for Personality Disorders" provides another description of this disorder (American Psychiatric Association, 2022). It is described as an impaired capacity for relationship and eccentricities in perception, cognition, and behavior associated with distorted self-image and incoherent goals involving suspiciousness and limited emotional expression.

Characteristic difficulties are noted in identify, self-direction, empathy, and intimacy, as well as suspiciousness, withdrawal, restricted affect, eccentricity, unusual beliefs and experiences, or cognitive and perceptual dysregulation.

Prototypic Presentation

A prototype is a brief description that captures the essence of how a particular disorder commonly presents. Prototypic descriptions are useful and convenient, and clinicians commonly rely on them rather than lists of behavioral criteria and core and instrumental beliefs (Westen, 2012). Here is a common prototypic description of the Schizotypal Personality Disorder: These individuals display disorganized behavior and speech and emotional blunting, but not the delusions and hallucinations associated with the diagnosis of Schizophrenia. Their characteristic eccentric thinking and behavior, strange beliefs, and unusual perceptual experiences are below the threshold of psychosis. These symptoms have an early onset and usually remain stable throughout life. It is also not uncommon for these individuals to be misdiagnosed as having Asperger's Disorder.

Associated Features

Prevalence. Schizotypal Personality Disorder has been identified in 1.3 percent of the general population and 5.7 percent in clinical practice (Torgersen, 2021).

Differential Diagnosis. Schizotypal Personality Disorder can be distinguished from schizophrenia, delusional disorder, and bipolar or depressive disorder with psychotic features since these disorders are characterized by a period of persistent psychotic symptoms of delusions and hallucinations.

To give the additional diagnosis of Schizotypal Personality Disorder, this personality disorder must have been present before the onset of psychotic symptoms and persist when the psychotic symptoms remit (American Psychiatric Association, 2022).

Development and Course. Schizotypal Personality Disorder appears to develop as a result of both genetics and childhood experiences. It may appear in childhood and adolescence with solitariness, social anxiety, underachievement, hypersensitivity, peculiar thoughts and language, bizarre fantasies, and poor peer relationship. As a result, they may be teased because of their oddness or eccentricity (American Psychiatric Association, 2022).

Culture, Sex, and Gender. Culturally determined characteristics regarding the supernatural or religious beliefs and practices like evil eye, voodoo, or speaking in tongues, can appear to be schizotypal to the uninformed clinicians. Schizotypal Personality Disorder appears to be slightly more common in males than females (American Psychiatric Association, 2022).

Alternative Model of Schizotypal Personality Disorder

The Alternative Model of Personality Disorders (AMPD) offers a clinically useful description of the Schizotypal Personality Disorder in terms of typical features and trait facets. Typical features are impairments in the capacity for social and close relationships, as well as eccentricities in cognition, perception, and behavior that are associated with distorted self-image and incoherent personal goals and accompanied by suspiciousness and restricted emotional expression. Trait facet criteria include cognitive and perceptual dysregulation, unusual beliefs and experiences, eccentricity, restricted affectivity, withdrawal, and suspiciousness. Four or more are required (American Psychiatric Association, 2022).

Conceptualizations of the Schizotypal Personality Disorder

Psychodynamic Case Conceptualizations

Gunderson (1988) admits that little is known about the dynamics of the Schizotypal Personality Disorder. Gabbard (1990) among other psychoanalytically oriented writers believes that except for a few symptoms suggestive of an attenuated form of schizophrenia, the schizoid personality and the schizotypal personality are inherently similar.

On the other hand, Kellerman and Burry (1989) believe that the dynamics of the two disorders are quite different. They classify the schizoid personality disorder as an emotion controlled character type—along with the paranoid and obsessive compulsive personality disorders—while they classify the Schizotypal Personality Disorder as an emotion avoidant character type—along with the borderline and avoidant personality disorders.

Kellerman and Burry believe that schizotypal individuals probably experienced consistent object contact in early childhood. However, their parents failed to provide sufficient emotional closeness and warmth and were probably punitive and critical. These factors probably account for the social hypersensitivity which serves as a defense against intense social anxiety noted in these individuals. Emotion is generally restricted but when expressed tends to be inappropriate. These individuals typically utilize a wide variety of defense mechanisms including projection to externalize fear and anger, preoccupational with magic thinking and intellectualization to reduce emotional overstimulation, and hysterical denial to screen out undesirable social interactions in order to rationalize them.

Biosocial Case Conceptualization

The schizotypal personality is viewed by Millon and Everly (1985) as a syndromal continuation of the schizoid and avoidant personality disorders. Thus, the etiological and developmental determinants of the schizotypal disorder will be similar as in the schizoid and avoidant disorders, but in greater intensity or chronicity. Biogenic factors in the schizotypal schizoid variant include a genetic predisposition at least as reported in one study (Torgerson, 1984). Millon and Everly suggest that schizotypal-schizoid individuals embody a passive infantile reaction pattern which probably initiated a sequence of impoverished infantile stimulation and consequent parental indifference. Further, they point out that a dampening of the ascending reticular activity system of the limbic system may result in the auto stimulation and fantasy of these individuals. Environmentally, a cold and formal family environment combined with fragmented parental communication probably interacts with biogenic factors to produce this personality pattern and disorder. The background of schizotypal-avoidant individuals is somewhat different. Genetically, these individuals are more likely to exhibit a "slow-to-warm-up" temperament (Thomas & Chess, 1974). These individuals tend to be apprehensive, tense and do not adapt quickly to new situations. Such behavior can precipitate parental tension and derogation where further aggravates this temperament. Socially, the developmental histories of these individuals typically show parental deprecation as well as peer and sibling humiliation which results in interpersonal mistrust and lowered self-esteem. Continuation of these derogating and humiliating attitudes eventually leads to self-criticism and self-deprecation.

The schizotypal personality is self-perpetuated by social isolation, overprotection, and self-insulation. While social isolation and overprotectiveness have immediate benefits, in the long run they are counterproductive as they deprive these individuals of opportunities to develop social school, besides fostering dependency. Furthermore, their tendency toward self-insulation serves to foster and further perpetuate the spiral of cognitive and social deterioration that typifies this disorder (Millon & Davis, 1996).

Cognitive Behavioral Case Conceptualizations

According to Beck (2015) individuals with schizotypal personality are odd and different from others. There are characteristics core, conditional, and instrumental beliefs noted in individuals with this disorder. Their *core belief* includes the world is uncaring and life is full of powerful forces that cannot be explained. Their *conditional belief* is that if they get close to normal people, they will be rejected; if others view them as different, they will be left alone; and if they use their special gifts, the powers will protect them. Their *instrumental belief* is to being different is protective. Underlying these various beliefs are their beliefs about self and the world. They tend to view themselves as different, special, gifted, or supernaturally attuned. They typically view others as unfriendly and hostile, untrustworthy, and unable to understand their specialness. Accordingly, their basic strategy is to cultivate unusual appearance or mannerisms, keep a distance from others, and use their special gifts or magical powers to protect themselves (Renton & Mankiewicz, 2015).

From a behavioral perspective, Turkat (1990) describe the Schizotypal Personality Disorder, but is unable to provide behavioral formulation for it. Instead, he notes that these individuals tend to be quite diverse in terms of behavioral presentation. This is consistent with the observation that schizotypal personality is a decompensation of either the avoidant personality or the schizoid personality (Millon & Everly, 1985; 2000; Millon & Davis, 2000).

Interpersonal Case Conceptualization

According to Benjamin (1995), persons diagnosed with Schizotypal Personality Disorder likely had parents who punished them for allegedly inappropriate customary talking, while their parents did the same. Thus, the absent father severely reprimands the child for not staying home. Essentially, such a parent modelled "mindreading", suggesting that even though not present, he "knew" something vitally important about the child. The adult consequence of this schizotypal modeling is that the individual imitates this pattern of "knowing" through special means such as telepathy, mind reading or "sixth" sense. Parents were also likely to place inappropriate reliance on children for performance of household duties with undue threat and duress. Thus, these children learned that proper behavior and obedience could avert bad outcomes. The adult consequence is the paradoxical tendency to submit to rituals that bring control. Severe abuse, often involving invasion of these children's' personal boundaries is common. Furthermore, it also is likely that strong injunctions against learning the home for peer play or other reasons, were levied by the parents. Such prohibitions interfered with the development of social feelings and skills, and reinforced social isolation as well as fantasy and autism. Finally, there is a fear of being attacked and controlled by humiliation. These individuals are prone to hostile withdrawal and self-neglect. Furthermore, they believe they can magically influence—from a distance—circumstances and individuals through telepathy or ritual. Although they may be aware of their aggressive feelings, they usually constrain them.

Integrative Case Conceptualizations

The following integrative formulation provides a biopsychosocial explanation for how the Schizotypal Personality Disorder is likely to develop and be maintained. Because this disorder is as a syndromal extension or deterioration of the Schizoid or the Avoidant Personality Disorders (Millon, 1981), the biological and temperamental features of both of these subtypes should be consulted. The schizoid subtype of a schizotypal personality is characterized with a passive infantile pattern, probably resulting from low autonomic nervous system reactivity and parental indifference that led to impoverished infantile stimulation. On the other hand, the avoidant subtype is characterized by the fearful infantile temperamental pattern (Millon, 1981). This probably resulted from the child's high autonomic nervous system reactivity combined with parental criticalness and depreciation that was further reinforced by sibling and peer depreciation. Both subtypes of the schizotypal personality have been noted to have impaired eye tracking motions which is a characteristic shared with schizophrenic individuals.

Psychologically, schizotypal individual view themselves, others, the world, and life's purpose in terms of the following themes. They tend to view themselves by some variant of the theme: "I'm on a different wave length than others." They commonly experience being selfless, that is, they experience feeling empathy, estranged, and disconnected or dissociated from the rest of life. Their world view is some variant of the theme: "Life is strange and unusual, and others have special magical intentions." As a result, they are likely to conclude "Therefore, observe caution while being curious about these special magical intentions of others." The most common defense mechanism utilized by them is undoing, the effort to neutralize "evil" deeds and thoughts by their eccentric and peculiar beliefs and actions.

Socially, predictable patterns of parenting and environmental factors can be noted for the Schizotypal Personality Disorder. The parenting patterns noted previously of the cold indifference of the schizoid subtype, or the deprecating and derogatory parenting style and family environment of the avoidant subtype are noted. In both cases, the level of functioning in the family of origin then would be noted in the Schizoid Personality Disorder or the Avoidant Personality Disorder. Fragmented parental communications are a feature common to both subtypes of the Schizotypal Personality Disorder. The parental injunction is likely to have been "You're a strange bird" (Sperry & Mosak, 1996; Sperry, 2015). Table 13.2 summarizes the characteristics of this disorder.

Table 13.2 Characteristics of Schizotypal Personality Disorder

Triggering Event(s)	Close interpersonal relationships
Behavioral Style:	Eccentric and peculiar behaviors
	Odd speech but not incoherent
	Depersonalization and/or dissociation
Interpersonal Style:	May relate to others with similar unusual interests
	Suspicious of others not in their like-minded group
	Indifferent to social convention
Cognitive Style:	Tangential and scattered thought processing
	Magical thinking and superstitious
Feeling Style:	Inappropriate or constricted affect
	Hypersensitive
Temperament:	*Schizoid types*: passive infantile pattern
	Avoidance type: fearful infantile pattern
Attachment Style	Fearful and dismissive
Parental Injunction:	"You're a strange bird"
Self-View:	"I'm on a different wavelength than others"
World View:	"Life is strange and unusual and others have special magic intentions. Therefore, observe caution while being curious"
Maladaptive Schemas	Alienation; abandonment; dependence; vulnerability to harm
Optimal Diagnostic Criteria	Thinking, speech, behavior or appearance that is odd, eccentric, or peculiar

Assessment of Schizotypal Personality Disorder

Several sources of information are useful in establishing a diagnosis and treatment plan for personality disorders. Observation, collateral information, and psychological testing are important adjuncts to the patient's self-report in the clinical interview. This section briefly describes some characteristic observations that the clinician makes and the nature of the rapport likely to develop in initial encounters with specific personality-disordered individuals. Characteristic response patterns on various objective personality tests (i.e., MMPI-2 and MCMI-IV) and projective test (i.e., Rorschach) are also described.

Interview Behavior and Rapport. Interviewing Schizotypal Personality Disordered individuals usually elicits surprising statements and peculiar ideas. Rapport is hampered as long as they feel the clinician cannot appreciate their experiences. To the extent the clinician is empathic and indicates understanding, they will be more willing to share their secret and autistic world. Unlike the schizoid, these individuals establish rapport easily and are usually willing to respond to all types of questions. The clinician will frequently need to ask for clarification of the impressions and constructions. Empathic listening together with continuation techniques is usually suffice in encouraging them to explain their experience. On the other hand, doubting questions or confronting their views will cause them to recoil. More intelligent individuals with this disorder may query the clinicians wanting to know whether the clinician had had experiences similar to their. Handling this situation is more a matter of rapport than an issue of formulating questions more effectively (Othmer & Othmer, 2002; Ackley, Mack, Beyer, & Erdberg, 2011).

Psychological Testing Data. The Minnesota Multiphase Personality Inventory (MMPI-2), the Millon Clinical Multiaxial Inventory (MCMI-IV), and the Rorschach Psychodiagnostic Test, can be useful in diagnosing the Schizotypal Personality Disorder as well as the Schizotypal Personality style or trait.

On the MMPI-2 a 2-7-8 (Depression-Psychasthenia-Schizophrenia) code is likely among these individuals (Edell, 1987). Scales F (Frequency) and O (social Introversion) are also likely to be elevated (Graham, 2011).

On the MCMI-IV elevations on S (Schizotypal), 2A (Avoidant), 7 (Compulsive), and 8A (Negativistic: passive aggressive) can be expected (Choca & Denburg, 1997; Millon et al., 2016).

On the Rorschach it might be expected that these individuals would respond much like those with Schizoid Personality Disorder. However, the responses of schizotypal individuals are more similar to schizophrenics and those with Borderline Personality Disorder then those with Schizoid Personality Disorder (Swiercinsky, 1985). The new Rorschach Performance Assessment System (R-PAS) is an improved method for scoring and interpreting the Rorschach Inkblot Test. Besides being evidence-based and internationally normed, it increases clinical utility and is easier to use than Exner's Comprehensive System (Mihura & Meyer, 2018).

Treatment Approaches and Interventions

Treatment Considerations

Included in the differential diagnosis of this disorder are three other personality disorders: Schizoid Personality Disorder, Avoidant Personality Disorder, and the Borderline Personality

Disorder. The most common symptom disorders associated with Schizotypal Personality Disorder are the Schizophrenias, particularly the Disorganized, Catatonic and Residual types. Other disorders noted are the Anxiety Disorders, the Somatic Symptom Disorders, and the Dissociative Disorders.

Individuals with this disorder find it difficult to engage and remain in psychotherapeutic relationship. Typically, they are on medication and may be referred for adjunctive psychotherapy. Accordingly, the focus of treatment is on "management" rather than on "treatment." Thus, instead of attempting personality restructuring, the realistic treatment goal for the schizotypal personality is to increase the individual's ability to function more consistently even though on the periphery of society. Specifically, successful management will likely incorporate psychoeducational or social skills training with supportive psychotherapeutic methods. Reid (1989) noted that if these patients can remain in long-term treatment, they may be able to increase their ability to function more consistently and with less disease. He reports that homogeneous groups can occasionally be a useful adjunct to individual treatment. In terms of medication, low dose neuroleptics have been found to be useful for the schizotypal personality even in the absence of psychotic features. Yet, it should be noted that medication compliance is particularly a problem with this disorder (Sperry, 2015).

Individual Psychotherapy

Psychodynamic Psychotherapy Approaches

Schizotypal personality-disordered individuals tend to be treated in office, clinics, and day treatment programs rather than in acute inpatient programs. They may profit from dynamically oriented psychotherapy, both expressive and supportive, depending on their level of functioning and treatment readiness. The basis for dynamic treatment is not interpretation of conflict, but rather internalization of a therapeutic relationship (Stone, 1985).

Essentially, the clinician's task is to "melt" the patient's frozen internal object relations by providing a correct emotional experience. Their style of relatedness results from inadequacies in early relationships with parental figures (Yeomans, Clarkin, & Levy, 2021). As a result, these patients go through life distancing themselves from others. Therapy must therefore provide a new relationship for internalization (Gabbard, 2000).

There has been relatively little psychodynamic research about this personality disorder, as noted by Perry, Presniak, & Olson (2013). They conducted a study that evaluated the defense mechanisms used by individuals with various personality disorders during videotaped therapy sessions. With schizotypal individuals, there was the least variance of defense mechanisms among the other disorders. Projection, splitting, passive aggression, and devaluation were the most common defenses used. Defenses specific to schizoid personality disorder included displacement and fantasy. Individuals with this disorder prefer to deal with others indirectly. Since their basic mode of functioning is non-relational, they find the task of therapy very challenging and difficult. Not surprisingly, they respond to the challenge with silence and emotional distancing. Clinicians need to adopt a permissive, accepting attitude, and must be exceedingly patient with these individuals. It is more helpful to understand silence as a nonverbal form of relating rather than as treatment resistance. By listening with a third ear, the clinician can learn much about these patients. Through projective identification they will evoke certain responses in that clinician that contain valuable diagnostic information regarding the patient's inner world (Gabbard, 1990). Dealing effectively with countertransference issues is critical in working with schizotypal patients. Accepting silent non-relatedness is foreign to the clinician's psychological predisposition and training. Thus, when silence is prolonged, the clinician must guard against acting out and projecting their own self and object representations onto the patient. Accepting the silence and refraining from interpreting it legitimizes the patient's private, noncommunicative core self. It may be the only viable technique for building a therapeutic alliance (Gabbard, 1990).

Long-Term vs. Short-Term Dynamic Therapy: Decisions about the type and frequency of dynamic therapy should be based on the patient's level of functioning and motivation and readiness for treatment. Higher functioning schizotypal patients who exhibit some depressive symptoms, or some capacity for empathy and emotional warmth tend to have better outcomes in dynamic psychotherapy (Stone, 1983). Similarly, patients with better ego functioning in terms of judgement, reality testing, and cognitive slippage, tend to do better than those with poorer ego functioning.

Those patients who are highly motivated for exploratory psychotherapy can make dramatic gains in intense, long-term treatment of two to three sessions per week over several years. On the other hand, long-term supportive psychotherapy is indicated for the majority of schizotypal patients who present with major ego deficits and personal eccentricities. The goal of such treatment is improved adaptive functioning in day-to-day living (Stone, 1989). Mehlum et al (1991) described a long-term day treatment program for Schizotypal Personality Disordered individuals based on psychodynamic principles.

Short term dynamic therapy is indicated for crisis issues and situational difficulties related to job or personal life. It may also serve as a follow-up to a previous course of long-term psychotherapy. Not surprisingly, there are few case reports of short-term dynamic individual treatment as curative intervention.

Cognitive Behavioral Therapy Approach

Stone (1989) indicates that for schizotypal patients who aspire to "fit in" better and feel less alienated may be necessary. For instance, referral to elocution lessons, or a Dale Carnegie course, or accompanying the patient to a clothing store to assist in selecting appropriate apparel for a job interview, etc. Stone has also found videotape feedback useful in pointing out the patient's awkwardness of gait, or gestures. Turkat (1990) recommends that anxiety management and modification of hypersensitivity and hypervigilance also may be necessary, depending on the case formulation.

Cognitive Therapy. Beck, Freeman, and associates (2004) briefly describe the Cognitive Therapy approach to working with Schizotypal Personality Disordered individuals. Developing a collaborative working relationship is the starting point for treatment with these individuals. Since these individuals hold a number of irrational beliefs about others, the importance of the therapeutic relationship should not be underestimated. Since these individuals desire social relationships and experience distress with social isolation, assisting them in increasing their social support network is an initial treatment goal. Increasing social appropriateness is a related goal. Social skills training as well as the therapist modelling appropriate behavior and speech are effective strategies. In combination with these behavioral strategies, the clinician works collaboratively with the individual to identify automatic thoughts and underlying schemas about social interactions. Role playing more appropriate behavior then becomes much more meaningful.

Perhaps the most critical aspect of treatment is helping the schizotypal individual seek out objective evidence in the environment to evaluate their thoughts, rather than relying on emotional responses. As they learn to disregard inappropriate thoughts, they are able to consider the consequences that responding emotionally or behaviorally to such thoughts would have and respond more rationally. The individual's eccentric and magical thoughts are perceived as symptoms, and predesigned coping statements such as "There I go again. Even though I have this thought, it doesn't mean it's true", are practiced. In addition to guided discovery and direct disputation of maladaptive beliefs, indirect strategies such as encouraging the schizotypal individual to keep track of the predictions they make, and the accuracy of these predictions is an effective but less threatening intervention. In addition to focusing on automatic thoughts and schemas, efforts to change the schizotypal's cognitive style are helpful. Since the communication patterns of these individuals tends to be circumstantial and idiosyncratic, collaborative experiments can be set up to modify this style. Furthermore, Beck and associates (1990) notes that provided the therapist has realistic treatment expectations, much can be accomplished, and the collaborative work can be a positive experience as these individuals are able to control portions of their inappropriate behaviors and thoughts.

Freeman et al. (1990) are not optimistic about the cognitive treatment of schizotypal individuals indicating that behavioral interventions: social skills training, are initially useful. It is only after these individuals can be more socially appropriate—that is they begin acting more like schizoid personalities—are their automatic thoughts and cognitive distortions amenable to cognitive methods.

Renton and Mankiewicz (2015) agree that establishing a collaborative and trusting therapeutic relationship is crucial to the successful treatment of these individuals. Typically, they present for help only when some external crisis forces them to do so. Schizotypal patients often harbor suspicions about the therapist, which may include magical thinking such as having their minds read against their will. Once trust is established and therapeutic goals have been identified, a number of cognitive interventions can be attempted. Developmental conceptualizations may be particularly useful in helping schizotypal individuals see how past events shape the beliefs and rules they currently hold about the world. However, these individuals may resist deeper examination into the origins of their belief systems and commonly terminate therapy once symptom relief is achieved or the presenting situation is resolved (Fowler, Orme, & Hart, 2021).

Schema Therapy. Schema Therapy is an elaboration of cognitive therapy that has been developed by Young (1994; 1999) specifically for personality disorders, and other difficult individual and couples problems. Schema Therapy involves identifying maladaptive schemas and planning specific strategies and interventions. Four main strategies are cognitive, experiential, behavioral and the therapeutic relationship itself. Cognitive restructuring, modification of maladaptive schemas, is an important cognitive strategy, but is combined with imagery exercises, empathic confrontation, homework assignments and "limited reparenting," i.e., a form of corrective emotional experience (Young, 1999).

Maladaptive schemas typically associated with Schizotypal Personality Disorder include: *abandonment,* i.e., the belief that significant others will not or cannot provide reliable and stable support; *alienation*, i.e., the belief that one must meet the needs of others at the expense of one's own gratification; *vulnerability to harm,* i.e., the exaggerated fear that imminent catastrophe will strike at any time and that one will be unable to prevent it; and *dependence* i.e., the belief that one is unable to competently everyday responsibilities without considerable help from others (Bernstein, 2002).

Interpersonal Approach

For Benjamin (2003) psychotherapeutic interventions with Schizotypal Personality Disordered individuals can be planned and evaluated in terms of whether they enhance collaboration, facilitate learning about maladaptive patterns and their roots block these patterns, enhance the will to change, and effectively encourage new patterns.

The therapist facilitates collaboration by deferring to the Schizotypal individuals' sensitivities. For example, at the beginning of therapy, the therapist may need to be quite tolerant about cancelled appointments and control over the course of sessions. If not allowed to maintain distance and control in this manner, these individuals will quickly terminate. Gradually the therapist should be able to engage these individuals through empathic listening, accurate mirroring and constancy. As treatment progresses, they may develop sufficient trust and insight to relinquish control by magic and ritual. Unlike parents, clinicians require no caregiving themselves. And unlike the parents of schizotypals, therapists can be consistent in mainstreaming focus and supportive attention. Such an experience is, therefore, emotionally corrective.

During the course of treatment, schizotypal individuals need to learn that the unrealistic responsibility is an abusive situation when they were helpless predisposed them to magical thinking. Such early experiences led these individuals to assume they had inordinate power and influence. Next, they are helped to recognize when and how they distort reality. At the same time, they are taught new self-talk that can keep them grounded in the here and now. Later, they are helped to understand the contribution of early experiences and learnings to their unrealistic thoughts. However, for reconstructive changes to occur, these individuals must change their wish to magically protect their self and others while maintaining loyalty to early abusers. For example, interpreting suicidal or other fantasies in relation to underlying wishes can lead to fuller awareness, allowing the individual an opportunity for a new choice. Accurate mirroring and empathy can assist these individuals in mobilizing their will to recover and visualize better ways of viewing self, the world and others. With these individuals, the therapist must remain cautious. There is a fragile balance between allowing the patient to continue to participate in maladaptive behaviors in order to keep them in therapy and blocking them when they occur to promote change. Benjamin is doubtful that major changes in learning patterns will occur, believing that this disorder is genetically mediated.

Group Therapy

Clinical reports of group therapy with schizotypal patients have been limited. Nevertheless, there is sufficient indication these patients may profit from supportive group therapy (Stone, 1989; Mehlum et al., 1991).

A reasonable outcome of goal of group therapy is increased awareness that other harbor fantasies and self-criticisms similar to schizotypals and that others may find them likeable despite their conviction of unlikability (Ogrodniczuk, Uliaszek, Lebow, & Kealy, 2021). Group therapy may impact such social alienating tendencies as standoffishness and peculiarities of speech. An ongoing heterogeneous group may be able to tolerate some degree of these tendencies. But beyond the limits of tolerability, these behaviors may so affect either the patient or other group members that therapeutic group process is mollified. Obviously, appropriate selection of which schizotypal patients will benefit from being in a group is an important task of the group leaders (Stone, 1989).

Marital and Family Therapy

Clinical reports of marital or family therapy with schizotypal patients have not yet appeared. In general, schizotypal individuals tend to remain single. Because of either their rejection sensitivity or insensitivity to others' feelings, these patients are likely to avoid committed relationships. Not surprisingly, schizotypals who do marry tend to have problems stemming either from insensitivity to the feelings of their partner or from over sensitivity to the partner's behavior. Therefore, in couples therapy, the clinician's first task is to assess the degree of and balance between these two tendencies. Typically, it is easier to assist in hypersensitive partner respond more appropriately, then to help an insensitive partner become more empathic (Stone, 1989).

Family therapy has been identified as a potentially beneficial intervention for adolescents with schizoid personality disorder (Ryan, Macdonald, & Walker, 2013). Because of the shared symptoms with schizophrenia and other schizophrenia spectrum disorders, family education interventions have been adapted to schizotypal personality disorder that enlist family members to support patient recovery (Ogrodniczuk, Uliaszek, Lebow, & Kealy, 2021). These include family education about the disorder, identification of relapse signs and development of action plans, and communication training to reduce stress within the family.

Medication

Currently, there are no psychotropic medications specifically indicated for treating this personality disorder (Silk & Feurino, 2012). Nevertheless, medications are used that target specific troubling symptoms associated with the disorder, such as depression, anxiety, or sleep problems. Generally, these medications are used as an adjunct to psychotherapy and skills training (Nelson & Tsheringld, 2021). Because troubling symptoms often respond to medications sooner than most psychological interventions, medications are usually prescribed at the onset of treatment. These include low dose neuroleptics which can be useful in decreasing anxiety associated with loss of control (Sperry, 1995b). In a randomized controlled trial, Risperdal (risperidone), an antipsychotic medication, has been shown to be effective with this disorder (Koenigsberg, Woo-Ming, & Siever, 2002; Silk & Feurino, 2012).

Combined and Integrative Treatment Approaches

Probably because of the impairing nature of this disorder, there is surprisingly little resistance to combining medication with psychological treatments, and tailoring treatment. Liebowitz et al. (1986) suggest beginning individual therapy and medication, where indicated, concurrently. Stone (1992) advocates beginning with medication or a behavioral intervention and adding a dimensional psychotherapy: a blending of supportive, exploratory, cognitive and behavioral elements to match the concurrent needs and circumstances of the patient. This, of course, represents the epitome of integrated, tailored treatment (Stanley, Brodsky, & Gratch, 2021).

Others have advocated social skills training as an adjunct to supportive psychotherapy (Liebowitz et al., 1986) or combining group therapy with individual dynamic psychotherapy (Gabbard, 1994). Mehlum et al. (1991) reports on the combining of several treatment modalities for schizotypal and borderline personality-disordered patients: individual psychodynamic psychotherapy, group therapy, community meetings, art therapy, awareness group therapy, and milieu therapy. This unique prospective study of a day treatment program showed that efficacy of this combined treatment approach held up an average of three years later. Major changes were noted in symptom reduction. However, social adjustments and employment were not as robust as with borderline patients. Nathanson, Connick, and Jamison (2011) present a case study with a 21-year-old US combat infantryman diagnosed with schizotypal personality disorder. His treatment involved selectively reinforcing positive self-statements, social skills training, and anxiety reduction, as well as pharmacological interventions. Ryan, Macdonald, & Walker (2013) note that many individuals with schizophrenia spectrum disorders also abuse cannabis, which can exacerbate psychotic symptoms. To address this issue, they discuss Motivational Interviewing as an effective option.

References

Accordino, M. P., Keat II, D. B., & Guerney, Jr., B. G. (2003). Using relationship enhancement therapy with an adolescent with serious mental illness and substance dependence. *Journal of Mental Health Counseling, 25*(2), 152–164.
Ackley, C., Mack, S., Beyer, K., & Erdberg, P. (2011). *Investigative and forensic interviewing: A personality-focused approach.* CRC Press.
Adler, A. (1956). Problems in psychotherapy. *American Journal of Individual Psychology, 12*, 12–24.
Adler, G. (1985). *Borderline psychopathology and its treatment.* Jason Aronson.
Ainsworth, M. D. S., Blehar, M. C., Waters, E., & Wall, S. (1978). *Patterns of attachment: A psychological study of the strange situation.* Erlbaum.
Akhtar, S. (1987). Schizoid personality disorder: A synthesis of developmental, dynamic, and descriptive features. *American Journal of Psychotherapy, 41*, 449–518.
Alden, L. (1989). Short-term structured treatment for avoidant personality disorder. *Journal of Consulting and Clinical Psychology, 57*, 756–764.
Alden, L. (1992). Cognitive-interpersonal treatment of avoidant personality disorder. In P. Keller & S. Heyman (Eds), *Innovations in clinical practice: A source book. Vol. 11* (pp. 5–22). Professional Resources Exchange.
Alexander, J. & Parsons, B. (1973). Short-term behavioral intervention with delinquent families: Impact on family process and recidivism. *Journal of Abnormal Psychology, 8*, 219–225.
Allen, J. & Fonagy, P. (Eds). (2006). *The handbook of mentalization-based treatment.* Wiley.
Allnutt, S. & Links, P. (1996). Diagnosing specific personality disorders and the optimal criteria. In P. Links (Ed.), *Clinical assessment and management of severe personality disorders* (pp. 21–48). American Psychiatric Press.
Allport, G. (1937). *Personality: A psychological interpretation.* Holt.
Alonso, A. (1992). The shattered mirror: Treatment of a group of narcissistic patients. *Group, 16*, 210–219.
Alonso, A. & Rutan, J. (1984). The impact of object relations theory on psychodynamic group therapy. *American Journal of Psychiatry, 141*, 1376–1380.
American Psychiatric Association. (2013). *Diagnostic and Statistical Manual of Mental Disorders, Fifth edition.* American Psychiatric Publishing.
American Psychiatric Association. (2022). *Diagnostic and statistical manual of mental disorders. Fifth edition. Text revision.* American Psychiatric Association.
Anderson, C. (1983). A psychoeducational program for families of patients with schizophrenia. In W. McFarlane (Ed). *Family therapy in schizophrenia* (pp. 99–116). Guilford Press.
Appel, G. (1974). An approach to the treatment of schizoid phenomena. *Psychoanalytic Review, 61*, 99–113.
Armstrong, R. (2002). Schizoid phenomena in substance abusers. *Journal of Addictive Diseases, 21*(3), 73–85.
Arntz, A. (2015). Borderline personality disorder. In A. Beck, D. Davis, & A. Freeman (Eds), *Cognitive therapy of personality disorders* (3rd ed., pp. 366–392). Guilford Press.
Azima, F. (1983). Group psychotherapy with personality disorders. In H. Kaplan & B. Sadock (Eds), *Comprehensive group psychotherapy* (2nd ed., pp. 262–268). Wilkins & Wilkins.

Babiak, P. & Hare, R. (2007). *Snakes in suits: When psychopaths go to work*. Harper.
Bach, B. & Mulder, R. (2022). Empirical foundation of the ICD-11 classification of personality disorders. In S. K. Huprich (Ed.), *Personality disorders and pathology: Integrating clinical assessment and practice in the DSM-5 and ICD-11 era* (pp. 27–52). American Psychological Association. https://doi.org/10.1037/0000310-003.
Bach, B. & Tracy, M. (2022). Clinical utility of the alternative model of personality disorders: A 10th year anniversary review. *Personality Disorders: Theory, Research, and Treatment, 13*(4), 369–379. https://doi.org/10.1037/per0000527.
Bailey, G. (1998). Cognitive-behavioral treatment of obsessive-compulsive personality disorder. *Journal of Psychological Practice, 4*, 51–59.
Balint, M. (1968). *The basic fault: Therapeutic aspects of regression*. Tavistock.
Balint, M., Ornstein, P., & Balint, E. (1972). *Focal psychotherapy*. Tavistock.
Baliousis, M., Khalifa, N., & Völlm, B. (2018). The neurobiology of antisocial personality disorders focusing on psychopathy. In C. Schmahl, K. L. Phan, R. O. Friedel (Eds). *Neurobiology of personality disorders* (pp. 319–358). Oxford University Press.
Barber, J., Morse, J., Krakauer, I., Chittams, J., & Crits-Christoph, K. (1997). Change in obsessive-compulsive and avoidant personality disorder following time-limited supportive-expressive therapy. *Psychotherapy, 34*, 133–143.
Barlow, D. & Waddell, M. (1985). Agoraphobia. In D. Barlow (Ed.), *Clinical handbook of psychological disorders: A step-by-step manual*. Guilford Press.
Bartholomew, K. (1990). Avoidance of intimacy: An attachment perspective. *Journal of Social and Personal Relationships, 7*, 147–178.
Bartholomew, K. & Horowitz, L. (1991). Attachment styles among young adults: A test of a four-category model. *Journal of Personality and Social Psychology, 61*, 226–244.
Bateman, A. W. (2022). Mentalization-based treatment. In S. K. Huprich (Ed.), *Personality disorders and pathology: Integrating clinical assessment and practice in the DSM-5 and ICD-11 era* (pp. 237–258). American Psychological Association. https://doi.org/10.1037/0000310-011.
Bateman, A. & Fonagy, P. (1999). Effectiveness of partial hospitalization in the treatment of borderline personality disorder: A randomized controlled trial. *American Journal of Psychiatry, 156*, 1563–1569.
Bateman, A. & Fonagy, P. (2001). Treatment of borderline personality disorder with psychoanalytically oriented partial hospitalization: An 18-month follow-up. *American Journal of Psychiatry, 158*, 36–42.
Bateman, A. & Fonagy, P. (2007). *Mentalization based treatment: A practical guide*. Oxford University Press.
Bateman, A. & Fonagy, P. (2009). Randomly controlled trial of outpatient mentalizing-based treatment versus structured clinical management for borderline personality disorder. *American Journal of Psychiatry, 166*, 1355–1364.
Bateman, A. & Fonagy, P. (2010). Mentalization based treatment for borderline personality disorder. *World Psychiatry, 9*(1), 11–15.
Beck, A. (2015). Theory of personality disorders. In A. Beck, D. Davis, & A. Freeman, A. (Eds) *Cognitive therapy of personality disorders* (3rd ed., pp. 19–62). Guilford Press.
Beck, A., Davis, D., & Freeman, A. (Eds) (2015) *Cognitive therapy of personality disorders* (3rd ed.). Guilford Press.
Beck, A., Freeman, A., & associates (1990). *Cognitive therapy of personality disorders*. Guilford Press.
Beck, A., Freeman, A., Davis, D., & associates (2004). *Cognitive therapy of personality disorders* (2nd ed.). Guilford Press.
Behary, W. & Davis, D. (2015). Narcissistic personality disorder. In A. Beck, D. Davis, & A. Freeman, A. (Eds), *Cognitive therapy of personality disorders* (3rd ed., pp. 299–324). Guilford Press.
Beitman, B. (2003). *Integrating psychotherapy and pharmacotherapy: Dissolving the mind-brain barrier*. Norton.
Beitman, B. & Yue, D. (1999). *Learning psychotherapy*. Norton.
Bellak, L. (1997). *The TAT, CAT and SAT in clinical use* (6th ed.). Allyn & Bacon.
Bellino, S., Rinaldi, C., & Bogetto, F. (2010). Adaptation of interpersonal psychotherapy to borderline personality disorder: a comparison of combined therapy and single pharmacotherapy. *Canadian Journal of Psychiatry, 55*, 74–81.

Bellino, S., Bozzatello, P., & Bogetto, F. (2015). Combined treatment of borderline personality disorder with interpersonal psychotherapy and pharmacotherapy: Predictors of response. *Psychiatry Research*, 226, 284–288.
Bender, D., Morey, L., & Skodol, A. (2011). Toward a model for assessing level of personality functioning in DSM–5, Part I: A review of theory and methods, *Journal of Personality Assessment*, 93(4), 332–346.
Benjamin, L. (1993). *Interpersonal diagnosis and treatment of personality disorders.* Guilford Press.
Benjamin, L. (2003a). *Interpersonal diagnosis and treatment of personality disorders* (2nd ed.). Guilford Press.
Benjamin, L. (2003b). *Interpersonal reconstructive therapy: Promoting change in nonresponders.* Guilford Press.
Benjamin, L. (2007). *Interpersonal reconstructive therapy: An integrative, personality-based treatment for complex cases.* Guilford Press.
Berger, P. (1987). Pharmacologic treatment for borderline personality disorder. *Bulletin of the Menninger Clinic*, 51, 277–284.
Berkowitz, D. (1985). Self-object needs and marital disharmony. *Psychoanalytic Review*, 72, 229–237.
Berkowitz, D., Shapiro, R., Zinner, J., & Shapiro, H. (1974). Concurrent family treatment of narcissistic disorders in adolescents. *International Journal of Psychoanalysis*, 3, 371–396.
Berman, E. (1983). The treatment of troubled couples. In L. Grinspoon (Ed.), *Psychiatric Updates, Vol. 2.* American Psychiatric Association.
Bernstein, D. (2002). Cognitive therapy of personality disorders in patients with histories of emotional abuse or neglect. *Psychiatric Annals*, 32, 618–628.
Binder, J. (1979). Treatment of narcissistic problems in time-limited psychotherapy. *Psychiatric Quarterly*, 51, 257–270.
Black, D., Zanarini, M., Romine, A., Shaw, M., Allen, J., & Schulz, S. (2014). Comparison of low and moderate doses of extended-release quetiapine in borderline personality disorder: A randomized, double-blind, placebo-controlled trial. *American Journal of Psychiatry*, 171, 1174–1182.
Bliton, C. F., Rosenstein, L. K., & Pincus, A. L. (2022). Trading patients: Applying the alternative model for personality disorders to two cases of DSM-5 borderline personality disorder over time and across therapists. *Frontiers in Psychology*, 13, 794624.
Blocher, D. (1974). *Developmental counseling.* Wiley.
Blocher, D. (2000). *Counseling: A developmental approach* (4th ed.). Wiley.
Bogdanoff, M. & Elbaum, P. (1978). Role lock: Dealing with monopolizers, isolates, helpful hannahs, and other associated characters in group psychotherapy. *International Journal of Group Psychotherapy*, 28, 247–281.
Bonime, W. (1959). The pursuit of anxiety-laden areas in therapy of the schizoid patient. *Psychiatry*, 22, 239–244.
Bornstein, R. (2012). Dependent personality disorder. In T. Widiger (Ed.), *The Oxford handbook of personality disorders* (pp. 505–526). Oxford University Press.
Bowlby, J. (1973). *Attachment and loss, Vol. 2, Separation.* Basic Books.
Brauer, L. & Reinecke, M. (2015). Dependent personality disorder. In A. Beck, D. Davis, & A. Freeman (Eds), *Cognitive therapy of personality disorders* (3rd ed., pp. 155–173). Guilford Press.
Brennan, K. & Shaver, P. (1998). Attachment styles and personality disorders: Their connection to each other and to parental divorce, parental death, and perceptions of parental caregiving. *Journal of Personality*, 66, 835–878.
Brown, E., Heimberg, R., & Juster, H. (1995). Social phobia subtype and avoidant personality disorder: Effects of severity of social phobia impairment and outcome of cognitive behavioral treatment. *Behavior Therapy*, 26, 467–486.
Buie, D. & Adler, G. (1982). The definitive treatment of the borderline personality. *International Journal of Psychoanalysis*, 9, 51–87.
Cain, N. M. & Mulay, A. L. (2022). The alternative *DSM-5* Model for Personality Disorders and its empirical support. In S. K. Huprich (Ed.), *Personality disorders and pathology: Integrating clinical assessment and practice in the DSM-5 and ICD-11 era* (pp. 9–26). American Psychological Association. https://doi.org/10.1037/0000310-002.
Caligor, E., Levy, K., & Yeomans, F. (2015). Narcissistic personality disorder: Diagnostic and clinical challenges. *American Journal of Psychiatry*, 172, 415–422.

Carlson, J. (2006). *Psychotherapy over time* [DVD]. Washington, DC: American Psychological Association.
Cass, D., Silvers, F., & Abrams, G. (1972). Behavioral group treatment of hysterics. *Archives of General Psychiatry, 26*, 42–50.
Chessick, R. (1982). Intensive psychotherapy of a borderline patient. *Archives of General Psychiatry, 39*, 413–419.
Chessick, R. (1985). *Psychology of the self and the treatment of narcissism*. Jason Aronson.
Choca, J. & Denburg, E. (1997). *Interpretative guide to the Millon Clinical Multiaxial Inventory* (Second edition). American Psychological Association.
Chodoff, P. (1989). Histrionic personality disorder. In T. Karasu (Ed.), *Treatment of psychiatric disorders* (pp. 2727–2735). American Psychiatric Press.
Clarkin, J., Cain, N., & Livesley, J. (2015). An integrated approach to patients with personality disorders. *Journal of Psychotherapy Integration, 25*, 3–12.
Clarkin, J., Foelsch, P., Levy, K., Hull, J., Delaney, J., & Kernberg, O. (2001). The development of a psychodynamic treatment for patients with borderline personality disorder: A preliminary study of behavior change. *Journal of Personality Disorders, 15*, 487–495.
Clarkin, J., Marziali, E., & Munroe-Blum, H. (1991). Group and family treatment of borderline personality disorder. *Hospital and Community Psychiatry, 42*, 1038–1043.
Clarkin, J., Yeomans, F., & Kernberg, O. (2015). *Transference-focused psychotherapy for borderline personality disorder: A clinical guide*. American Psychiatric Publishing.
Clinical Psychiatry News (1991). Better personality disorders therapies foreseen. *Clinical Psychiatry News*, September, 26.
Cloninger, C. (2004). *Feeling good: The science of well-being*. Oxford University Press.
Cortright, B. (1997). *Psychotherapy and spirit*. State University of New York Press.
Costa, P. & McCrae, R. (1990). Personality disorders and the five-factor model of personality. *Journal of Personality Disorders, 4*, 362–371.
Costello, C. (Ed.). (1996). *Personality characteristics of the personality disordered*. New York: Wiley.
Cramer Azima, F. (1983). Group psychotherapy with personality disorders. In H. Kaplan & B. Sadock (Eds), *Comprehensive group psychotherapy*. Williams & Wilkins.
Crits-Christoph P. & Barber, J. (2002). Psychological treatment for personality disorders. In P. Nathan & J. Gorman (Eds), *A guide to treatments that work* (2nd ed., pp. 611–624). Oxford Press.
Davidson, K., Halford, J., Kirkwood, L., Newton-Howes, G., Sharp, M., & Tata, P. (2010). CBT for violent men with antisocial personality disorder: Reflections on the experience of carrying out therapy in MASCOT, a pilot randomized controlled trial. *Personality and Mental Health, 4*, 86–95.
Davidson, K., Tyrer, P., Tata, P., Cooke, D., Gumley, A., Ford, I., et al. (2009). Cognitive behaviour therapy for violent men with antisocial personality disorder in the community: An exploratory randomized controlled trial. *Psychological Medicine, 39*, 569–577.
Day, M. & Semrad, E. (1971). Group therapy with neurotics and psychotics. In H. Kaplan & B. Sadock (Eds), *Comprehensive group psychotherapy* (pp. 566–580). Williams and Wilkins.
Diamond, R. (2009). *Instant psychopharmacology* (3rd ed.). W. W. Norton.
Dimaggio, G., Catania, D., Salvatore, G., Carcione, A., & Nicolo, G. (2006). Psychotherapy of paranoid personality disorder from the perspective of dialogical self-theory. *Counseling Psychology Quarterly, 19*, 69–87.
Dimaggio, G., D'Urzo, M., Pasinetti, M., Salvatore, G., Lysaker, P. H., Catania, D., & Popolo, R. (2015). Metacognitive interpersonal therapy for co-occurrent avoidant personality disorder and substance abuse. *Journal of Clinical Psychology, 71*(2), 157–166.
Dolan, M. & Park, I. (2002). The neuropsychology of antisocial personality disorder. *Psychological Medicine, 32*, 417–427.
Dorfman, W. I. (2000). Histrionic personality disorder. In H. E. Hersen & M. Biaggio (Eds), *Effective brief therapies: A clinician's guide* (pp. 355–370). Academic Press.
Dowgwillo, E. A., Molina, J., & Forche, K. R. (2022). Principles of psychological assessment for personality disorders. In S. K. Huprich (Ed.), *Personality disorders and pathology: Integrating clinical assessment and practice in the DSM-5 and ICD-11 era* (pp. 77–108). American Psychological Association. https://doi.org/10.1037/0000310-005.
Driscoll, K., Cukrowicz, K., Reardon, M., & Joiner, T. (2004). *Simple treatments for complex problems: A flexible cognitive behavior analysis system approach to psychotherapy*. Lawrence Erlbaum Associates.

Eells, T. (2007). Comparing the methods. Where is the common ground? In T. Eells (Ed.), *Handbook of psychotherapy case formulation* (2nd ed., pp. 412–432). Guilford Press.
Eells, T. (2010). The unfolding case formulation: The interplay of description and inference. *Pragmatic Case Studies in Psychotherapy, 6*(4), 225–254.
Eikenaes, I., Gude, T., & Hoffart, A. (2006). Integrated wilderness therapy for avoidant personality disorder. *Nordic Journal of Psychiatry, 60*, 275–281.
Edell, W. (1987). Relationship of borderline syndrome disorders to early schizophrenia on the MMPI. *Journal of Clinical Psychology, 43*, 163–174.
Ekleberry, S. (2014). *Treating co-occurring disorders: A handbook for mental health and substance abuse professionals*. Routledge.
Epstein, L. (1984). An interpersonal-object relations perspective working with destructive aggression. *Contemporary Psychoanalysis, 20*, 651–662.
Erdman, P. & Caffery, T. (Eds). (2003). *Attachment and family systems: Conceptual, empirical and therapeutic relatedness*. Brunner/Routledge.
Eskedal, G. & Demetri, J. (2006). Etiology and treatment of cluster C personality disorders. *Journal of Mental Health Counseling, 28*, 1–18.
Everett, S., Halperin, S., Volgy, S., & Wissler, A. (1989). *Treating the borderline family: A systematic approach*. Allyn & Bacon.
Exner, J. (1986). *The Rorschach: A comprehensive system* (2nd ed.). John Wiley.
Fairburn, W. (1954). *An object-relations theory of the personality*. Basic Books.
Farrell, J. & Shaw, I. A. (2022). Schema therapy: Conceptualization and treatment of personality disorders. In S. K. Huprich (Ed.), *Personality disorders and pathology: Integrating clinical assessment and practice in the DSM-5 and ICD-11 era* (pp. 281–304). American Psychological Association. https://doi.org/10.1037/0000310-013.
Fawcett, J. (2002). Schemas or traits and states: Top down or bottom up? *Psychiatric Annals, 32*, 567.
Fay, A. & Lazarus, A. (1993). Cognitive-behavior group therapy. In A. Alonso & H. Willer (Eds), *Group therapy in clinical practice* (pp. 449–469). American Psychiatric Press.
Fenichel, O. (1945). *The psychoanalytic theory of the neurosis*. Norton.
Fernandez, S. (2010). Complex case Carmen: Histrionic personality disorder and psychotherapy. *Personality and Mental Health, 4*, 146–152.
Fernando, J. (1998). The etiology of the narcissistic personality disorder. *Psychoanalytic Study of the Child, 53*, 141–158.
Finn, B. & Shakir, S. (1990). Intensive group psychotherapy of borderline patients, *Group, 14*, 99–110.
Fiore, D., Dimaggio, G., Giuseppe, N., Semerari, A., & Carcione, A. (2008). Metacognitive interpersonal therapy in a case of obsessive-compulsive and avoidant personality disorders. *Journal of Clinical Psychology: In Session, 64*, 168–180.
Flegenheimer, W. (1982). *Techniques of brief therapy*. Jason Aronson.
Fossatti, A., Madeddu, F., & Maffei, C. (1999). Borderline personality disorder and childhood sexual abuse: A meta-analytic study. *Journal of Personality Disorders, 13*, 2268–2280.
Fowler, J. C., Orme, W. H., & Hart, J. M. (2021). Cognitive-behavioral therapy. In A. E. Skodol & J. M. Oldham (Eds). *American Psychiatric Association Publishing textbook of personality disorders, Third edition*. (pp. 383–406). American Psychiatric Publishing.
Fraiberg, S. (1969). Libidinal object constancy and mental representation. *Psychoanalytic Study of the Child, 24*, 9–47.
Frances, A. (2013). *Essentials of psychiatric diagnosis: Responding to the challenge of DSM-5* (rev. ed.). Guilford Press.
Frances, A., Clarkin, J., & Perry, S. (1984). *Differential therapeutics in psychiatry: The art and science of treatment selection*. Brunner/Mazel.
Freeman, A., Pretzer, J., Fleming, B., & Simon, K. (1990). *Clinical application of cognitive therapy*. Plenum.
Freud, S. (1914/1976). On narcissism: An introduction. *Complete psychological works, standard edition, Vol. 14* (pp. 69–102). Hogarth Press.
Friedel, R. O., Schmahl, C., & Distel, M. (2018). The neurobiological basis of borderline personality disorder. In C. Schmahl, K. L. Phan, R. O. Friedel (Eds). *Neurobiology of personality disorders* (pp. 279–317). Oxford University Press.
Gabbard, G. (1989). On "doing nothing" in the psychoanalytic treatment of the refractory borderline patient. *International Journal of Psychoanalysis, 70*, 527–534.

Gabbard, G. (1990). *Psychodynamic psychiatry in clinical practice*. American Psychiatric Press.
Gabbard, G. (1994). *Psychodynamic psychiatry in clinical practice: The DSM-IV edition*. American Psychiatric Press.
Gabbard, G. (2000). *Psychodynamic psychiatry in clinical practice* (3rd ed.). American Psychiatric Press.
Gabbard, G. (2014). *Psychodynamic psychiatry in clinical practice* (5th ed.). American Psychiatric Press.
Gamache, D. & Diguer, L. (2012). The film enthusiast: Reflections on the treatment of schizoid personality disorder. *Mental Health in Quebec, 37*, 135–155.
Gilbert, S. & Gordon, K. (2012). Interpersonal psychotherapy informed treatment for avoidant personality disorder with subsequent depression. *Clinical Case Studies, 12*, 111–127.
Gilles, G. & Wienclaw, R. (2008). Schizoid personality disorder. In L. Fundukian & J. Wilson (Eds), *The Gale encyclopedia of mental health* (2nd ed., pp. 990–993). The Gale Group.
Glantz, K. & Goisman, R. (1990). Relaxation and merging in the treatment of personality disorders. *American Journal of Psychotherapy, 44*, 405–413.
Glueck, S. & Glueck, E. (1950). *Unraveling juvenile delinquency*. Harvard University Press.
Goldberg, A. (1973). Psychotherapy of narcissistic injuries. *Archives of General Psychiatry, 28*, 722–726.
Goldberg, A. (1989). Self psychology and the narcissistic personality disorders. *Psychiatric Clinics of North America, 12*, 731–739.
Gomez, R., Watson, S., & Stavropoulos, V. (2020). Personality inventory for DSM–5, Brief Form: Factor structure, reliability, and coefficient of congruence. *Personality Disorders: Theory, Research, and Treatment, 11*(1), 69–74.
Graham, J. (2012). *MMPI-2: Assessing personality and psychopathology* (5th ed.). Oxford University Press.
Graybar, S. & Boutilier, L. (2002). Nontraumatic pathways to borderline personality disorder. *Psychotherapy: Theory/Research/Practice/Training, 39*(2), 152–162.
Greist, J. & Jefferson, J. (1992). *Panic disorder and agoraphobia: A guide*. Anxiety Disorders Center and Information Centers.
Groth-Marnat, G. (2009). *Handbook of Psychological Assessment* (5th ed.). Wiley.
Grotjahn, M. (1984). The narcissistic person in analytic group psychotherapy. *International Journal of Group Psychotherapy, 30*, 299–318.
Guerney, B. (1977). *Relationship enhancement: Skill-training programs for therapy, problem prevention, and enrichment*. Jossey-Bass.
Guidano, V. & Liotti, G. (1983). *Cognitive processes and emotional disorders*. Guilford Press.
Gunderson, J. (1986). Pharmacotherapy for patients with borderline personality disorders. *Archives of General Psychiatry, 43*, 698–700.
Gunderson, J. (1988). Personality disorders. In A. Nicholi (Ed.), *The new Harvard guide to psychiatry* (pp. 337–357). Harvard University Press.
Gunderson, J. (1989). Borderline personality disorder. In T. Karasu (Ed.), *Treatments of Psychiatric Disorders* (pp. 2749–2758). American Psychiatric Press.
Gunderson, J. (1996). Introduction to section IV: Personality disorders. In T. Widiger, A. Frances, H. Pincus, R. Ross, M. First, W. Davis, et al. (Eds), *DSM IV Sourcebook* (pp. 647–664). American Psychiatric Association.
Gurman, A. & Kniskern, D. (1981). Family therapy outcomes research: Known and unknown. In A. Gorman & D. Kniskern (Eds), *Handbook of family therapy* (pp 742–776). Brunner/Mazel.
Haley, J. (1978). *Problem solving therapy*. Jossey-Bass.
Haley, J. & Hoffman, L. (1976). *Techniques of family therapy*. Basic Books.
Halleck, S. (1978). *The treatment of emotional disorders*. Jason Aronson.
Harbir, H. (1981). Family therapy with personality disorders. In J. Lion (Ed.), *Personality disorders: Diagnosis and management* (2nd ed.). Williams & Wilkins.
Hare, R., Neumann, C., & Widiger, T. (2012). Psychopathy. In T. Widiger (Ed.), *The Oxford handbook of personality disorders* (pp. 478–504). Oxford University Press.
Harman, M. & Waldo, M. (2001). Family treatment of borderline personality disorder through relationship enhancement therapy. In M. MacFarlane (Ed.), *Family therapy and mental health: Innovations in theory and practice* (pp. 215–235). Haworth Clinical Practice Press.

Harper, R. (2004). *Personality-guided therapy in behavioral medicine.* American Psychological Association.
Harris, G. & Rice, M. (2006). Treatment of psychopathy: A review of empirical findings. In C. Patrick (Ed.), *Handbook of psychopathy* (pp. 555–572), Guilford Press.
Harwood, I. (1992). Advances in group psychotherapy and self-psychology: An interobjective approach with narcissistic and borderline patients. *Group, 16,* 220–232.
Hatchett, G. (2015). Treatment guidelines for clients with antisocial personality disorder. *Journal of Mental Health Counseling, 37*(1), 15–27.
Havens, J., Cornelius, L., Ricketts, E., Latkin, C., Bishai, D., Lloyd, J., et al. (2007). The effect of a case management intervention on drug treatment entry among treatment-seeking injection drug users with and without comorbid antisocial personality disorder. *Journal of Urban Health, 84*(2), 267–271.
Havens, L. (1976). Discussion: How long the Tower of Babel? *Proceedings of American Psychopathological Association, 64,* 62–73.
Hayes, S., Follette, V. & Linehan, M. (Eds). (2004). *Mindfulness and acceptance: Expanding the cognitive-behavioral tradition.* Guilford Press.
Hazan, C. & Shaver, P. (1987). Romantic love conceptualized as a attachment process. *Journal of Personality and Social Psychology, 52,* 511–524.
Hend, S., Baker, J., & Williamson, D. (1991). Family environment characteristics and dependent personality disorder. *Journal of Personality Disorders, 5,* 256–263.
Herpertz, S. C. & Bertsch, K. (2022). Neuroscience and personality disorders. In S. K. Huprich (Ed.), *Personality disorders and pathology: Integrating clinical assessment and practice in the DSM-5 and ICD-11 era* (pp. 323–349). American Psychological Association. https://doi.org/10.1037/0000310-015.
Herpertz, S. C., Schneider, I., Renneberg, B., & Schneider, A. (2022). Patients with personality disorders in everyday clinical practice: Implications of the ICD-11. *Deutsches Ärzteblatt International, 119*(1-2), 1–7.
Hill, D. (1970). Outpatient management of passive dependent women. *Hospital and Community Psychiatry, 21,* 402–405.
Hoch, J., O'Reilly, R., & Carscadden, J. (2006). Relationship management therapy for patients with borderline personality disorder. *Psychiatric Services 57*(2), 179–181.
Hopwood, C. J. (2018). A framework for treating DSM-5 alternative model for personality disorder features. *Personality and Mental Health, 12*(2), 107–125.
Hopwood, C. J., Kaurin, A., & Pincus, A. L. (2024). Call for papers: Revitalizing the future of personality disorders science and practice: A call for innovation. www.apa.org/pubs/journals/abn/revitalizing-future-personality-disorders.
Hopwood, C. J., Mulay, A. L., & Waugh, M. H. (Eds). (2019). *The DSM-5 Alternative Model for Personality Disorders: Integrating multiple paradigms of personality assessment.* Routledge.
Hopwood, C. & Thomas, K. (2012). Paranoid and Schizoid Personality Disorders. In T. Widiger (Ed.), *The Oxford handbook of personality disorders* (pp. 582–602). Oxford University Press.
Horowitz, L. (1977). Group psychotherapy of the borderline. In P. Hartocollis (Ed.), *Borderline personality disorder* (pp. 399–422). International Universities Press.
Horowitz, L. (1980). Group psychotherapy for borderline and narcissistic patients. *Bulletin of the Menninger Clinic, 4,* 181–200.
Horowitz, L. (1987). Indications for group psychotherapy with borderline and narcissistic patients. *Bulletin of the Menninger Clinic, 51,* 248–318.
Horowitz, L. (1997). Psychotherapy of histrionic personality disorder. *Journal of Psychotherapy Practice and Research, 6*(2), 93–107.
Horowitz, M. (1988). *Introduction to psychodynamics: A new synthesis.* Basic Books.
Horowitz, M. & Lerner, U. (2010). Treatment of Histrionic Personality Disorder. In J. F. Clarkin, P. Fonagy, & G. O. Gabbard (Eds), *Psychodynamic psychotherapy for personality disorders: A clinical handbook* (pp. 289–309). American Psychiatric Publishing, Inc.
Horowitz, M., Marmar, C., Krupnick, J., Wilner, N., Kaltreider, N., & Wallerstein, R. (1984). *Personality styles and brief psychotherapy.* Basic Books.
Hulse, W. (1958). Psychotherapy with ambulatory schizophrenic patients in mixed analytic groups. *Archives of Neurology and Psychiatry, 79,* 681–687.

Huprich, S. K. (2022a). Introduction: The changing landscape of personality disorders. In S. K. Huprich (Ed.), *Personality disorders and pathology: Integrating clinical assessment and practice in the DSM-5 and ICD-11 era* (pp. 3–6). American Psychological Association. https://doi.org/10.1037/0000310-001.

Huprich, S. K. (2022b). Principles of treating personality pathology. In S. K. Huprich (Ed.), *Personality disorders and pathology: Integrating clinical assessment and practice in the DSM-5 and ICD-11 era* (pp. 135–158). American Psychological Association. https://doi.org/10.1037/0000310-007.

Imbesi, E. (2000). On the etiology of narcissistic personality disorder. *Issues in Psychoanalytic Psychology*, 22(2), 3–58.

Jenike, M., Baer, L., & Minichiello, W. (1998). *Obsessive-compulsive disorders: Theory and management* (3rd ed.). St. Louis, MO: Mosby.

Jones, S. (1987). Family therapy with borderline and narcissistic patients. *Bulletin of the Menninger Foundation*, 51, 285–295.

Kabat-Zinn, J., Massion, A., Kristeller, J., Peterson, L., Fletcher, K., Ebert, L., et al. (1992). Effectiveness of a meditation-based stress reduction intervention in the treatment of anxiety disorders. *American Journal of Psychiatry*, 149, 936–943.

Kagan, J., Resnick, J., & Snidman, N. (1988). Biological basis of childhood shyness. *Science*, 240, 167–171.

Kalojera, I., Jacobson, G., Hoffman, G., Hoffman, P., Raffe, I., White, H., & Leonard-White, L. (1998). The narcissistic couple. In J. Carlson & L. Sperry (Eds), *The disordered couple* (pp. 207–238). Brunner/Mazel.

Kantor, M. (1992). *Diagnosis and Treatment of the Personality Disorders*. Ishiyaku EuroAmerica.

Kavaler-Adler, S. (2004). Anatomy of regret: A developmental view of the depressive position and a critical turn toward love and creativity in the transforming schizoid personality. *American Journal of Psychoanalysis*, 64(1), 39–76.

Keller, M., McCullough, J., Klein, D., Arnow, B., et al. (2000). A comparison of nefazodone, the cognitive behavioral analysis system or psychotherapy, and their combination for the treatment of chronic depression. *New England Journal of Medicine*, 342, 1462–1470.

Kellerman, H. & Burry, A. (1989). *Psychopathology and differential diagnosis: Vol. 2, Diagnostic primer*. Columbia University Press.

Kellett, S. (2007). A time series evaluation of the treatment of histrionic personality disorder with cognitive analytic therapy. *Psychology and Psychotherapy: Theory, Research and Practice*, 80(3), 389–405.

Kellett, S. & Hardy, G. (2014). Treatment of Paranoid Personality Disorder with cognitive analytic therapy: A mixed methods single case experimental design. *Clinical Psychology & Psychotherapy*, 21(5), 452–464.

Kellner, R. (1986). Personality disorders. *Psychotherapy and Psychosomatics*, 46(1–2), 58–66.

Kernberg, O. (1975). *Borderline conditions and pathological narcissism*. Jason Aronson.

Kernberg, O. (1984). *Severe personality disorders: Psychotherapeutic strategies*. Yale University Press.

Kernberg, O. (2010). Narcissistic personality disorder. In J. Clarkin, P. Fonagy, & G. Gabbard (Eds), *Psychodynamic psychotherapy for personality disorders: A clinical handbook* (pp. 289–309). American Psychiatric Publishing.

Khan, M. (1975). Grudge and the hysteric. *International Journal of Psychoanalysis and Psychotherapy*, 4, 349–357.

Klein, P., Fairweather, A. K., & Lawn, S. (2022). The impact of educational interventions on modifying health practitioners' attitudes and practice in treating people with borderline personality disorder: an integrative review. *Systematic Reviews*, 11(1), 108, 1–19.

Klein, R. (1989a). Diagnosis and treatment of the lower-level borderline patient. In J. Masterson & R. Klein (Eds), *Psychotherapy of disorders of the self* (pp. 147–168). Brunner/Mazel.

Klein, R. (1989b). Shorter-term psychotherapy of the personality disorders In J. Masterson & R. Klein (Eds), *Psychotherapy of disorders of the self* (pp. 90–109). Brunner/Mazel.

Koenigsberg, H. (1993). Combining psychotherapy and pharmacotherapy in the treatment of borderline patients. In J. Oldham, M. Riba, & A. Tasman. (Eds), *American Psychiatric Press Review of Psychiatry, Vol. 12* (pp. 541–564). American Psychiatric Press.

Koenigsberg, H., Woo-Ming, A., & Siever, L. (2002). Pharmacological treatment for personality disorders. In P. Nathan & J. Gorman (Eds), *A guide to treatments that work* (2nd ed., pp. 625–641). Oxford University Press.

Kohut, H. (1971). *The analysis of the self*. International Universities Press.
Kohut, H. (1977). *The restoration of the self*. International Universities Press.
Kristeller, J. & Hallet, B. (1999). An exploratory study of meditation-based intervention for binge eating disorder. *Journal of Health Psychology, 4*(3), 357–363.
Krueger, R. (2019). Criterion B of the AMPD and the interpersonal, multivariate, and empirical paradigms of personality assessment. In C. J. Hopwood, A. L. Mulay, & M. H. Waugh. *The DSM-5 Alternative Model for Personality Disorders: Integrating multiple paradigms of personality assessment* (pp. 60–76). Routledge.
Kvarstein, E. H., Frøyhaug, M., Pettersen, M. S., Carlsen, S., Ekberg, A., Fjermestad-Noll, J., ... & Pedersen, G. A. (2023). Improvement of personality functioning among people treated within personality disorder mental health services. A longitudinal, observational study. *Frontiers in Psychiatry, 14*, 1163347, 1–17.
Kwapil, T. & Barrantes-Vidal, N. (2012). Schizotypal personality disorder: An integrative review. In T. Widiger (Ed.), *The Oxford handbook of personality disorders* (pp. 437–477). Oxford University Press.
Kyrios, M. (1999). A cognitive-behavioral approach to the understanding and of obsessive-compulsive personality disorder. In C. Perris & P. McGorry (Eds), *Cognitive psychotherapy of psychotic and personality disorders* (pp. 351–378). Wiley.
Lachar, D. (1974). *The MMPI: Clinical assessment and automated interpretation*. Western Psychological Services.
Lachkar, J. (1986). Narcissistic/borderline couples: Implications for medication. *Conciliation Courts Review, 24*, 31–38.
Lachkar, J. (1992). *The narcissistic/borderline couple: A psychoanalytic perspective on marital treatment*. Brunner/Mazel.
Lachkar, J. (1999). Narcissistic/borderline couples: A psychodynamic approach to conjoint treatment. In J. Carlson & L. Sperry (Eds), *The disordered couple* (pp. 259–284). Brunner/Mazel.
Landucci, J., & Foley, G. (2014). Couples therapy: Treating selected personality-disordered couples within a dynamic therapy framework. *Innovations in Clinical Neuroscience, 11*(3–4), 29–36.
Lasch, C. (1991). *The culture of narcissism*. Norton.
Lazarus, A. (1981). *The practice of multimodal therapy*. McGraw-Hill.
Lazarus, A. (Ed.). (1985). *Casebook of multimodal therapy*. Guilford Press.
Lazarus, L. (1982). Brief psychotherapy of narcissistic disturbances. *Psychotherapy: Theory, Research and Practice, 19*, 228–236.
Leszcz, M. (1989). Group psychotherapy of the characterologically difficult patient. *International Journal of Group Psychotherapy, 39*, 311–335.
Levy, K. (2012). Subtypes, dimensions, levels, and mental states in narcissism and narcissistic personality disorder. *Journal of Clinical Psychology, 68*, 886–897.
Levy, K. N., Ehrenthal, J. C., & Martin, J. A. (2022). Borderline personality disorder. In S. K. Huprich (Ed.), *Personality disorders and pathology: Integrating clinical assessment and practice in the DSM-5 and ICD-11 era* (pp. 353–373). American Psychological Association. https://doi.org/10.1037/0000310-016.
Levy, K. N., Yeomans, F. E., & Spina, D. S. (2022). Transference-focused psychotherapy. In S. K. Huprich (Ed.), *Personality disorders and pathology: Integrating clinical assessment and practice in the DSM-5 and ICD-11 era* (pp. 211–235). American Psychological Association. https://doi.org/10.1037/0000310-010.
Liberman, R. P., DeRisi, W. J., & Mueser, K. T. (1989). *Social skills training for psychiatric patients*. Pergamon Press.
Liebowitz, M. & Klein, D. (1981). Interrelationship of hysteroid dysphoria and borderline personality disorder. *Psychiatric Clinics of North America, 4*, 67–87.
Liebowitz, M., Stone, M., & Turkat, I. (1986). Treatment of personality disorders. In A. Frances & R. Hales (Eds), *Psychiatric Update, American Psychiatric Association, Annual Review, Vol. 5* (pp. 356–393). American Psychiatric Press.
Linehan, M. (1983). *Dialectical behavior therapy for treatment of parasuicidal women: Treatment manual*. University of Washington.
Linehan, M. (1987). Dialectical behavior therapy: A cognitive behavioral approach to parasuicide. *Journal of Personality Disorders, 1*, 328–333.
Linehan, M. (1993). *Cognitive-behavioral treatment for borderline personality disorder*. Guilford Press.

Linehan, M. (1994). Acceptance and change. The central dialectic in psychotherapy. In S. Hayes, N. Jacobson, V. Follette, & M. Dougher (Eds), *Acceptance and change: Content and context in psychotherapy* (pp. 73–86). Context Press.

Linehan, M. (2015). *DBT skills training manual* (2nd ed.). Guilford Press.

Linehan, M., Armstrong, H., Suarez, A., Allmon, D., & Heard, H. (1991). Cognitive-behavioral treatment of chronically parasuicidal borderline patients. *Archives of General Psychiatry*, 48(12), 1060–1064.

Linehan, M., Heard, H., & Armstrong, H. (1993). Naturalistic follow-up of a behavioral treatment for chronically parasuicidal borderline patients. *Archives of General Psychiatry* 50(12), 971–974.

Links, P., Stockwell, M., & MacFarlane, M. (2004a). Indications for couple therapy: The paradox of the histrionic/obsessive-compulsive couple. *Journal of Family Psychotherapy*, 15(4), 73–88.

Links, P., Stockwell, M., & MacFarlane, M. (2004b). Is couples therapy indicated for patients with dependent personality disorder? *Journal of Family Psychotherapy*, 15(3), 63–79.

Livesley, W. J. (2012). Integrated treatment: a conceptual framework for an evidence-based approach to the treatment of personality disorder. *Journal of Personality Disorders*, 26(1), 17–42.

Luborsky, L. & Crits-Christoph, P. (1990). *Understanding transference: The Core Conflictual Relationship Theme method*. Basic Books.

Lyddon, W. & Sherry, A. (2001). Developmental personality styles: An attachment theory conceptualization of personality disorders. *Journal of Counseling and Development*, 79(4), 405–414.

Lynch T. & Cuper, P. (2012). Dialectical behavior therapy of borderline and other personality disorders. In T. Widiger (Ed.), *The Oxford handbook of personality disorders* (pp. 785–793). Oxford University Press.

Lynch, T., Trost, W., Salsman, N., & Linehan, M. (2007). Dialectical behavior therapy for borderline personality disorders. *Annual Review of Clinical Psychology*, 3, 181–205.

Mackinnon, R. & Michels, R. (1971). *The psychiatric interview in clinical practice*. Saunders.

MacNamara, A., Phan, K. L., Schmahl, C., & Friedel, R. O. (2018). Neurocircuitry of affective, cognitive, and regulatory systems. In C. Schmahl, K. L. Phan & R. O. Friedel (Eds). *Neurobiology of personality disorders.* (pp. 3–38). Oxford University Press.

Main, M., Goldwyn, R., & Hesse, E. (1998). Adult attachment scoring and classification system. Unpublished manuscript, University of California at Berkeley.

Main, M. & Solomon, J. (1990). Procedures for identifying infants as disorganized/disoriented during the Ainsworth Strange Situation. In M. T. Greenberg, D. Cicchetti, & E. M. Cummings (Eds), *Attachment in the Preschool Years* (pp. 121–160). University of Chicago Press.

Malan, D. (1976). *The frontier of brief psychotherapy*. Plenum.

Malancharuvil, J. (2012). Empathy deficit in antisocial personality disorder: A psychodynamic formulation. *American Journal of Psychoanalysis*, 72(3), 242–250.

Malinow, K. (1981). Dependent personality. In J. Lion (Ed.), *Personality disorders: Diagnosis and management* (2nd ed., pp. 79–91). Williams & Wilkins.

Manduchi, K., & Schoendorff, B. (2012). First steps in FAP: Experiences of beginning Functional Analytic Psychotherapy therapist with an obsessive-compulsive personality disorder client. *International Journal of Behavioral Consultation and Therapy*, 7(2–3), 72.

Mann, J. (1973). *Time-limited psychotherapy*. Harvard University Press.

Mann, J. (1984). Time-limited psychotherapy. In L. Grinspoon (Ed.), *Psychiatry Update, Vol. 3*. American Psychiatric Association.

Marin, L. K., Foster, C., & Goodman, M. (2022). Pharmacotherapy for personality disorders. In S. K. Huprich (Ed.), *Personality disorders and pathology: Integrating clinical assessment and practice in the DSM-5 and ICD-11 era* (pp. 305–321). American Psychological Association. https://doi.org/10.1037/0000310-014.

Mark, D., Roy, S., Walsh, H., & Neumann, C. S. (2022). Antisocial personality disorder. In S. K. Huprich (Ed.), *Personality disorders and pathology: Integrating clinical assessment and practice in the DSM-5 and ICD-11 era* (pp. 391–411). American Psychological Association. https://doi.org/10.1037/0000310-018.

Markowitz, J., Bleiberg, K., Pessin, H., & Skodol, A. (2007). Adapting interpersonal psychotherapy for borderline personality disorder. *Journal of Mental Health*, 16, 103–116.

Marlatt, G. (1994). Addiction, mindfulness and acceptance. In S. Hayes, N. Jacobson, V. Follette, & M. Dougher (Eds), *Acceptance and change: Content and context in psychotherapy* (pp. 175–197). Context Press.

Marlatt. G. & Kristeller, J. (1999). Mindfulness and meditation. In. W. Miller (Ed.), *Integrating spirituality into treatment: Resources for practitioners* (pp. 67–84). American Psychological Association.

Marmar, C. & Freeman, M. (1988). Brief dynamic psychotherapy of post-traumatic stress disorders: Management of narcissistic regression. *Journal of Traumatic Stress*, 1, 323–337.

Marra, T. (2005). *Dialectic behavior therapy in private practice: A practical and comprehensive guide*. New Harbinger Publications.

Martin, J. (1997). Mindfulness: A proposed common factor. *Journal of Psychotherapy Integration*, 7, 291–312.

Masterson, J. (1976). *Psychotherapy of the borderline adult: A developmental approach*. Brunner/Mazel.

Masterson, J. (1981). *The narcissistic and borderline disorders*. Brunner/Mazel.

Masterson, J. & Klein, R. (Eds) (1989). *Psychotherapy of the disorders of the self*. Brunner/Mazel.

McCormack, C. (1989). The borderline/schizoid marriage: The holding environment as an essential treatment construct. *Journal of Marital and Family Therapy*, 15, 299–309.

McCommon, B., Sowislo, J. F., & Caligor, E. (2022). Higher level personality disorders. In S. K. Huprich (Ed.), *Personality disorders and pathology: Integrating clinical assessment and practice in the DSM-5 and ICD-11 era* (pp. 413–434). American Psychological Association. https://doi.org/10.1037/0000310-019.

McCullough, J. (2000). *Treatment for chronic depression: Cognitive behavioral analysis system of psychotherapy*. Guilford Press.

McCullough, J. (2002). What kind of questions are we trying to answer with our psychotherapy research? *Clinical Psychology: Science and Practice*, 9, 447–452.

McCullough, J., Schramm, E., & Penberthy, J. (2015). *CBASP as a distinctive treatment for persistent depressive disorder: Distinctive features*. Routledge.

McGauley, G., Yakeley, J., Williams, A., & Bateman, A. (2011). Attachment, mentalization, and antisocial personality disorder: The possible contribution of mentalization-based treatment. *European Journal of Psychotherapy & Counselling*, 13(4), 371–393.

McMain, S., Boritz, T., & Leybman, M. (2015). Common strategies for cultivating a positive therapy relationship in the treatment of borderline personality disorder. *Journal of Psychotherapy Integration*, 25(1), 20–29.

McMain, S., Links, P., Gnam, W., Guimond, T., Cardish, R., Korman, L., & Streiner, D. (2009). A randomized trial of dialectical behavior therapy versus general psychiatric management for borderline personality disorder. *American Journal of Psychiatry*, 166(12), 1365–1374.

Meares, R., Stevenson, J., & Comerford, A. (1999). Psychotherapy with borderline personality patients: A comparison between treated and untreated cohorts. *Australian & New Zealand Journal of Psychiatry*, 33, 467–472.

Megargee, E. & Bohn, M. (1979). *Classifying criminal offenders*. Sage.

Mehlum, L., Fris, S., Irion, T., Johns, S., Karterud, S., Vaglum, P., et al. (1991). Personality disorders 2–5 years after treatment: A prospective follow-up study. *Acta Psychiatrica Scandinavia*, 84, 72–77.

Meichenbaum, D. (1977). *Cognitive-behavioral modification: An integrated approach*. Plenum.

Meissner, W. (1978). *The paranoid process*. Jason Aronson.

Meissner, W. (1986). *Psychotherapy and the paranoid process*. Jason Aronson.

Meissner, W. (1989). Paranoid personality disorder. In T. Karasu (Ed.), *Treatments of psychiatric disorders* (pp. 2705–2711). American Psychiatric Press.

Meloy, J. (1988). *The psychopathic mind: Origins, dynamics, and treatment*. Jason Aronson.

Meloy, J. & Yakeley, J. (2010). Psychodynamic treatment of antisocial personality disorder. In J. Clarkin, P., Fonagy, & G. Gabbard (Eds), *Psychodynamic psychotherapy for personality disorders: A clinical handbook* (pp. 289–309). American Psychiatric Publishing.

Messina, N., Farabee, D., & Rawson, R. (2003). Treatment responsivity to cocaine-dependent patients with antisocial personality disorder to cognitive-behavioral and contingency management interventions. *Journal of Consulting and Clinical Psychology*, 71(2), 320–329.

Messina, N., Wish, E., Hoffman, J., & Nemes, S. (2002). Antisocial personality disorder and TC treatment outcomes. *American Journal of Drug and Alcohol Abuse*, 28(2), 197–212.

Meyer, R. (1995). *The clinician's handbook: Integrated diagnostics, assessment, and intervention in adult and adolescent psychotherapy* (4th ed.). Allyn & Bacon.

Mihura, J. L. & Meyer, G. J. (2018). Principles of R-PAS interpretation. In G. J. Meyer (ed.). *Using the Rorschach Performance Assessment System (R-PAS)* (pp. 23–45). Guilford Press.

Miller, W. & Rollnick, S. (2013). *Motivational Interviewing: Helping People Change* (3rd ed.). Guilford Press.
Millon, T. (1981). *Disorders of personality: DSM-III Axis II*. Wiley.
Millon, T. (1990). *Toward a new personology: An evolutionary model*. Wiley.
Millon, T. & Davis, R. (1996). *Disorders of personality: DSM-IV and Beyond* (2nd ed.). Wiley.
Millon, T. & Davis, R. (2000). *Personality disorders in modern life*. John Wiley & Sons.
Millon, T. & Everly, G. (1985). *Personality and its disorders: A biosocial learning approach*. Wiley.
Millon, T., Millon, C., Grossman, S., Boice, A., & Sinsabaugh, K. (2015). *MCMI-IV manual*. Pearson.
Minuchin, S. (1974). *Families and family therapy*. Harvard University Press.
Minuchin, S. & Montalvo, B. (1967). Techniques for working with disorganized low socioeconomic families. *American Journal of Orthopsychiatry, 37*(5), 880.
Mitchell, D., Tafrate, R., & Freeman, A. (2015). Antisocial personality disorder. In A. Beck, D. Davis, & A. Freeman, A. (Eds), *Cognitive therapy of personality disorders* (3rd ed., pp. 346–365). Guilford Press.
Möhler, E. (2022). Personality disorders and development. *Brain Sciences, 12*(8), 983, 1–4.
Montgomery, J. (1971). Treatment management of passive-dependent behavior. *International Journal of Social Psychiatry, 17*, 311–319.
Morey, L., Skodol, A., & Oldham J. (2014). Clinician judgments of clinical utility: A comparison of DSM-IV-TR personality disorders and the alternative model for DSM-5 personality disorders. *Journal of Abnormal Psychology, 123*, 398–405.
Mulder, R. (2012). Cultural aspects of personality disorders. In T. Widiger (Ed.), *The Oxford handbook of personality disorders* (pp. 260–274). Oxford University Press.
Mulder, R. & Bach, B. (2022). Assessment and treatment of personality disorders within the *ICD-11* framework. In S. K. Huprich (Ed.), *Personality disorders and pathology: Integrating clinical assessment and practice in the DSM-5 and ICD-11 era* (pp. 183–208). American Psychological Association. https://doi.org/10.1037/0000310-009.
Nachmani, G. (1984). Hesitation, perplexity, and annoyance at opportunity. *Contemporary Psychoanalysis, 20*, 448–457.
Nathanson, B. & Jamison, S. (2011). Psychotherapeutic and pharmacologic treatment of schizotypal personality disorder: The heuristic utility of stressing function over form. *Clinical Case Studies, 10*(5), 395–407.
Nehls, N. (1991). Borderline personality disorder and group therapy. *Archives of Psychiatric Nursing, 5*, 137–146.
Nehls, N. & Diamond, R. (1993). Developing a systems approach to caring for persons with borderline personality disorder. *Community Mental Health Journal, 29*, 161–172.
Nelson, S. M., Cawood, C. D., Suzuki, T., Chapman, E., & Lusk, R. (2022). Dialectical behavior psychotherapy. In S. K. Huprich (Ed.), *Personality disorders and pathology: Integrating clinical assessment and practice in the DSM-5 and ICD-11 era* (pp. 259–280). American Psychological Association. https://doi.org/10.1037/0000310-012.
Nelson, K. J. & Tsheringld, S. (2021). Pharmacological management. In A. E. Skodol & J. M. Oldham (Eds), *American Psychiatric Association Publishing textbook of personality disorders*, Third edition (pp. 465–492). American Psychiatric Publishing.
Nichols, W. (1996). Persons with antisocial and histrionic personality disorders in relationships. In F. Kaslow (Ed.), *Handbook of relational diagnosis and dysfunctional family patterns* (pp. 287–299). Wiley.
Nurse, A. (1998). The dependent/narcissistic couple. In J. Carlson & L. Sperry (Eds), *The disordered couple* (pp. 315–332). Brunner/Mazel.
O'Donohue, W., Fowler, K., & Lilienfeld, S. (2007). *Personality Disorders: Toward the DSM-V*. Sage.
O'Leary, K., Turner, E., Gardner, D., & Cowdry, R. (1991). Homogeneous group therapy or borderline personality disorder. *Group, 15*, 56–64.
Oldham, J. & Skodol, A. (2000). Charting the future of Axis II. *Journal of Personality Disorders, 14*, 17–29.
Ogloff, J., Talevski, D., Lemphers, A., Wood, M., & Simmons, M. (2015). Co-occurring mental illness, substance use disorders, and antisocial personality disorder among clients of forensic mental health services. *Psychiatric Rehabilitation Journal, 1*, 16–23.

Ogrodniczuk, J. S., Uliaszek, A. Lebow, J., & Kealy, D. (2021). Group, family, and couples therapies. In A. E. Skodol & J. M. Oldham (Eds). *American Psychiatric Association Publishing textbook of personality disorders, Third edition.* (pp. 439–464). American Psychiatric Publishing.

Osterbaan, D., van Balkom, A., Spinhoven, P., de Meij, T., & van Dyck, R. (2002). The influence of treatment gain on comorbid avoidant personality disorder in patients with social phobia. *Journal of Nervous and Mental Disease, 190*(1), 41–43.

Othmer, E. & Othmer, S. (2002). *The clinical interview using DSM-IV, Vol. 1, Fundamentals.* American Psychiatric Press.

Padesky, C. & Beck, J. (2015). Avoidant personality disorder. In A. Beck, D. Davis, & A. Freeman, A. (Eds), *Cognitive therapy of personality disorders* (3rd ed., pp. 174–202). Guilford Press.

Parsons, B. & Alexander, J. (1973). Short-term family interventions: A therapy outcome study. *Journal of Abnormal Psychology, 8,* 219–225.

PDM Task Force (2006). *Psychodynamic diagnostic manual (PDM).* Alliance of Psychoanalytic Organizations.

Perry, J., Francis, A., & Clarkin, J. (1990). *A DSM-III-R casebook of treatment selection.* Brunner/Mazel.

Perry, J. C., Presniak, M., & Olson, T. (2013). Mechanisms in schizotypal, borderlines, antisocial, and narcissistic personality disorders. *Psychiatry, 76*(1), 32–52.

Phillips, K. & Stein, D. (Eds). (2015). *Handbook on obsessive-compulsive and related disorders.* American Psychiatric Publishing.

Pies, R. (1992). The psychopharmacology of personality disorders. *Psychiatric Times,* February, 23–24.

Pincus, A., Wright, A., & Cain, N. (2014). Narcissistic grandiosity and narcissistic vulnerability in psychotherapy. *Personality Disorders: Theory, Research, and Treatment, 5*(4), 439–443.

Pines, M. (1975). Group psychotherapy with difficult patients. In L. Wolberg & M. Aronson (Eds), *Group therapy 1975: An overview.* Stratton Intercontinental Medical Books.

Porcerelli, J., Dauphin, V., Ablon, J., Leitman, S., & Bambery, M. (2007). Psychoanalysis with avoidant personality disorder: A systemic case study. *Psychotherapy: Theory, Research, Practice, Training, 44*(1), 1–13.

Pretzer, J. (1988). Paranoid personality disorder: A cognitive view. *International Cognitive Therapy Newsletter, 4*(4), 10–12.

Pucker, H. E., Temes, C. M., & Zanarini, M. C. (2019). Description and prediction of social isolation in borderline patients over 20 years of prospective follow-up. *Personality Disorders: Theory, Research, and Treatment, 10*(4), 383–388. https://doi.org/10.1037/per0000337.

Quality Assurance Project (1991). Treatment outlines for borderline, narcissistic and histrionic personality disorders. *Australian & New Zealand Journal of Psychiatry, 25,* 392–403.

Regier, D., Boyd, J., Burke, J., Rae, D., Myers, J., Kramer, M., et al. (1988). One-month prevalence in mental disorders in the United States. *Archives of General Psychiatry, 45,* 977–986.

Reich, J. (2002). Drug treatment of personality disorder traits. *Psychiatric Annals, 32*(10), 590–600.

Reich, J. (2005). State and trait in personality disorders. In J. Reich (Ed.), *Personality Disorders: Current Research and Treatments* (pp. 3–20). Routledge.

Reid, W. (1989). *The treatment of psychiatric disorders. Revised for the DSM-III-R.* Brunner/Mazel.

Rennenberg, B., Goldstein, A., Phillips, D., & Chambliss, D. (1990). Intensive behavioral group treatment of avoidant personality disorder. *Behavior Therapy, 21,* 363–377.

Renton, J. & Mankiewicz, P. (2015). Paranoid, schizotypal, and schizoid personality disorders. In A. Beck, D. Davis, & A. Freeman, A. (Eds), *Cognitive therapy of personality disorders* (3rd ed., pp. 244–275). Guilford Press.

Rentrop, M., Zilker, T., Lederle, A., Birkhofer, A., & Horz, S. (2014). Psychiatric comorbidity and personality structure in patients with polyvalent addiction. *Psychopathology, 47*(2), 133–140.

Rinsley, D. (1982). *Borderline and other self disorders.* Jason Aronson.

Roche, M., Pincus, A. Lukowitsky, R., Ménard, K., & Conroy, D. (2013). An integrative approach to the assessment of narcissism. *Journal of Personality Assessment, 9*(3), 237–248.

Rodriguez-Seijas, C., Ruggero, C., Eaton, N. R., & Krueger, R. F. (2019). The DSM-5 alternative model for personality disorders and clinical treatment: A review. *Current Treatment Options in Psychiatry, 6,* 284–298.

Roemer, L. & Orsillo, S. (2002). Expanding our conceptualization of and treatment for generalized anxiety disorder: Integrating mindfulness/acceptance-based approaches with existing cognitive-behavioral models. *Clinical Psychology: Science and Practice. 9*(1), 54–68.

Ronningstam, E. (2011). Narcissistic personality disorder: A clinical perspective. *Journal of Psychiatric Practice, 17*, 89–99.

Ronningstam, E. (2012). Narcissistic personality disorder: The diagnostic process. In T. Widiger (Ed.), *The Oxford handbook of personality disorders* (pp. 527–548). Oxford University Press.

Ronningstam, E. (2022). Narcissistic personality disorder. In S. K. Huprich (Ed.), *Personality disorders and pathology: Integrating clinical assessment and practice in the DSM-5 and ICD-11 era* (pp. 375–389). American Psychological Association. https://doi.org/10.1037/0000310-017.

Rosell, D. R. & Siever, L. J. (2018). The neurobiology and genetics of schizotypal personality disorder. In C. Schmahl, K. L. Phan, & R. O. Friedel (Eds), *Neurobiology of personality disorders.* (pp. 301–319). Oxford University Press.

Rutan, J. S., Stone, W., & Shay, J. (2014). *Psychodynamic group psychotherapy* (5th ed.). Guilford Press.

Ryan, A., Macdonald, A., & Walker, E. (2013). Treatment of adolescents with schizotypal personality disorder and related conditions: A practice-oriented review of the literature. *Clinical Psychology: Science and Practice, 20*(4), 408–424.

Ryle, A. (2004). The contribution of cognitive analytic therapy to the treatment of borderline personality disorder. *Journal of Personality Disorders, 18*(1), 3–35.

Sadoff, R. & Collins, D. (1968). Passive dependency in sufferers. *American Journal of Psychiatry, 124*, 1127–1136.

Salkovskis, P. & Kirk, J. (1989). Obsessional disorders. In K. Hawton, P. Salkovskis, J. Kirk, & D. Clark (Eds), *Cognitive behavior therapy for psychiatric problems* (pp. 129–168). Oxford University Press.

Salvatore, G., Russo, B., Russo, M., Popolo, R., & Dimaggio, G. (2012). Metacognition-oriented therapy for psychosis: The case of a woman diagnosed with delusional disorder and paranoid personality disorder. *Journal of Psychotherapy Integration, 22*(4), 314–329.

Salzman, L. (1980). *Treatment of the obsessive personality*. Jason Aronson.

Salzman, L. (1989). Compulsive personality disorder. In T. Karasu (Ed.), *Treatment of psychiatric disorders* (pp. 2771–2782). American Psychiatric Press.

Samuels, J. & Costa, P. (2012). Obsessive-compulsive personality disorder. In T. Widiger (Ed.), *The Oxford handbook of personality disorders* (pp. 566–581). Oxford University Press.

Sanislow, C., da Cruz, K., Gianoli, M., & Reagan, E. (2012). Avoidant Personality Disorder, Traits, and Type. In T. Widiger (Ed.), *The Oxford handbook of personality disorders* (pp. 549–565). Oxford University Press.

Schanche, E., Stiles, T., McCullough, L., Svartberg, M., & Nielsen, G. (2011). The relationship between activating affects, inhibitory affects, and self-compassion in patients with Cluster C personality disorders. *Psychotherapy, 48*, 293–303.

Schane, M. & Kovel, V. (1988). Family therapy in severe borderline personality disorder. *International Journal of Family Psychiatry, 9*, 241–258.

Scheidlinger, S. & Porter, K. (1979). Group therapy combined with individual therapy. In T. B. Karasu and L. Bellak (Eds), *Specialized Techniques in Psychotherapy* (pp. 201–224). Brunner/Mazel.

Scheidlinger, S. & Porter, K. (1980). Group therapy combined with individual psychotherapy. In T. Karasu & L. Bellak (Eds), *Specialized Techniques in Individual Psychotherapy* (pp. 426–440). Brunner/Mazel.

Schwartz, J. & Begley, S. (2002). *The mind and the brain: Neuroplasticity and the power of mental force*. HarperCollins.

Segal, Z., Williams, J., & Teasdale, J. (2002). *Mindfulness-based cognitive therapy of depression*. Guilford Press.

Segal, Z., Williams, J., Teasdale, J., & Williams, M. (2004). Mindfulness-based cognitive therapy: Theoretical and empirical status. In S. Hayes, V. Follette, & M. Linehan (Eds), *Mindfulness and acceptance: Expanding the cognitive-behavioral tradition* (pp. 45–65). Guilford Press.

Shafer, R. (1954). *Psychoanalytic interpretation in Rorschach testing*. Grune and Stratton.

Shapiro, D. (1965). *Neurotic styles*. Basic Books.

Shapiro, E. (1982). The holding environment and family therapy for acting out adolescents. *International Journal of Psychoanalysis, 9*, 209–226.
Sharoff, K. (2002). *Cognitive coping therapy*. Brunner/Routledge.
Sharp, C., Cano, K., Bo, S., & Hutsebaut, J. (2022). The assessment of personality function in adolescents. In S. K. Huprich (Ed.), *Personality disorders and pathology: Integrating clinical assessment and practice in the DSM-5 and ICD-11 era* (pp. 109–134). American Psychological Association. https://doi.org/10.1037/0000310-006.
Sheldon, W., Dupertius, C., & McDermott, E. (1954). *A guide for somatotyping the adult male at all ages. Atlas of men* (2nd ed.). Harper Brothers.
Shostrum, E. (1976). *Actualizing therapy: Foundations for a scientific ethic*. EdITS Publishers.
Shulman, B. (1982). An Adlerian interpretation of the borderline personality. *Modern Psychoanalysis, 7*, 137–153.
Siefert, C. J., Porcerelli, J., Meehan, K. B., & Dauphin, B. (2022). Clinical utility of proposed dimensional personality disorder models: Considerations and opportunities. In S. K. Huprich (Ed.), *Personality disorders and pathology: Integrating clinical assessment and practice in the DSM-5 and ICD-11 era* (pp. 53–73). American Psychological Association. https://doi.org/10.1037/0000310-004.
Siegel, D. (1999). *The developing mind*. Guilford Press.
Siever, L. J. & Weinstein, L. N. (2009). The neurobiology of personality disorders: implications for psychoanalysis. *Journal of the American Psychoanalytic Association, 57*(2), 361–398.
Sifneos, P. (1972). *Short-term psychotherapy and emotional crisis*. Harvard University Press.
Sifneos, P. (1984). The current status of short-term dynamic psychotherapy and its future: An overview. *American Journal of Psychotherapy, 38*, 472–487.
Silk, K. & Feurino, L. (2012). Psychopharmacology of personality disorders. In T. Widiger (Ed.), *The Oxford handbook personality disorders* (pp. 713–726). Oxford University Press.
Simon, W. (2009). Follow-up psychotherapy outcome of patients with dependent, avoidant and obsessive–compulsive personality disorders: A meta-analytic review. *International Journal of Psychiatry in Clinical Practice, 13*, 153–165.
Simon, K. (2015). Obsessive-compulsive personality disorder. In A. Beck, D. Davis, & A. Freeman (Eds), *Cognitive therapy of personality disorders* (3rd ed., pp. 203–222). Guilford Press.
Singer, M. T. & Larson, D. G. (1981). Borderline personality and the Rorschach test. *Archives of General Psychiatry, 38*(6), 693–698.
Skodol, A. E. (2021a). Personality disorders: Recent history and new directions. In A. E. Skodol & J. M. Oldham (Eds), *The American Psychiatric Publishing textbook of personality disorders, Third edition*. (pp. 3–12). American Psychiatric Publishing.
Skodol, A. E. (2021b). Manifestations, assessment, diagnosis, and differential diagnosis. In A. E. Skodol, A. E. & J. M. Oldham (Eds), *The American Psychiatric Publishing textbook of personality disorders, Third edition*. (pp. 105–142). American Psychiatric Publishing.
Skodol, A. E., Bender, D., Gunderson, J., & Oldham, J. (2014). Personality disorders. In R. Hales, S. Yudofsky, & L. Weiss (Eds), *The American Psychiatric Publishing Textbook of Psychiatry* (pp. 851–894). American Psychiatric Publishing.
Skodol, A. E., Bender, D. S., & Oldham, J. M (2019). Personality pathology and personality disorders. In L W. Roberts (Ed.). *The American Psychiatric Association publishing textbook of psychiatry*. (pp. 711–748). American Psychiatric Publishing
Slavik, S., Sperry, L., & Carlson, J. (1992). The schizoid personality disorder: A review and an Adlerian view and treatment. *Individual Psychotherapy, 7*, 137–154.
Slavson, S. (1939). *Dynamics of group psychotherapy*. Jason Aronson.
Slavson, S. (1964). *A textbook in analytic group psychotherapy*. International Universities Press.
Snyder, M. (1994). Couple therapy with narcissistically vulnerable clients: Using the relationship enhancement model. *Family Journal: Counseling and Therapy for Couples and Families, 2*, 27–35.
Soloff, P., Lynch, K., & Kelly, T. (2002). Childhood abuse as a risk factor for suicidal behavior in borderline personality disorder. *Journal of Personality Disorders, 16*(3), 201–214.
Solomon, M. (1989). *Narcissism and Intimacy: Love and Marriage in an Age of Confusion*. Norton.
Solomon, M. (1999), Treating narcissistic and borderline couples. In J. Carlson & L. Sperry (Eds), *The disordered couple* (pp. 239–258). New York: Brunner/Mazel.
Sperry, L. (1989). Integrative case formulations: What they are and how to write them. *Journal of Individual Psychology, 45*, 500–507.

Sperry, L. (1990). Personality disorders: Biopsychosocial descriptions and dynamics. *Journal of Individual Psychology*, 46, 193–202.
Sperry, L. (1992). Demystifying the psychiatric case formulation. *Jefferson Journal of Psychiatry*, 10(2), 12–19.
Sperry, L. (1995a). *Handbook of the diagnosis and treatment of DSM-IV personality disorders*. Brunner/Mazel.
Sperry, L. (1995b). *Psychopharmacology and psychotherapy: Strategies for maximizing treatment outcomes*. Brunner/Mazel.
Sperry, L. (1988). Biopsychosocial therapy: An integrative approach for tailoring treatment. *Journal of Individual Psychology*, 44, 225–235.
Sperry, L. (2000). Biopsychosocial therapy: Essential strategies and tactics. In J. Carlson & L. Sperry (Eds), *Brief therapy with individuals and couples*. Zeig, Tucker & Theisen.
Sperry, L. (2002). From psychopathology to transformation: Retrieving the developmental focus in psychotherapy. *Journal of Individual Psychology*, 58, 398–421.
Sperry, L. (2003). *Handbook of the diagnosis and treatment of DSM-IV-TR personality disorders* (Second edition). Brunner-Routledge.
Sperry, L. (2005). Case conceptualization: The missing link between theory and practice. *The Family Journal: Counseling and Therapy for Couples and Families*, 13, 71–76.
Sperry, L. (2006a). *Cognitive behavior therapy of DSM-IV-TR Personality disorders: Highly effective interventions for the most common personality disorders* (2nd ed.). Brunner/Mazel.
Sperry, L. (2006b). *Psychological treatment of chronic illness: The biopsychosocial therapy approach*. Brunner/Mazel.
Sperry, L. (2010). *Core competencies in counseling and psychotherapy: Becoming a highly competent and effective therapist*. Routledge.
Sperry, L. (2014). Effecting change: The centrality of the case conceptualization. In L. Sperry & J. Carlson. *How master therapists work: Effecting change from the first through the last session and beyond* (pp. 74–99). Routledge.
Sperry, L. (2015). Personality disorders. In L. Sperry, J. Carlson, J. Duba-Sauerheber, & J. Sperry (Eds), *Psychopathology and psychotherapy: DSM-5 diagnosis, case conceptualization and treatment* (3rd ed., pp. 27–61). Routledge.
Sperry, L. (2016). Educating the next generation of psychotherapists: Considering the future of theory and practice in Adlerian Psychotherapy. *Journal of Individual Psychology*, 72, 4–11.
Sperry, l. (2022a). *Highly effective therapy: Effecting deep change in counseling and psychotherapy. Second edition*. Routledge.
Sperry, L. (2022b). Adlerian case conceptualization and therapy: The Pattern focused approach. *Journal of Individual Psychology*, 78(4), 465–478.
Sperry, L. (2024a). Optimizing clinical decision-making with pattern-focused case conceptualizations. *Journal of Individual Psychology*, 80(3), 229–238.
Sperry, L. (2024b). Adlerian case conceptualization. In L. Sperry, J. Sperry, & M. Bluvshtein (Eds). *Psychopathology and psychotherapy: DSM-5-TR, Diagnosis, case conceptualization and treatment. Fourth edition* (pp. 6–15). Routledge.
Sperry, L., Blackwell, B., Gudeman, J. & Faulkner, L. (1992). *Psychiatric case formulations*. American Psychiatric Press.
Sperry, L., Brill, P., Howard, K., & Grissom, G. (1996). *Treatment outcomes in psychotherapy and psychiatric interventions*. Brunner/Mazel.
Sperry, L. & Carlson, J. (2014). *How master therapists work: Effecting change from the first to the last session and beyond*. Routledge.
Sperry, L., Gudeman, J., Blackwell, B., & Faulkner, L. (1992). *Psychiatric case formulations*. American Psychiatric Press.
Sperry, L. & Maniacci, M. (1996). The histrionic-obsessive couple. In J. Carlson & L. Sperry (Eds), *The disordered couple* (pp. 187–205). Brunner/Mazel.
Sperry, L. & Mosak, H. (1996). Personality disorders. In L. Sperry & J. Carlson (Eds), *Psychopathology and psychotherapy: From diagnosis to treatment* (2nd ed., pp. 279–336). Accelerated Development/Taylor & Francis.
Sperry, L. & Sperry, J. (2012). *Case conceptualization: Mastering this competency with ease and confidence*. Routledge.

Sperry, L. & Sperry, J. (2016). *Cognitive behavior therapy of DSM-5 Personality Disorders* (3rd ed.). Routledge.
Sperry, L. & Sperry, J. (2020). *Case conceptualization: Mastering this competency with ease and confidence. Second edition*. Routledge.
Spotnitz, H. (1975). The borderline schizophrenic in group psychotherapy. *International Journal of Group Psychotherapy*, 7, 155–174.
Stanley, B., Brodsky, B., & Gratch, I. (2021). Dialectical behavior therapy. In A. E. Skodol & J. M. Oldham (Eds). *American Psychiatric Association Publishing textbook of personality disorders, Third edition* (pp. 361–382). American Psychiatric Publishing.
Stern, B., Yeomans, F., & Diamond, D. (2013). Transference-focused psychotherapy (TFP) for narcissistic personality disorder. In J. Ogrodniczuk (Ed.), *Understanding and treating pathological narcissism* (pp. 235–252). American Psychological Association.
Stevenson, J. & Meares, R. (1992). An outcome study of psychotherapy for patients with borderline personality disorder. *American Journal of Psychiatry*, 149, 144–150.
Stone, M. (1983). Psychotherapy with schizotypal borderline patients. *Journal of the American Academy of Psychoanalysis*, 11, 87–111.
Stone, M. (1985). Schizotypal personality: Psychotherapeutic aspects. *Schizophrenia Bulletin*, 11, 576–589.
Stone, M. (1989). Schizotypal personality disorder. In T. Karasu (Ed.), *Treatment of psychiatric disorders* (pp. 2719–2726). American Psychiatric Press.
Stone, M. (1992). Treatment of severe personality disorders. In A. Tasman & M. Riba (Eds), *American Psychiatric Press Review of Psychiatry. Vol. 2* (pp. 98–115). American Psychiatric Press.
Stone, M. (1993). *Abnormalities of personality: Within and beyond the realm of treatment*. Norton.
Stone, W. & Whiteman, R. (1980). Observation and empathy in group psychotherapy. In L. Wolberg & M. Aronson (Eds), *Group and Family Therapy*. Brunner/Mazel.
Stone, M. & Weissman, R. (1984). Group therapy with borderline patients. In H. Slavinska (Ed.), *Contemporary perspectives in group psychotherapy*. Routledge & Kegan Paul.
Stout, M. (2005). *The sociopath next door*. Broadway Books.
Strauss, J., Hayes, A., Johnson, S., Newman, C., Brown, G., Barber, J., et al. (2006). Early alliance, alliance ruptures, and symptom change in a nonrandomized trial of cognitive therapy for avoidant and obsessive-compulsive personality disorders. *Journal of Consulting and Clinical Psychology*, 74, 337–345.
Stravynski, A., Grey, S., & Elie, R. (1987). Outline of the therapeutic process in social skills training with socially dysfunctional patients. *Journal of Consulting and Clinical Psychology*, 55, 224–228.
Stravynski, A., Marks, I., & Yule, W. (1982). Social skills problems in neurotic outpatients. *Archives of General Psychology*, 39, 1378–1383.
Strupp, H. & Binder, J. (1984). *Psychotherapy in a new key: A guide to time-limited dynamic psychotherapy*. Basic Books.
Sungar, M. & Gunduz, A. (2015). Histrionic personality disorder. In A. Beck, D. Davis, & A. Freeman, A. (Eds), *Cognitive therapy of personality disorders* (3rd ed., pp. 325–345). Guilford Press.
Svartberg, M., Stiles, T., & Seltzer, M. (2004). Randomized control trial of the effectiveness of short-term dynamic therapy and cognitive therapy for Cluster C personality disorders. *American Journal of Psychiatry*, 161(5), pp. 810–817.
Swiercinsky, D. (Ed.). (1985). *Testing adults*. Test Corporation of America.
Symington, N. (1980). The response aroused by the psychopath. *International Review of Psychoanalysis*, 7, 291–298.
Tacbacnik, N. (1965). Isolation, transference, splitting and combined treatment. *Comprehensive Psychiatry*, 6, 336–346.
Tarrier, N. (Ed.). (2006). *Case formulation in cognitive behaviour therapy. The treatment of challenging and complex cases*. Routledge.
Teasdale, J., Segal, Z. Williams, J., Mark, G., Ridgeway, V., Soulsby, J, et al. (2000). Prevention of relapse/recurrence in depression by mindfulness-based cognitive therapy. *Journal of Consulting and Clinical Psychology*, 68, 615–623.
Thomas, A. & Chess, S. (1977). *Temperament and development*. Brunner/Mazel.
Thylstrup, B. & Hesse, M. (2009). "I am not complaining"—Ambivalence construct in schizoid personality disorder. *American Journal of Psychotherapy*, 63(2), 147–167.

Toman, W. (1961). *Family constellation: Theory and practice of a psychological game*. Springer.
Torgersen, S. (1984). Genetic and nosological aspects of schizotypal and borderline personality disorders: A twin study. *Archives of General Psychiatry, 41*, 546–554.
Torgersen, S. (2009). Prevalence, sociodemographics, and functional impairment. In J. Oldham, J. Skodol, & D. Bender (Eds), *Essentials of personality disorders* (pp. 83–102). American Psychiatric Publishing.
Torgersen, S. (2012). Epidemiology. In T. Widiger (Ed.), *The Oxford handbook of personality disorders* (pp. 186–205). Oxford University Press.
Torgersen, S. (2021). Prevalence, sociodemographics, and functional impairment. In A. E. Skodol & J. M. Oldham (Eds). *American Psychiatric Association Publishing textbook of personality disorders, Third edition.* (pp. 143–163). American Psychiatric Publishing.
Trujillo, M. (2013). Treating pathological narcissism with short term dynamic psychotherapy. In J. Ogrodniczuk (Ed.), *Understanding and treating pathological narcissism* (pp. 269–284). American Psychological Association.
Turkat, I. (1990). *The personality disorders: A psychological approach to clinical management*. Pergamon.
Turkat, L. & Maisto, S. (1985). Application of the experimental method to the formulation and modification of personality disorders. In D. Barlow (Ed.), *Clinical handbook of psychological disorders* (pp. 503–570). New York: Guilford Press.
Vaccani, J. (1989). Borderline personality and alcohol abuse. *Archives of Psychiatric Nursing, 3*, 113–119.
Valliant, G. & Perry, J. (1985). Personality disorders. In H. Kaplan & B. Sadock (Eds), *Comprehensive textbook of psychiatry* (4th ed.). Williams & Wilkins.
Van der Kolk, B. A., Perry, J. C., & Herman, J. L. (1991). Childhood origins of self-destructive behavior. *American Journal of Psychiatry, 148*(12), 1665–1671.
Van Gelder, K. (2010). *The Buddha and the borderline: A memoir*. New Harbinger.
Vaughn, B. & Bost, K. (1999). Attachment and temperament: Redundant, independent, or interacting influences on interpersonal adaptation and personality development? In P. Cassidy & P. Shaver (Eds), *Handbook of attachment: Theory, research and clinical applications* (pp. 198–225). Guilford Press.
Vinogradov, S. & Yalom, I. (1989). *Concise guide to group psychotherapy*. American Psychiatric Press.
Wagner, E. & Wagner, C. (1981). *The interpretation of psychological test data*. Charles Thomas.
Waldinger, R. (1986). Intensive psychodynamic psychotherapy with borderline patients: An overview. *American Journal of Psychiatry, 144*, 267–274.
Waldo, M. & Harman, M. (1993). Relationship enhancement therapy with borderline personality. *Family Journal, 1*, 25–30.
Waldo, M. & Harman, M. (1998). Borderline personality disorder and relationship enhancement marital therapy. In J. Carlson & L. Sperry (Eds), *The disordered couple* (pp. 285–298). Brunner/Mazel.
Walker, R. (1992). Substance abuse and B-cluster disorders: Treatment recommendations. *Journal of Psychoactive Drugs, 24*, 233–241.
Wallerstein, R. (1986). *Forty-two lives in treatment: A study of psychoanalysis and psychotherapy*. Guilford Press.
Walsh, A. & Wu, H. H. (2008). Differentiating antisocial personality disorder, psychopathy, and sociopathy: Evolutionary, genetic, neurological, and sociological considerations. *Criminal Justice Studies, 21*(2), 135–152.
Waugh, M. H., Ridenour, J. M., & Lewis, K. C. (2022). The alternative *DSM* Model for Personality Disorders in psychological assessment and treatment. In S. K. Huprich (Ed.), *Personality disorders and pathology: Integrating clinical assessment and practice in the DSM-5 and ICD-11 era* (pp. 159–182). American Psychological Association. https://doi.org/10.1037/0000310-008.
Weeks, G. & L'Abate, L. (1982). *Paradoxical psychotherapy: Theory and practice with individuals, couples, and families*. Brunner/Mazel.
Weissman, M., Markowitz, J., & Klerman, G. (2000). *Comprehensive guide to interpersonal psychotherapy*. Basic Books.
Weissman, M., Markowitz, J., & Klerman, G. (2007). *Clinician's quick guide to interpersonal psychotherapy*. Oxford University Press.

Wells, M., Glickauf-Hughes, C., & Buzzell, V. (1990). Treating obsessive-compulsive personalities in psychoanalytic/interpersonal group therapy. *Psychotherapy, 27*, 366–379.

Westen, D. (2012). Prototypic diagnosis of psychiatric syndromes. *World Psychiatry, 11*(1), 16–21.

Wilberg, T., Karterud, S., Urnes, O., Pedersen, G., & Friis, S. (1999). One-year follow-up of day treatment for poorly functioning patients with personality disorders. *Psychiatric Services, 50*(10), 1326–1330.

Wilberg, T. & Silk, K. (2018). The Neurobiological Basis of Avoidant Personality Disorder. In C. Schmahl, K. L. Phan, & R. O. Friedel (Eds). *Neurobiology of personality disorders* (pp. 359–384). Oxford University Press.

Williams, J. (1988). Cognitive intervention for a paranoid personality disorder. *Psychotherapy, 25*, 570–575.

Williams, P. (2010). Psychotherapeutic treatment of Cluster A personality disorders. In J. Clarkin, P. Fonagy, & G. Gabbard (Eds), *Psychodynamic psychotherapy for personality disorders: A clinical handbook* (pp. 289–309). American Psychiatric Publishing.

Winer, J. & Pollock, G. (1989). Psychoanalysis and dynamic therapy. In T. Karasu (Ed.), *Treatments of psychiatric disorders* (pp. 2639–2648). American Psychiatric Press.

Winkeller, V. & Schlesinger, A.B. (2021). Collaborative treatment. In A. E. Skodol & J. M. Oldham (Eds). *American Psychiatric Association Publishing textbook of personality disorders, Third edition*. (pp. 493–518). American Psychiatric Publishing.

Winston, A. & Pollack, J. (1991). Brief adaptive psychotherapy. *Psychiatric Annals, 21*, 415–418.

Woody, G., McLellan, A., Luborsky, L., & O'Brien, C. (1985). Sociopathy and psychotherapy outcome. *Archives of General Psychiatry, 42*(11), 1081–1086.

Wright, A., Hallquist, M., Morse, J, Scott, L., Stepp, S., Nolf, K, et al. (2013). Clarifying interpersonal heterogeneity in borderline personality disorder using latent mixture modeling. *Journal of Personality Disorders, 27*(2), 125–143.

Wurmser, L. (1981). *The mask of shame*. Johns Hopkins University Press.

Yalch, M. M., Ceroni, D. B., & Dehart, R. M. (2023). Influence of child abuse and neglect on histrionic personality pathology. *Journal of Trauma & Dissociation, 24*(1), 111–124.

Yalom, I. (1995). *The theory and practice of group psychotherapy* (4th ed.). Basic Books.

Yeomans, F.E., Clarkin, J. F. & Levy, K. N. (2021). Psychodynamic psychotherapies. In A. E. Skodol & J. M. Oldham (Eds). *American Psychiatric Association Publishing textbook of personality disorders, Third edition*. (pp. 335–360). American Psychiatric Publishing.

Young, J. (1994). *Cognitive therapy for personality disorders: A schema-focused approach* (rev. ed.). Professional Resource Exchange.

Young, J. (1999). *Cognitive therapy for personality disorders: A schema-focused approach* (3rd ed.). Professional Resource Press.

Young, J., Klosko, J., & Weishaar, M. (2003). *Schema therapy: A practitioner's guide*. Guilford Press.

Young, P. (1990). *Cognitive therapy for personality disorders: A schema-focused approach*. Professional Resource Exchange.

Zanarini, M., Frankenburg, F., Reich, D., & Fitzmaurice, G. (2010). Time-to-attainment of recovery from borderline personality disorder and stability of recovery: A 10-year prospective follow-up study. *American Journal of Psychiatry, 167*, 663–667.

Zanarini, M. C., Temes, C. M., Frankenburg, F. R., Reich, D. B., & Fitzmaurice, G. M. (2018). Description and prediction of time-to-attainment of excellent recovery for borderline patients followed prospectively for 20 years. *Psychiatry Research, 262*, 40–45.

Zimbardo, P. (1977). *Shyness*. Jove/Berkeley Publishing Group.

Zimmerman, M., Rothschild, L., & Chelminski, I. (2005). The prevalence of DSM-IV personality disorders in outpatients. *American Journal of Psychiatry, 162*, 1911–1918.

Index

abandonment 15, 64, 105, 225
abandonment depression 92
Accordino, M. P. 109
acculturation 6, 41
Ackley, C. 59, 97, 191, 206, 222
Adler, A. 205
Adler, G. 89, 92, 99, 173
affective/emotional style: Antisocial Personality Disorder 53–4; Avoidant Personality Disorder 70; Borderline Personality Disorder 89; Dependent Personality Disorder 114; Histrionic Personality Disorder 131; Narcissistic Personality Disorder 148; Obsessive-Compulsive Personality Disorder 166; Paranoid Personality Disorder 184; Schizoid Personality Disorder 201; Schizotypal Personality Disorder 216
agoraphobia 127
Ainsworth, M. 3, 26
Akhtar, S. 203
Alden, L. 82–84
Alexander, J. 66, 122
alienation 225–226
Allen, J. 155
Allnutt, S. 27, 54, 71, 90, 114, 131, 148, 167, 185, 201, 217
Allport, G. 4
Alonso, A. 178
Alternative Model for Personality Disorders 28–37; Antisocial Personality Disorder 54; Borderline Personality Disorder 91; components 30–37; Dependent Personality Disorder 116; Histrionic Personality Disorder 133; Narcissistic Personality Disorder 149–150; Obsessive-Compulsive Personality Disorder 168; Paranoid Personality Disorder 186; prevalence 55; prototypic presentation 54–55; rationale for 28–31; Schizoid Personality Disorder 203; Schizotypal Personality Disorder 218
American Psychiatric Association 1–2; Alternative Model for Personality Disorders 30; Antisocial Personality Disorder 54; Avoidant Personality Disorder 71–72; Borderline Personality Disorder 90; Dependent Personality Disorder 115; Histrionic Personality Disorder 132; Narcissistic Personality Disorder 148–149; Obsessive-Compulsive Personality Disorder 167; Paranoid Personality Disorder 185; Schizoid Personality Disorder 202; Schizotypal Personality Disorder 217
American Psychological Association 12, 98
Anderson, C. 212
antidepressants 44, 111, 137, 144, 173, 180, *see also* monoamine oxidase inhibitors (MAOIs); selective serotonin reuptake inhibitors (SSRIs)
antipsychotics 110, 198, 207, 212, 227
Antisocial Personality Disorder 50–68; affective/emotional style 53–54; Alternative Model for Personality Disorders 54; assessment 58–60; attachment style 54; behavioral style 53; biosocial case conceptualizations 56; and Borderline Personality Disorder 60, 67; case studies 51; characteristics 59; cognitive style 53; cognitive-behavioral case conceptualizations 57; description 50–55; DSM-5 description 54; fearful-dismissing attachment style 4; and Histrionic Personality Disorder 67, 143; integrative case conceptualization 58; interpersonal case conceptualizations 57; interpersonal style 53; interview behavior and rapport 58–59; medication strategies 143–144; and Narcissistic Personality Disorder 60, 154; optimal diagnostic criterion 54; and Paranoid Personality Disorder 60, 188, 192; psychodynamic case conceptualizations 55–56; psychological testing data 59–60; and Psychopathic Personality Disorder 52, 53; and Sociopathic Personality Disorder 53; style vs. disorder 50–51; treatment 60–68; triggering event 53
antisocial personality style 50–52, 59, 86

anxiety: Avoidant Personality Disorder 75, 79; Borderline Personality Disorder 88; Generalized Anxiety Disorder 192; Obsessive-Compulsive Personality Disorder 173; separation anxiety 88, 98, 122; Social Anxiety Disorder 72, 83, 120, 137, 173
Appel, G. 211
approval-seeking 80, 124–125, 140, 195
Armstrong, R. 213
Arntz, A. 94
Asperger's Disorder 217
assertiveness training 105, 123, 124, 126
assessment: Antisocial Personality Disorder 58–60; Avoidant Personality Disorder 76–77; Borderline Personality Disorder 97–98; Dependent Personality Disorder 118–120; Histrionic Personality Disorder 136–137; integrative *see* integrative assessment; Narcissistic Personality Disorder 153–154; Obsessive-Compulsive Personality Disorder 171–173; Paranoid Personality Disorder 190–191; Schizoid Personality Disorder 206–207; Schizotypal Personality Disorder 222
attachment behaviors 18
attachment style 2–4, 26; Antisocial Personality Disorder 54; Avoidant Personality Disorder 70; Borderline Personality Disorder 89; Dependent Personality Disorder 114; dismissing 4; disorganized 4; fearful 4; fearful–dismissing 4; Histrionic Personality Disorder 131; insecure 3; meaning of attachment 2; Narcissistic Personality Disorder 148; Obsessive-Compulsive Personality Disorder 166–167; Paranoid Personality Disorder 184–185; preoccupied 3; preoccupied–fearful 4; Schizoid Personality Disorder 201; Schizotypal Personality Disorder 217
attention-seeking, Histrionic Personality Disorder 135
automatic thoughts 8, 63, 170, 176, 194, 225; challenging 79–80, 139–140, 209, *see also* Schema Therapy
autonomy 57, 65, 160, 178, 193; Borderline Personality Disorder 94, 99; Dependent Personality Disorder 117, 123
Avoidant Personality Disorder 69–85; affective/emotional style 70; anxiety-based 75, 79; assessment 76–77; attachment style 70; behavioral style 69–70; biosocial case conceptualizations 74; case studies 71; cognitive style 70; cognitive-behavioral case conceptualizations 74–75; and Dependent Personality Disorder 120; description 69–71; DSM-5 description 71–72; interpersonal case conceptualizations 75, 75–76; interpersonal style 70; interview behavior and rapport 76; medication strategies 19, 82; and Obsessive-Compulsive Personality Disorder 175; optimal diagnostic criterion 71; preoccupied–fearful attachment style 4, 70; prototypic presentation 72; psychodynamic case conceptualizations 73–74; psychological testing data 77; and Schizotypal Personality Disorder 219–221; and social phobia 80; style vs. disorder 69–70; treatment 19, 77–85; triggering event 69
avoidant personality style 69–71, 77
Axis I 8

Babiak, P. 52
Bach, B. 30, 31
Baer, L. 173
Baker, J. 116
Balint, E. 193
Balint, M. 203
Barber, J. 175, 192
Barlow, D. 127, 128
Barrantes-Vidal, N. 214
Bartholomew, K. 3
Bateman, A. 17–18, 62, 92, 99–100, 102
Beck, A. 8, 23, 57, 63, 64, 74, 75, 79, 83, 84, 93, 102, 117, 123, 127, 134, 139, 140, 152, 158–159, 170, 175, 187, 194, 204, 209–210, 219, 224–225
Begley, S. 13
Behary, W. 152, 159
Behavior Therapy 7
behavioral case conceptualizations 170
behavioral style 24; Antisocial Personality Disorder 53; Avoidant Personality Disorder 69–70; Borderline Personality Disorder 88; Dependent Personality Disorder 113; Histrionic Personality Disorder 130; Narcissistic Personality Disorder 148; Obsessive-Compulsive Personality Disorder 166; Paranoid Personality Disorder 184; Schizoid Personality Disorder 200; Schizotypal Personality Disorder 216
Beitman, B. 19, 40
beliefs: conditional 57, 152, 187, 204, 220; core *see* core beliefs; instrumental *see* instrumental beliefs
Bellak, L. 60, 98, 120, 137, 154, 173, 191
Bellino 111
Bender, D. 50, 69, 86, 112, 129, 145, 164, 182, 199, 214
Benjamin, L. 23–24, 57, 64–65, 75, 81–83, 94–95, 105–106, 117, 125, 134, 140–141, 152, 159–160, 170, 177–178, 179, 188, 195–196, 197, 204, 210, 220, 226

Berger, P. 111
Berkowitz, D. 161
Bernstein, D. 64, 80, 90, 105, 125, 140, 159, 177, 195, 210, 226
Bertsch, K. 6, 7
Binder, J. 83, 121, 122, 157
Biopsychosocial Therapy 12
biosocial case conceptualizations: Antisocial Personality Disorder 56; Avoidant Personality Disorder 74; Borderline Personality Disorder 93; Dependent Personality Disorder 116–117; Histrionic Personality Disorder 133–134; Narcissistic Personality Disorder 151; Obsessive-Compulsive Personality Disorder 169; Paranoid Personality Disorder 188–189; Schizoid Personality Disorder 203–204; Schizotypal Personality Disorder 219
Bipolar Disorder 19, 55, 60, 137, 192, 207, 218
Black, D. 19, 110
Bliton, C. F. 34
Blocher, D. 18, 19, 181
Bo, S. 2
Bogdanoff, M. 211
Bogetto, F. 111
Bohn, M. 60
Bonime, W. 208
Borderline Personality Disorder 86–111; affective/emotional style 89; Alternative Model for Personality Disorders 91; and Antisocial Personality Disorder 60, 67; assessment 97–98; attachment style 89; behavioral style 88; biosocial case conceptualizations 93; borderline-dependent individuals 93; borderline-histrionic individuals 93; borderline-passive aggressive individuals 93; case studies 87–88; and categorical model 29; characteristics 96; childhood abuse 90; Cognitive Behavior Analysis System of Psychotherapy 11; cognitive style 89; cognitive-behavioral case conceptualizations 93–94; description 86–90; disorganized attachment style 4; DSM-5 description 90–91; DSM-IV-TR criteria 29; individual psychotherapy 98–106; integrative case conceptualization 95–96; interpersonal case conceptualizations 94–95; interpersonal style 88–89; interview behavior and rapport 97; medication strategies 109–110; mentalization approach 92, 99–100; optimal diagnostic criterion 89–90; prevalence 91; prototypic presentation 90–91; psychodynamic case conceptualizations 91–93; psychological testing data 97–98; and Schizotypal Personality Disorder 219, 222; severe borderline pathology 109; Structural Analysis of Social Behavior 94–95, 106; style vs. disorder 86–87; treatment 98–111; triggering event 88
borderline personality style 86–88, 97
Boritz, T. 111
Bornstein, R. 112, 122
Bost, K. 5
bottom-up strategies 14
Boutilier, L. 5, 26, 90
Bowlby, J. 3
Bozzatello, P. 111
Brauer, L. 117, 124
Brennan, K. 6
Brief Adaptive Psychotherapy (BAP) 138–139
brief dynamic psychotherapy: Histrionic Personality Disorder 138–139; Paranoid Personality Disorder 193–194
brief psychoanalytically oriented psychotherapy 157–158
Brill, P. 12, 40
Brodsky, B. 103, 228
Brown, E. 80
Buddha and the Borderline (Van Gelder) 48
Buie, D. 99
Burry, A. 133, 186, 203, 218–219
Buzzel, V. 178

Caffery, T. 26
Cain, N. 2, 28, 30, 111, 163
Caligor, E. 7, 146, 147, 155
Cano, K. 2
carbamazepine 109
Carlson, J. 39, 48, 211, 213
Carscadden, J. 108
case conceptualizations 38–49; Antisocial Personality Disorder 55–58; Avoidant Personality Disorder 73–76; biosocial *see* biosocial case conceptualizations; Borderline Personality Disorder 91–95; case of Aimee 46–48; case of Geri 42–44; case of Kiera 44–46; clinical formulation 39; cognitive-behavioral *see* cognitive-behavioral case conceptualizations; commentary on cases 48; concise 42; definition/components 38–42; Dependent Personality Disorder 116–118; diagnostic formulation 39; elements 40; Histrionic Personality Disorder 133–135; integrative *see* integrative case conceptualization; interpersonal *see* interpersonal case conceptualizations; Narcissistic Personality Disorder 150–153; Obsessive-Compulsive Personality Disorder 168–171; Paranoid Personality Disorder 186–190; premises 40; psychodynamic *see* psychodynamic case conceptualizations;

Schizoid Personality Disorder 203–205;
Schizotypal Personality Disorder 218–221;
strengths and protective factors 40–41
"Case of Mrs. A" 173
Cass, D. 142
CAT *see* Cognitive Analytic Therapy (CAT)
catastrophizing 117, 170
categorical model of personality disorders *see*
    DSM-IV-TR Model of Personality Disorders
    (categorical model)
Cawood, C. D. 8, 9, 10
CBT *see* Cognitive Behavioral Therapy
Chapman, E. 8, 9, 10
character 5–6
Chess, S. 5, 56, 58, 75, 93, 95, 219
Chessick, R. 99, 156
childhood abuse, Borderline Personality
    Disorder 90
Choca, J. 60, 77, 97, 120, 136, 154, 173, 191, 222
Chodoff, P. 138
Clarkin, J. 16, 24, 61, 78, 92, 98–99, 100, 102,
    108, 110–111, 121, 138, 155, 174, 178–179,
    192, 196, 207, 223
clinical formulation 39; case
    conceptualizations 39
Clinical Psychiatry News 1
Clinically Relevant Behaviors (CRBs) 181
Cloniger, C. 5
Cognitive Analytic Therapy (CAT) 139,
    193–194
Cognitive Behavior Analysis System of
    Psychotherapy (CBASP) 7, 10–11; and
    Pattern-Focused Therapy 12; theory 11;
    treatment 11–12
Cognitive Behavioral Therapy 7–8; Antisocial
    Personality Disorder 63–64; Avoidant
    Personality Disorder 79–80; Borderline
    Personality Disorder 93–94, 102–105;
    Dependent Personality Disorder 123–125;
    Histrionic Personality Disorder 139–140;
    Narcissistic Personality Disorder 158–159;
    Obsessive-Compulsive Personality Disorder
    175–177; Paranoid Personality Disorder
    194–195; Schizoid Personality Disorder
    209–210; Schizotypal Personality Disorder
    224–226; traditional treatment 7–8
Cognitive Coping Therapy 105, 124
cognitive distortions 93, 107, 117, 134, 158,
    170, 225
cognitive restructuring 9, 13, 64, 80, 105, 124,
    140, 159, 176, 195, 198, 207, 210, 225
cognitive style 24; Antisocial Personality
    Disorder 53; Avoidant Personality Disorder
    70; Borderline Personality Disorder 89;
    Dependent Personality Disorder 114;
Histrionic Personality Disorder 131;
    Narcissistic Personality Disorder 148;
    Obsessive-Compulsive Personality Disorder
    166; Paranoid Personality Disorder
    184; Schizoid Personality Disorder 201;
    Schizotypal Personality Disorder 216
Cognitive Therapy 7–10; Borderline Personality
    Disorder 93–94, 102; Narcissistic Personality
    Disorder 159–160; Paranoid Personality
    Disorder 194–195; Schizoid Personality
    Disorder 209–210; Schizotypal Personality
    Disorder 224–225
cognitive-behavioral case conceptualizations:
    Antisocial Personality Disorder 57; Avoidant
    Personality Disorder 74–75; Borderline
    Personality Disorder 93–94; Dependent
    Personality Disorder 117; Histrionic
    Personality Disorder 134; Narcissistic
    Personality Disorder 152; Paranoid
    Personality Disorder 187–188; Schizoid
    Personality Disorder 204; Schizotypal
    Personality Disorder 219–220
collaboration 105, 141, 177
Collins, D. 126
collusion 62
combined and integrated treatment methods
    19; Antisocial Personality Disorder 67–68;
    Avoidant Personality Disorder 83–85;
    Borderline Personality Disorder 110–111;
    Dependent Personality Disorder 128;
    Histrionic Personality Disorder 144;
    Narcissistic Personality Disorder 163;
    Obsessive-Compulsive Personality Disorder
    180–181; Paranoid Personality Disorder
    198; Schizoid Personality Disorder 213;
    Schizotypal Personality Disorder 227–228
Comerford, A. 102
comorbidity 29, 80, 83
Compulsive Personality Disorder 172, 188,
    see also Obsessive-Compulsive Personality
    Disorder
conditional beliefs 57, 152, 187, 204, 220
Conduct Disorder 55
Conversion Disorders 120, 173
core beliefs 55, 57, 72, 115, 132, 167, 176, 185,
    187, 202, 217
Core Conflictual Relationship Theme (CCRT)
    122
Cortright, B. 19
Costa, P. 164
Costello, C. 6
counseling 101
countertransference issues 122, 154, 174, 178,
    192–193, 208, 224; Antisocial Personality
    Disorder 61, 62, 63; Borderline Personality
    Disorder 98, 106, 111

couples therapy: Avoidant Personality Disorder 77, 81, 83; Dependent Personality Disorder 127; Histrionic Personality Disorder 137, 143; Narcissistic Personality Disorder 160, 161; Obsessive-Compulsive Personality Disorder 177; Paranoid Personality Disorder 197; Schizotypal Personality Disorder 227
Cramer Azima, F. 82
Crits-Christoph, P. 122, 192
Cukrowicz, K. 11
cultural formulation 39
cultural identity 39
culture, sex, and gender 6; Antisocial Personality Disorder 55; Avoidant Personality Disorder 72; Borderline Personality Disorder 91; Dependent Personality Disorder 115–116; Histrionic Personality Disorder 132–133; Narcissistic Personality Disorder 149; Obsessive-Compulsive Personality Disorder 168; Paranoid Personality Disorder 186; Schizoid Personality Disorder 202; Schizotypal Personality Disorder 218
Cuper, P. 8, 10

Davidson, K. 64
Davis, D. 23, 152, 159
Davis, R. 74, 83, 88, 93, 117, 127, 133, 151, 162, 169, 188, 203, 219, 220
Day, M. 107
DBT *see* Dialectical Behavior Therapy
decatastrophizing 79, 140
defectiveness 27, 64, 80, 103, 105, 124, 140, 159, 192, 195, 210
defense mechanisms 5, 58, 76, 153, 157, 187, 205, 219, 221, 223
Delusional Disorders 154–155, 192, 202, 218
Demetri, J. 74
Denburg, E. 60, 77, 97, 154, 173, 191, 222
Dependent Personality Disorder 112–128; affective/emotional style 114; Alternative Model for Personality Disorders 116; assessment 118–120; attachment style 114; and Avoidant Personality Disorder 120; behavioral style 113; biosocial case conceptualizations 116–117; case studies 113; characteristics 119; cognitive style 114; cognitive-behavioral case conceptualizations 117; description 112–115; DSM-5 description 115; and Histrionic Personality Disorder 120, 137; integrative case conceptualization 118; interpersonal case conceptualizations 117–118; interpersonal style 113; interview behavior and rapport 119; and Narcissistic Personality Disorder 127; and Obsessive-Compulsive Personality Disorder 173; optimal diagnostic criterion 114; parental overprotection 116; prevalence 115; prototypic presentation 115; psychodynamic case conceptualizations 116; psychological testing data 119–120; style vs. disorder 112, 114; treatment 120–128; triggering event 113
dependent personality style 112–114, 119, 199
Depersonalization Disorder 207
depression: abandonment depression 92; Dysthymic Disorder 11, 95; Major Depressive Disorder 11, 36, 43; and mindfulness 13; Paranoid Personality Disorder 192; Persistent Depressive Disorder 95, 120, 137, 155; unipolar 11
DeRisi, W. J. 14
development and course: Antisocial Personality Disorder 55; Avoidant Personality Disorder 72; Borderline Personality Disorder 91; Dependent Personality Disorder 115; Histrionic Personality Disorder 132; Narcissistic Personality Disorder 149; Obsessive-Compulsive Personality Disorder 168; Paranoid Personality Disorder 186; Schizoid Personality Disorder 202; Schizotypal Personality Disorder 218
developmental mourning 208
developmental therapy 7, 18–19, 180–181; developmental levels of personality 20–21
diagnosis of personality disorders 2–7
Diagnostic and Statistical Manual of Mental Disorders, 5th edition (DSM-5): Alternative Model for Personality Disorders *see* Alternative Model for Personality Disorders; Antisocial Personality Disorder 54; Avoidant Personality Disorder 71–72; Borderline Personality Disorder 90–91; categorical model of personality disorders 28–29; Dependent Personality Disorder 115; Histrionic Personality Disorder 132; Narcissistic Personality Disorder 148–149; Obsessive-Compulsive Personality Disorder 167; Paranoid Personality Disorder 185; pathological functioning vs. normal functioning 19; Schizoid Personality Disorder 202; Schizotypal Personality Disorder 217
diagnostic formulation 39
Dialectical Behavior Therapy 8–10; Borderline Personality Disorder 94, 103–105; case study 45; compared to traditional CBT 8–9; core strategies 10, 104; practicing 10; research support 10; stages of treatment 9–10; theory 8–9; treatment 9–10
Dialogical Self Theory (DST) 193
Diamond, R. 110, 111
Dick, B. M. 108

differential diagnosis: Antisocial Personality Disorder 55; Avoidant Personality Disorder 72; Borderline Personality Disorder 91; Dependent Personality Disorder 115; Histrionic Personality Disorder 132; Narcissistic Personality Disorder 149; Obsessive-Compulsive Personality Disorder 168; Paranoid Personality Disorder 185–186; Schizoid Personality Disorder 202; Schizotypal Personality Disorder 218
Diguer, L. 209
Dimaggio, G. 81, 82, 95, 193
dismissing attachment style 4, 201
disorganized attachment style 4
Dissociative Disorders 223
Dolan, M. 53
dopaminergic postsynaptic receptors 203, 205
Dorfman, W. I. 144
Dowgwillo, E. A. 2
Driscoll, K. 11
DSM-5 *see Diagnostic and Statistical Manual of Mental Disorders*, 5th edition (DSM-5)
DSM-I 5
DSM-II 5, 53
DSM-III 28, 30
DSM-IV-TR Model of Personality Disorders (categorical model): attachment styles 3–4; compared to Alternative Model for Personality Disorders 28; concerns/reasons for replaced 28–29, *see also* Alternative Model for Personality Disorders
Dupertius, C. 205
Dysfunctional Thought Record 124, 176, 209
Dysthymic Disorder 11, 95

Early Maladaptive Schema 14, 94
Eaton, N. R. 34
Eells, T. 38, 40
Eikenaes, I. 85
Ekleberry, S. 128
Elbaum, P. 211
Elie, R. 82
emotion skills 105, 124
emotional deprivation 64, 105, 140, 159
emotional inhibition 177
emotional regulation, compared to maladaptive thought process 8
emotional/affective style 26; Antisocial Personality Disorder 53; Avoidant Personality Disorder 70; Borderline Personality Disorder 89; Dependent Personality Disorder 114; Histrionic Personality Disorder 131; Narcissistic Personality Disorder 148; Obsessive-Compulsive Personality Disorder 166; Paranoid Personality Disorder 184; Schizoid Personality Disorder 201; Schizotypal Personality Disorder 216
empathy 62–63, 160, 177
entitlement 64, 159
Epstein, L. 192
Erdman, P. 26
erotic transference 138
Eskedal, G. 74
Everett, S. 108
Everly, G. 56, 74, 93, 116, 133, 135, 151, 188, 203, 219
explanatory power 41

Factitious Disorders 60, 120
Fairberg, S. 92
Fairburn, W. 203
Fairweather, A. K. 22
family therapy *see* marital and family therapy
Farrell, J. 14
Fay, A. 124
fearful attachment style 4, 184
fearful–dismissing attachment style 4, 148, 217
Fenichel, O. 78
Fernandez, S. 138
Fernbach, B. 62
Feurino, L. 67, 83, 127–128, 143, 163, 180, 198, 207, 212–213, 227
Finn, B. 107
Fiore, D. 81, 82
Flegenheimer, W. 122
fluoxetine 109
Foley, G. 143, 162, 179
Follette, V. 8
Fonagy, P. 17, 62, 92, 99, 100, 102, 155
Forche, K. R. 2
Fossatti, A. 90
Foster, C. 19
Fowler, J. C. 63, 79, 103, 123, 139, 158, 175, 194, 209, 225
Fowler, K. 138
Frances, A. 126, 178, 179
Freeman, A. 23, 24, 57, 63, 64, 79, 83, 84, 102, 140, 158, 175, 194, 205, 224, 225
Freeman, M. 158
Freud, S. 150, 156, 173
Functional Analytic Psychotherapy (FAP) 181

Gabbard, G. 60, 61, 62, 73, 74, 78, 107, 116, 121, 122, 133, 137, 138, 142, 175, 178, 186, 187, 207–208, 213, 218, 223–224, 228
GAF *see* Global Assessment of Functioning (GAF)
Gamache, D. 209
Generalized Anxiety Disorder 192
Gertsley, L. 61–63
Gilbert, S. 81

Giles, G. 211
Glantz, K. 62, 128
Glickhauf-Hughes, C. 178
Global Assessment of Functioning (GAF) 110
Glueck, E. 66
Glueck, S. 66
Goisman, R. 62, 128
Goldberg, A. 156
Goldwyn, R. 3
Goodman, M. 19
Gordon, K. 81
Graham, J. 60, 77, 97, 120, 136, 154, 173, 191, 206, 222
grandiosity trait, in Narcissistic Personality Disorder 29, 145, 150
Gratch, I. 103, 228
Graybar, S. 5, 26, 90
Greist, J. 80
Grey, S. 82
Grissom, G. 12, 40
Groth-Marnat, G. 59, 77, 97, 119, 136, 172, 191
Grotjahn, M. 160
group therapy: Antisocial Personality Disorder 65–66; Avoidant Personality Disorder 81–82; Borderline Personality Disorder 106–108; Dependent Personality Disorder 125–126; Histrionic Personality Disorder 141–142; Narcissistic Personality Disorder 160–161; Obsessive-Compulsive Personality Disorder 177–179; Paranoid Personality Disorder 196–197; Schizoid Personality Disorder 211; Schizotypal Personality Disorder 226–227
Gude, T. 85
Guerney, B. 109
Guidano, V. 170
guided discovery 9, 79, 102, 123, 139, 194, 210, 225
Gunderson, J. 29, 67, 98, 99, 110, 122, 218
Gunduz, A. 134, 140
Gurman, A. 83

Haley, J. 80, 179
Halleck, S. 142
Hallet, B. 13
Harbir, H. 66, 126, 142, 143, 179, 197
Hardy, G. 193
Hare, R. 51, 52, 61
Harman, M. 109
Harper, R. 82
Hart, J. M. 63, 79, 103, 123, 139, 158, 175, 194, 209, 225
Harwood, I. 107
Hatchett, G. 61
Havens, J. 68
Havens, L. 138

Hayes, S. 8
Hend, S. 116
Herman, J. L. 90
Herpertz, S. 6, 7, 30
Hesse, M. 207
heterogeneous group treatment modality 24
Hill, D. 122
Histrionic Personality Disorder 129–144; affective/emotional style 131; Alternative Model for Personality Disorders 133; and Antisocial Personality Disorder 67, 143; assessment 136–137; attachment style 131; attention-seeking 133; behavioral style 130; biosocial case conceptualizations 133–134; case studies 130; characteristics 135; cognitive style 131; cognitive-behavioral case conceptualizations 134; and Dependent Personality Disorder 120, 137; description 129–133; DSM-5 description 132; gender dynamics 141; integrative case conceptualization 134–135; interpersonal case conceptualizations 134; interpersonal style 131; interview behavior and rapport 136; and Narcissistic Personality Disorder 137, 155; and Obsessive-Compulsive Personality Disorder 143, 179; optimal diagnostic criterion 131; preoccupied attachment style 3; prevalence 132; prototypic presentation 132; psychodynamic case conceptualizations 133; psychological testing data 136–137; style vs. disorder 129–130, 130; treatment 137–144; triggering event 130
histrionic personality style 129–131, 136
Hoch, J. 108
Hoffart, A. 85
Hoffman, L. 179
holding environment 107, 122, 162, 211
homogeneous group treatment modality 24
Hopwood, C. 21, 30, 34, 182
Horowitz, L. 3, 107, 110, 138, 144, 160, 161, 169
hostile autonomy 65
How Master Therapists Work (Sperry and Carlson) 48
Howard, K. 12, 40
Hulse, W. 107
Huprich, S. K. 1, 7, 30
hurting sociopath 57, 61
Hutsebaut, J. 2
Hypochondriasis 172, 191

Imbesi, E. 151
impulsivity, Borderline Personality Disorder 89
individuation developmental theory 91–92
insight-oriented psychotherapy 6, 61, 144, 173

instrumental beliefs 57, 167; Narcissistic Personality Disorder 152; Paranoid Personality Disorder 185, 187; Schizoid Personality Disorder 202, 204; Schizotypal Personality Disorder 217, 219–220

integrative case conceptualization: Antisocial Personality Disorder 58; Avoidant Personality Disorder 75–76; Borderline Personality Disorder 95–96; Histrionic Personality Disorder 134–135; Narcissistic Personality Disorder 153; Obsessive-Compulsive Personality Disorder 171; Paranoid Personality Disorder 189–190; Schizoid Personality Disorder 204–205; Schizotypal Personality Disorder 220–221

interpersonal case conceptualizations: Antisocial Personality Disorder 57; Avoidant Personality Disorder 75; Borderline Personality Disorder 94–95; Dependent Personality Disorder 117–118, 118; Histrionic Personality Disorder 134; Narcissistic Personality Disorder 152–153; Obsessive-Compulsive Personality Disorder 170–171; Paranoid Personality Disorder 188; Schizoid Personality Disorder 204; Schizotypal Personality Disorder 220

interpersonal psychotherapy approach 95

interpersonal style 24; Antisocial Personality Disorder 53; Avoidant Personality Disorder 70; Borderline Personality Disorder 88–89; Dependent Personality Disorder 113; Histrionic Personality Disorder 131; Narcissistic Personality Disorder 148; Obsessive-Compulsive Personality Disorder 166; Paranoid Personality Disorder 184; Schizoid Personality Disorder 200–201; Schizotypal Personality Disorder 216

interpersonal therapy: Antisocial Personality Disorder 64–65; Avoidant Personality Disorder 81; Borderline Personality Disorder 95, 105–106; Dependent Personality Disorder 125; Histrionic Personality Disorder 140–141; Narcissistic Personality Disorder 159–160; Obsessive-Compulsive Personality Disorder 177–178; Paranoid Personality Disorder 195–196; Schizoid Personality Disorder 210; Schizotypal Personality Disorder 226

interview behavior and rapport: Antisocial Personality Disorder 58–59; Avoidant Personality Disorder 76; Borderline Personality Disorder 97; Dependent Personality Disorder 119; Histrionic Personality Disorder 136; Narcissistic Personality Disorder 153–154; Obsessive-Compulsive Personality Disorder 171–172; Paranoid Personality Disorder 191; Schizoid Personality Disorder 206; Schizotypal Personality Disorder 222, *see also* Motivational Interviewing (MI)

Jamison, S. 228
Jefferson, J. 80
Jenike, M. 173
Joiner, T. 11
Jones, S. 161

Kabat-Zinn, J. 13
Kalojera, I. 162
Kantor, M. 122, 156–157, 208
Kaurin, A. 21
Kavaler-Adler, S. 208
Kealy, D. 66, 67, 81, 83, 106, 109, 125, 127, 142, 143, 160, 161, 178, 179, 196, 197, 211–212, 226, 227
Keller, M. 11
Kellerman, H. 133, 186, 203, 218–219
Kellner, R. 64–68
Kelly, T. 90
Kernberg, O. 16, 56, 91–92, 99–101, 111, 147, 151, 156–157
Khan, M. 138
Kirk, J. 180
Klein, D. 144
Klein, P. 22
Klein, R. 92, 99, 101, 157–158
Klerman, G. 95
Klosko, J. 14, 80, 94, 105, 124, 140, 176, 195, 210
Kniskern, D. 83
Koenigsberg, H. 111, 212, 227
Kohut, H. 92, 151, 156, 161
Kovel, V. 109
Kristeller, J. 13
Krueger, R. F. 28, 34
Kwapil, T. 214
Kyrios, M. 175

L'Abate, L. 80
Lachar, D. 206
Lachkar, J. 109, 161, 162
Landucci, J. 143, 162, 179
Lawn, S. 22
Lazarus, A. 111, 124, 126, 128, 157
Lebow, J. 66, 67, 81, 83, 106, 109, 125, 127, 142, 143, 160, 161, 178, 179, 196, 197, 211–212, 226, 227
Lerner, U. 138
Leszcz, M. 160, 211
Level of Personality Functioning Scale 31, 34, 35, 36, 42–43, 45–47
Levy, K. 16, 17, 61, 78, 99, 121, 138, 146–147, 155, 174, 192, 207, 223

Leybman, M. 111
Lieberman, M. 14
Liebowitz, M. 65, 144, 227–228
Lilienfeld, S. 138
Linehan, M. 8–10, 13, 34, 94, 98, 103–104, 107–108, 155
Links, P. 27, 54, 71, 90, 114, 127, 131, 143, 148, 167, 185, 201, 217
Liotti, G. 170
lithium 109
Livesley, W. J. 111
LPFS *see* Level of Personality Functioning Scale
Luborsky, L. 122
Lusk, R. 8, 9, 10
Lyddon, W. 3, 70, 89, 114, 201
Lynch, K. 90
Lynch, T. 8, 10, 98

Macdonald, A. 227, 228
Mackinnon, R. 78
Madeddu, F. 90
Maffei, C. 90
Main, M. 3
Maisto, S. 140, 170, 176, 194, 198
Major Depressive Disorder 11, 36, 43
maladaptive patterns 12, 40
maladaptive schemas 27; Antisocial Personality Disorder 64; Avoidant Personality Disorder 80; Borderline Personality Disorder 94, 105; Dependent Personality Disorder 124–125; Histrionic Personality Disorder 140; Schizoid Personality Disorder 210; Schizotypal Personality Disorder 225, *see also* Schema Therapy
Malan, D. 122, 138, 193
Malancharuvil, J. 62
malignant narcissism 147, 150
Malinow, K. 127
Manduchi, K. 181
Maniacci, M. 143, 179
Mankiewicz, P. 187, 195, 204, 210, 220, 225
Mann, J. 122
Marin, L. K. 19
marital and family therapy: Antisocial Personality Disorder 66–67; Avoidant Personality Disorder 83; Borderline Personality Disorder 108–109; Dependent Personality Disorder 126–127; Histrionic Personality Disorder 142–143; Narcissistic Personality Disorder 161–162; Obsessive-Compulsive Personality Disorder 179; Paranoid Personality Disorder 197; Schizoid Personality Disorder 211–212; Schizotypal Personality Disorder 227
Markowitz, J. 95
Marks, I. 82

Marlatt, G. 13
Marmar, C. 158
Marra, T. 8, 9, 10, 103, 104
Martin, J. 13
Masterson, J. 92, 99, 101–102, 156–157, 162
McCommon, B. 7
McCormack, C. 212, 213
McCrae, R. 6
McCullough 10, 11, 12, 175
McDermott, E. 205
McGauley, G. 62
McMain, S. 108, 111
Meares, R. 102
medication strategies 11, 19; Antisocial Personality Disorder 67; Avoidant Personality Disorder 19, 82; Borderline Personality Disorder 109–110; Dependent Personality Disorder 127–128; Histrionic Personality Disorder 143–144; Narcissistic Personality Disorder 163; Obsessive-Compulsive Personality Disorder 180; Paranoid Personality Disorder 198; Schizoid Personality Disorder 212–213; Schizotypal Personality Disorder 227
Megargee, E. 60
Mehlum, L. 224, 226, 228
Meichenbaum, D. 102
Meissner, W. 192–193, 196, 197
Meloy, J. 55, 56, 61, 62, 66
Menninger Outcome Study 101
Mentalization-Based Treatment (MBT) 17–18; Borderline Personality Disorder 92, 99–100; Narcissistic Personality Disorder 155
Messina, N. 66, 68
metacognition-oriented therapy 193
methadone 68
Meyer, G. J. 60, 77, 98, 120, 137, 154, 173, 191, 206, 222
Meyer, R. 77, 97, 120, 136, 154, 173, 191
Michels, R. 78
Mihura, J. L. 60, 77, 98, 120, 137, 154, 173, 191, 206, 222
Miller, W. 12, 63
Millon, T. 23, 56, 58–60, 74, 75, 77, 83, 88, 89, 93, 95, 97, 116, 117, 119, 120, 127, 133, 135–137, 151, 153, 162, 169, 173, 188, 189, 191, 201, 203, 205, 206, 219, 220–221, 222
Millon Clinical Multiaxial Inventory (MCMI-IV): Antisocial Personality Disorder 60; Avoidant Personality Disorder 77; Borderline Personality Disorder 97; Dependent Personality Disorder 120; Histrionic Personality Disorder 136; Narcissistic Personality Disorder 154; Obsessive-Compulsive Personality Disorder 173; Paranoid Personality Disorder 191;

Schizoid Personality Disorder 206; Schizotypal Personality Disorder 222
mindfulness 13–14
Mindfulness-Based Cognitive Therapy (MBCT) 7, 13
Minichiello, W. 173
Minnesota Multiphase Personality Inventory (MMPI-2): Antisocial Personality Disorder 60; Avoidant Personality Disorder 77; Borderline Personality Disorder 97; Dependent Personality Disorder 120; Histrionic Personality Disorder 136; Narcissistic Personality Disorder 154; Obsessive-Compulsive Personality Disorder 172; Paranoid Personality Disorder 191; Schizoid Personality Disorder 206; Schizotypal Personality Disorder 222
Minuchin, S. 179
mistrust/abuse 64, 105, 195
Mitchell, D. 57, 63
MMPI-2 see Minnesota Multiphase Personality Inventory (MMPI-2)
Möhler, E. 6, 7
Molina, J. 2
Montgomery, J. 126
Mosak, H. 23, 58, 153, 190, 205, 221
Motivational Interviewing (MI) 12, 34, 63, 213, 228
Mueser, K. 14
Mulay, A. 2, 28, 30
Mulder, R. 6, 30, 31

Nachmani, G. 203
narcissistic injury 151
Narcissistic Personality Disorder 145–163; affective/emotional style 148; Alternative Model for Personality Disorders 149–150; and Antisocial Personality Disorder 60, 154; assessment 153–154; attachment style 148; behavioral style 148; biosocial case conceptualizations 151; case studies 146; characteristics 150; cognitive style 148; cognitive-behavioral case conceptualizations 152; covert type 147; and Dependent Personality Disorder 127; description 145–150; DSM-5 description 148–149; fearful–dismissing attachment style 4; grandiosity trait 29, 145, 150; and Histrionic Personality Disorder 137, 155; integrative case conceptualization 153; interpersonal case conceptualizations 152–153; interpersonal style 148; interview behavior and rapport 153–154; malignant type 147; optimal diagnostic criterion 148; overt type 146–147; and Paranoid Personality Disorder 155, 188, 192; parental overindulgence 151, 153; prevalence 149; prototypic presentation 149; psychodynamic case conceptualizations 150–151; psychological testing data 154; style vs. disorder 145–146; treatment 154–163; triggering event 147
narcissistic personality style 145–147, 154
Nathanson, B. 228
nefazodone 11
Nehls, N. 107, 111
Nelson, K. J. 67, 83, 109, 128, 143, 163, 180, 198, 212, 227
Nelson, S. M. 8, 9, 10
Neumann, C. S. 51, 61
neurophysiological brain deficits, and early life relational deficits 2
Nichols, W. 67, 143
Nurse, A. 127, 162

object relations theory 16–17, 60; Narcissistic Personality Disorder 161, 162
Obsessive-Compulsive Personality Disorder 164–181; affective/emotional style 166; Alternative Model for Personality Disorders 168; assessment 171–173; attachment style 166–167; and Avoidant Personality Disorder 175; behavioral style 166; biosocial case conceptualizations 169; case studies 165–166; characteristics 172; cognitive style 166; and Dependent Personality Disorder 173; description 164–168; DSM-5 description 167; and Histrionic Personality Disorder 143, 179; integrative case conceptualization 171; interpersonal case conceptualizations 170–171; interpersonal style 166; interview behavior and rapport 171–172; optimal diagnostic criterion 167; and Paranoid Personality Disorder 192; preoccupied attachment style 3; prevalence 167; prototypic presentation 167; psychodynamic case conceptualizations 168–169; psychological testing data 172–173; and Schizoid Personality Disorder 207; and Schizotypal Personality Disorder 219; style vs. disorder 164–165; treatment 173–181; triggering event 166
obsessive-compulsive personality style 165–166, 180, 191
OCD see Obsessive-Compulsive Personality Disorder
O'Donohue, W. 138
Ogloff, J. 68
Ogrodniczuk, J. S. 66, 67, 81, 83, 106, 109, 125, 127, 142, 143, 160, 161, 178, 179, 196, 197, 211, 212, 226, 227
Oldham, J. 30, 50, 69, 86, 112, 129, 145, 158, 164, 182, 192, 214

O'Leary, K. 107
Olson, T. 223
open-ended questions 97, 154, 171, 206
optimal diagnostic criterion 27; Antisocial Personality Disorder 54; Avoidant Personality Disorder 71; Borderline Personality Disorder 89–90; Dependent Personality Disorder 114; Histrionic Personality Disorder 131; Narcissistic Personality Disorder 148; Obsessive-Compulsive Personality Disorder 167; Paranoid Personality Disorder 185; Schizoid Personality Disorder 201; Schizotypal Personality Disorder 217
orbitofrontal cortex 2–3, 7
Orcutt, C. 162
O'Reilly, R. 108
Orme, W. H. 63, 79, 103, 123, 139, 158, 175, 194, 209, 225
Ornstein, P. 112, 122
Orsillo, S. 13
Osterbaan, D. 80
Other Specified Personality Disorder 2, 37
Othmer, E. and S. 24, 53, 59, 69, 76, 88, 97, 113, 119, 130, 136, 147, 153, 166, 172, 183, 191, 200, 206, 215, 222

Pakesky, C. 75, 79
Panic Disorder 120, 173, 192
paradoxical intention 80
Paranoid Personality Disorder 182–198; affective/emotional style 184; Alternative Model for Personality Disorders 186; and Antisocial Personality Disorder 60, 188, 192; assessment 190–191; attachment style 184–185; behavioral style 184; biosocial case conceptualizations 188–189; case studies 183; characteristics 190; cognitive style 184; cognitive-behavioral case conceptualizations 187–188; and Compulsive Personality Disorder 188; description 182–186; DSM-5 description 185; fearful attachment style 4, 184; integrative case conceptualization 189–190; interpersonal case conceptualizations 188; interpersonal style 184; interview behavior and rapport 191; and Narcissistic Personality Disorder 155, 188; and Obsessive-Compulsive Personality Disorder 192; optimal diagnostic criterion 185; prevalence 185; prototypic presentation 185; psychodynamic case conceptualizations 186–187; psychological testing data 191; style vs. disorder 182–183, 184; treatment 192–198; triggering event 183
paranoid personality style 182–184
paranoid schizophrenia 182, 198

parental injunction, characteristics of personality disorders 26
parental overprotection 116
Park, I. 53
Parsons, B. 66, 67
Passive-Aggressive Personality Disorder 93, 95, 96, 173
pathological personality traits 2, 31–33
pattern recognition and change 40
Pattern-Focused Psychotherapy 12; practice 12–13; theory 12
patterns 12
Penberthy, J. 10
perceptual skills 105, 124
perfectionism 32, 47–48, 81, 164, 166–171, 176–177, 179–180, 190
perpetuants 40
Perry, J. 61, 90, 98, 178, 179, 196, 223
Perry, S. 24
Persistent Depressive Disorder 95, 120, 137, 155
Personality Disorder Not Otherwise Specified 2, 37
personality disorders: antisocial see Antisocial Personality Disorder; attachment 2–4, 6; diagnosis and treatment 2–20; DSM-5 section on 1–2; temperament 4–6; trends in diagnosis 2–7
personality functioning 2, 31–32, 37, see also Level of Personality Functioning Scale
pharmacotherapy see medication strategies
physiological skills 105, 124
Pies, R. 144
pimozide 198
Pincus, A. 21, 163
Pines, M. 107
Pollock, G. 138
Porcerelli, J. 28, 79
Porter, K. 142, 144
predictive power 38, 41–42, 48
preoccupied attachment style 3; Dependent Personality Disorder 114; Histrionic Personality Disorder 131; Obsessive-Compulsive Personality Disorder 166–167
preoccupied–fearful attachment style 4; Avoidant Personality Disorder 70
Presniak, M. 223
Pretzer, J. 94
prevalence: Avoidant Personality Disorder 72; Borderline Personality Disorder 91; characteristics 73; Dependent Personality Disorder 115; Histrionic Personality Disorder 132; Narcissistic Personality Disorder 149; Obsessive-Compulsive Personality Disorder 167; Paranoid Personality Disorder 185; Schizoid Personality Disorder 202; Schizotypal Personality Disorder 218

prevalence of personality disorder types, Alternative Model for Personality Disorders 55
projective identification 89, 95, 97, 107, 153, 156, 161, 187, 208, 213, 223
projective techniques 60
prototypic presentation: Antisocial Personality Disorder 54–55; Avoidant Personality Disorder 72; Borderline Personality Disorder 90–91; Dependent Personality Disorder 115; Histrionic Personality Disorder 132; Narcissistic Personality Disorder 149; Obsessive-Compulsive Personality Disorder 167; Paranoid Personality Disorder 185; prevalence 72; Schizoid Personality Disorder 202; Schizotypal Personality Disorder 217
psychoanalysis 156
psychoanalytic psychotherapy 99, 156–157
psychodynamic case conceptualizations: Antisocial Personality Disorder 55–56; Avoidant Personality Disorder 73–74; Borderline Personality Disorder 91–93; Dependent Personality Disorder 116; Histrionic Personality Disorder 133; Narcissistic Personality Disorder 150–151; Obsessive-Compulsive Personality Disorder 168–169; Paranoid Personality Disorder 186–187; Schizoid Personality Disorder 203; Schizotypal Personality Disorder 218–219
Psychodynamic Diagnostic Manual (PDM) 52
psychodynamic psychotherapy: Antisocial Personality Disorder 61–63; Avoidant Personality Disorder 78–79; Borderline Personality Disorder 99; Dependent Personality Disorder 121–122; Histrionic Personality Disorder 137–138; long-term vs. short-term dynamic therapy 209, 224; Narcissistic Personality Disorder 155–156; Obsessive-Compulsive Personality Disorder 174–175; Paranoid Personality Disorder 192–193; research support 101–102; Schizoid Personality Disorder 207–208; Schizotypal Personality Disorder 223–224; supportive therapy 100–101, 157, 208
psychoeducational group therapy 66
psychological testing data: Antisocial Personality Disorder 59–60; Avoidant Personality Disorder 77; Borderline Personality Disorder 97–98; Dependent Personality Disorder 119–120; Histrionic Personality Disorder 136–137; Narcissistic Personality Disorder 154; Obsessive-Compulsive Personality Disorder 172–173; Paranoid Personality Disorder 191; Schizoid Personality Disorder 206–207; Schizotypal Personality Disorder 222
psychometric tests 31, *see also* psychological testing data

Psychopathic Personality Disorder 50, 51, 52, 53
psychotherapy, individual: Antisocial Personality Disorder 61–65; Avoidant Personality Disorder 78–82; Borderline Personality Disorder 98–106; brief dynamic psychotherapy 138–139, 193–194; brief psychoanalytically oriented psychotherapy 157–158; Dependent Personality Disorder 121–125; Histrionic Personality Disorder 137–141; insight-oriented 6, 61, 144, 173; Narcissistic Personality Disorder 155–160; Obsessive-Compulsive Personality Disorder 174–177; Paranoid Personality Disorder 192–196; psychoanalytic psychotherapy 99, 156–157; psychodynamically oriented psychotherapy 192–193; reconstructive 101; Relationship Management Psychotherapy 108; Schizoid Personality Disorder 207–210; Schizotypal Personality Disorder 223–226; short-term dynamic psychotherapy 101; short-term-anxiety-provoking psychotherapy 138; supportive 100–101; time-limited dynamic psychotherapy 122–123
psychotherapy groups 66
punitiveness 177

Quality Assurance Project 138
quetiapine 110

"Rat Man" case 173
Reardon, M. 11
Reich, J. 19, 86, 109–110
Reid, W. 223
Reinecke, M. 117
rejection, Avoidant Personality Disorder 74–76
Relationship Enhancement Therapy 162
Relationship Management Psychotherapy 108
relaxation exercises 62
Rennenberg, B. 30, 82
Renton, J. 187, 195, 204, 210, 220, 225
Rentrop, M. 85
Rinaldi, C. 111
Rinsley, D. 156
Roche, M. 163
Rodriguez-Seijas, C. 34
Roemer, L. 13
role lock 211
Rollnick, S. 12, 63
Ronningstam, E. 145, 155
Rorschach Psychodiagnostic Test 23; Antisocial Personality Disorder 60; Avoidant Personality Disorder 77; Borderline Personality Disorder 97–98; Dependent Personality Disorder 120; Histrionic Personality Disorder 136–137; Narcissistic Personality Disorder 154;

Obsessive-Compulsive Personality Disorder 173; Paranoid Personality Disorder 191; Schizoid Personality Disorder 206; Schizotypal Personality Disorder 222
Rosell, D. R. 7
Ruggero, C. 34
Rutan, J. 142, 161, 178, 196
Ryan, A. 227, 228
Ryle, A. 139, 193

Sadoff, R. 126
Salkovskis, P. 180
Salvatore, G. 193
Salvson, S. 107, 141
Salzman, L. 168, 174, 175, 176, 178, 179, 180, 192
Sameuls, J. 164
Sanislow, C. 69
Scheidlinger, S. 142
Schema Therapy 14, 15; Antisocial Personality Disorder 64; Avoidant Personality Disorder 80; Borderline Personality Disorder 94, 105; Dependent Personality Disorder 124–125; Histrionic Personality Disorder 140; Narcissistic Personality Disorder 159; Obsessive-Compulsive Personality Disorder 176–177; Paranoid Personality Disorder 195; Schizoid Personality Disorder 210; Schizotypal Personality Disorder 225–226
Schizoid Personality Disorder 199–213; affective/emotional style 201; Alternative Model for Personality Disorders 203; assessment 206–207; attachment style 201; behavioral style 200; biosocial case conceptualizations 203–204; case studies 200; characteristics 205; cognitive style 201; cognitive-behavioral case conceptualizations 204; description 199–203; dismissing attachment style 4, 201; DSM-5 description 202; integrative case conceptualization 204–205; interpersonal case conceptualizations 204; interpersonal style 200–201; interview behavior and rapport 206; and Obsessive-Compulsive Personality Disorder 207; optimal diagnostic criterion 201; prevalence 202; prototypic presentation 202; psychodynamic case conceptualizations 203; psychological testing data 206–207; and Schizotypal Personality Disorder 219, 220, 221; style vs. disorder 199–200, 201; treatment 207–213; triggering event 200
schizoid personality style 199–201, 206
schizophrenias 55, 207, 214, 217, 223, 227
Schizotypal Personality Disorder 214–228; affective/emotional style 216; Alternative Model for Personality Disorders 218; assessment 222; attachment style 217; and Avoidant Personality Disorder 219–221; behavioral style 216; biosocial case conceptualizations 219; and Borderline Personality Disorder 219, 222; case studies 215; characteristics 221; cognitive style 216; cognitive-behavioral case conceptualizations 219–220; description 214–218; DSM-5 description 217; fearful-dismissing attachment style 4; integrative case conceptualization 220–221; interpersonal case conceptualizations 220; interpersonal style 216; interview behavior and rapport 222; and Obsessive-Compulsive Personality Disorder 219; optimal diagnostic criterion 217; prevalence 218; prototypic presentation 217; psychodynamic case conceptualizations 218–219; psychological testing data 222; and Schizoid Personality Disorder 219, 220, 221; style vs. disorder 214–215, 216; treatment 222–228; triggering event 215
schizotypal personality style 214–216, 222
Schneider, A. 30
Schneider, I. 30
Schoendorff, B. 181
Schramm, E. 10
Schwartz, J. 13
Segal, Z. 8, 13
selective serotonin reuptake inhibitors (SSRIs): Antisocial Personality Disorder 67; Avoidant Personality Disorder 83; Borderline Personality Disorder 110
self, working models 3
self-control, insufficient 64, 105, 159
self-harm 44, 110
self-help programs 128
self-object transferences 151
self-other schema, characteristics of personality disorders 26–27
self-psychology 101, 109; Narcissistic Personality Disorder 156, 160, 161, 162
self-sacrifice 80, 125
Seltzer, M. 78
Semrad, E. 107
separation anxiety 88, 98, 122
separation-individuation process 56, 208
sequential diagrammatic reformulation (SDR) 139, 193
serotonergic agents 109–110
serotonin 56, 198
sertraline 83, 109
Serzone 11
Shapiro, D. 169, 186, 187
Shapiro, E. 161, 212
Sharoff, K. 105, 124
Sharp, C. 2
Shaver, P. 3, 6
Shaw, I. A. 14

Shay, J. 142, 161, 178, 196
Sheldon, W. 205
Sherry, A. 3, 70, 89, 114, 201
short-term dynamic psychotherapy 101
short-term-anxiety-provoking psychotherapy (STAPP) 138
Shostrum, E. 19
Shulman, B. 89, 95
Siegel, D. 2, 4, 89
Siever, L. 6, 7, 212, 227
Sifneos, P. 122, 138
Silk, K. 7, 19, 67, 83, 127, 128, 143, 163, 180, 198, 207, 212–213, 227
Simon, K. 170, 176
Simon, W. 112
Simple Phobia 120, 173
Singer, M. T. 97
Skodol, A. 30, 31, 50, 69, 73, 77, 86, 95, 112, 116, 129, 133, 145, 164, 182, 186, 199, 203, 214
Slavik, S. 211, 213
Smucker, M. 105
Snyder, M. 162
Social Anxiety Disorder 72, 83, 120, 137, 173
social distancing 203, 204
social isolation 64, 80, 105, 210
social phobia 80
Sociopathic Personality Disorder 53–54; behavioral style 53; triggering event 53
Soloff, P. 90, 154
Solomon, J. 3
Solomon, M. 109, 162
Somatic Symptom Disorders 60, 97, 120, 136, 155, 173, 207
Sowislo, J. F. 7
Sperry, J. 12, 14, 15, 23, 38, 39, 40, 42, 44, 78
Sperry, L. 1, 12, 13, 14, 15, 16, 19, 23, 27, 34, 38, 39, 40, 42, 44, 48, 58, 61, 67, 72, 76, 78, 96, 118, 120, 128, 135, 137, 143, 153, 163, 171, 173, 179, 180–181, 190, 192, 205, 211, 213, 221, 223, 227
Spina, D. S. 16, 17
splitting: Borderline Personality Disorder 89, 93, 95, 97, 98, 107, 109, 111; Histrionic Personality Disorder 137; Narcissistic Personality Disorder 156, 160; Schizoid Personality Disorder 203, 213; Schizotypal Personality Disorder 223
sports heroes, as role models 65
SSRIs *see* selective serotonin reuptake inhibitors (SSRIs)
standards, unrelenting 159, 177
Stanley, B. 103, 228
Stern, B. 155
Stevenson, J. 102
Stiles, T. 78
Stockwell, M. 127, 143

Stone, M. 5, 107, 144, 207, 209, 212, 213, 223, 224, 226, 227
Stone, W. 142, 161, 178, 196–197
stranger self-object 55
Strauss, J. 175
Stravynski, A. 82
Structural Analysis of Social Behavior (SASB) 94–95, 106
structured treatment interventions 7, 14–16
Strupp, H. 83, 121, 122
subjugation 210
Substance Use Disorders 8, 36, 55, 60, 68, 85, 128
suicide attempts 29, 44, 91, 100, 134
Sungar, M. 134
support groups 65
supportive therapy 100–101, 157, 208
Suzuki, T. 8, 9, 10
Svartberg, M. 78, 175
Swiercinsky, D. 97, 222

Tacbacnik, N. 110
Tafrate, R. 67, 73
tailoring power 41, 42, 48
Tarrier, N. 38
TAT *see* Thematic Apperception Test (TAT)
Teasdale, J. 8, 13
temperament 5–6; characteristics of personality disorders 26; definitions 4, 13; and personality disorders 6
Thematic Apperception Test (TAT): Antisocial Personality Disorder 60; Borderline Personality Disorder 98; Dependent Personality Disorder 120; Histrionic Personality Disorder 136; Narcissistic Personality Disorder 155; Obsessive-Compulsive Personality Disorder 173; Paranoid Personality Disorder 191; Schizoid Personality Disorder 207
therapeutic community, Antisocial Personality Disorder 66
"third wave" behavior therapy 8
Thomas, A. 5, 56, 58, 75, 93, 95
Thomas, K. 182, 199
thought processes, maladaptive, compared to emotional regulation 8
Thylstrup, B. 207
time-limited dynamic psychotherapy 122–123
time-limited supportive-expressive psychotherapy 175
Toman, W. 169
Torgerson, S. 219
transference process 17, 78
Transference-Focused Psychotherapy (TFP) 16–17; Borderline Personality Disorder 92–93, 100
Treating the Borderline Family (Everett et al) 108
treatment as usual (TAU) 64

treatment of personality disorders: Antisocial Personality Disorder 60–68; Avoidant Personality Disorder 19, 77–85; Borderline Personality Disorder 98–111; case conceptualizations *see* case conceptualizations; Cognitive Behavioral Therapy *see* Cognitive Behavioral Therapy; combined methods *see* combined and integrated treatment methods; Dependent Personality Disorder 120–128; developmental therapy 39–40, 180–181; Dialectical Behavior Therapy 9–10; formulation *see* combined and integrated treatment methods; goals 60; Histrionic Personality Disorder 137–144; medication strategies *see* medication strategies; Mentalization-Based Treatment 17–18; mindfulness 13–14; Narcissistic Personality Disorder 154–163; Obsessive-Compulsive Personality Disorder 173–181; Pattern-Focused Psychotherapy 12–13; patterns 12; psychodynamic psychotherapy *see* psychodynamic psychotherapy; Schema Therapy 14; Schizoid Personality Disorder 207–213; Schizotypal Personality Disorder 222–228; structured interventions 14–16; Transference-Focused Psychotherapy 16–17; trends 17–21, *see also* group therapy; marital and family therapy

triggering event 24; Antisocial Personality Disorder 53; Avoidant Personality Disorder 69; Borderline Personality Disorder 88; Dependent Personality Disorder 113; Histrionic Personality Disorder 130; Narcissistic Personality Disorder 147; Obsessive-Compulsive Personality Disorder 166; Paranoid Personality Disorder 183; Schizoid Personality Disorder 200; Schizotypal Personality Disorder 215

Trujillo, M. 158
Tsheringld, S. 67, 83, 109, 128, 143, 163, 180, 198, 212, 227
Turkat, I. 23, 24, 57, 61, 75, 80, 103, 117, 124, 127, 134, 140, 152, 170, 176, 187, 188, 194, 198, 204, 220, 224

Uliaszek, A. 66, 67, 81, 83, 106, 109, 125, 127, 142, 143, 160, 161, 178, 179, 196, 197, 211–212, 226, 227
undeveloped self 210
Unspecified Personality Disorder 2, 37
"untreatable" conditions 1

Vaccani, J. 111
Valliant, G. 61
Van der Kolk, B. 90
Van Gelder, K. 48

Vaughn, B. 5
verbal holding 196
Vinogradov, S. 196
vulnerability to harm 226

Waddell, M. 127, 128
Wagner, C. 60
Wagner, E. 60
Waldinger, R. 98
Waldo, M. 109
Walker, E. 227, 228
Walker, R. 65, 66
Wallerstein, R. 101, 122
Walsh, A. 51
Waugh, M. H. 30
Weeks, G. 80
Weishaar, M. 14, 80, 94, 105, 124, 140, 176, 195, 210
Weissman, M. 95
Weissman, R. 107
Wells, M. 178, 180
Westen, D. 55, 72, 115, 132, 149, 167, 185, 202, 217
Whiteman, R. 161
Wienclaw, R. 211
Wilberg, T. 7, 82
wilderness survival training 65, 67, 85
Williams, A. 62
Williams, J. 8, 13, 195, 198
Williams, M. 8
Williams, P. 193
Williamson, D. 116
Winer, J. 138
Winston, A. 138
Wolberg, L. 122
Woody, G. 61, 67
Woo-Ming, A. 212, 227
World Health Organization 30
Wright, A. 29, 163
Wu, H. H. 51
Wurmser, L. 73

Yakeley, J. 62, 66
Yalom, I. 65, 81, 126, 178, 196, 211
Yeomans, F. 16, 17, 61, 78, 92, 99, 121, 138, 146, 147, 155, 174, 192, 207, 223
Young, J. 14, 27, 64, 80, 94, 105, 124, 140, 155, 159, 175, 176, 177, 195, 210, 225
Young, P. 14, 94
Yue, D. 40
Yule, W. 82

Zanarini, M. 19, 86, 90, 110
Zimbardo, P. 84
Zoloft 83